Aromatherapy

KT-430-247

£3.49
48

Aromatherapy

THE ENCYCLOPEDIA OF
PLANTS AND OILS
AND HOW THEY HELP YOU

DANIELE RYMAN

PIATKUS

To my dear friend Barbara Brittingham

Aromatherapy is a form of complementary medicine. However, you should always consult your doctor before replacing any existing medication with an aromatherapeutic treatment.

If you are in any doubt about your health, consult a doctor before having treatment. Your attention is also drawn to the information on pages 12 – 13 and 27 – 28 of this book.

The author and publisher disclaim all responsibility for any adverse reaction caused by inappropriate use of, or poor quality, essential oils.

Copyright © 1991 Danièle Ryman

First published in 1991 by
Judy Piatkus (Publishers) Ltd
5 Windmill Street, London W1P 1HF

First paperback edition published 1992
Reprinted 1992, 1993 (three times)

The moral right of the author has been asserted

A catalogue record for this book is
available from the British Library

ISBN 0 – 7499 – 1080 – 1
ISBN 0 – 7499 – 1156 – 5 (Pbk)

Designed by Paul Saunders
Illustrations by Paul Saunders
Edited by Susan Fleming

Typeset in Compugraphic Baskerville by
Action Typesetting Ltd, Gloucester
Printed and bound in Great Britain by
Butler & Tanner Ltd, Frome and London

CONTENTS

ACKNOWLEGEMENTS

It gives me great pleasure to thank my friend and distiller Christian Remy and to acknowledge his dynamic team, especially his wife Monique Remy, *Ingenieur Chimiste*, for all the information and help they have passed on to me in the last three years.

I also wish to thank Professeur Rouzet of l'Université de Nantes, Professeur Derbesy of l'Université de Marseilles, and Docteur Jalil Belkamel for the research and information they gave me. Also Docteur Perron from Marseilles and the late Docteur Maury from Grasse for their sound advice. Also John Middleton, Toxicologist, for having taken the time to check on the toxicity of essential oils.

Many thanks to Susan Fleming for the great help in organising all my work and without whose cooperation it would have been difficult for me to finish this voluminous book. Also to Heather Rocklin, Editor at Piatkus Books, for her precious help, and Gill Cormode and Judy Piatkus who have a strong belief in the book and who encouraged me to finish it on time!

In addition I would like to thank Barbara Freeth and Molly McCreadie, who met my awkward and time consuming demands with unfailing patience. And F S Kahn for his enthusiasm and encouragement.

And finally my son Nicolas who insisted that I finish this book quickly.

FOREWORD

This is the first truly comprehensive book on aromatherapy, and it has taken a great deal of time to complete. I have practised this therapy for 26 years, and I feel it is now time to give an honest account of my experiences using plants and essential oils. So, here is an introduction and guide to the undeniable benefits of aromatherapy.

Aromatherapy has been a part of my life for as long as I can remember, assisting and comforting me at different phases of my life. My very first memory is the smell of roses when, as a child, my mother gave me her last kiss goodnight. As she bent close I could smell her favourite scent – rose. Ever after the fragrance of roses has always instilled in me a feeling of security and love.

The smell of pine is for me the smell of freedom and long hot summers. When I was a teenager I would spend the summer at my grandfather's house in France. There was a pine forest behind his garden, and as the pine needles literally cracked under the hot sun they released their fresh aroma. Today the freedom and happiness of those holidays is rekindled each time I walk through pine trees or smell the fragrance.

Lily of the valley always bring me joy and remind me of the time my son was born, 15 years ago, and my room was filled with the sweet smelling flowers.

Aromatherapy involves more than fragrance. Plant essential oils have therapeutic powers in addition to beneficial fragrance, and all are antiseptic in different degrees. In the plane on my way to India a few years ago, my index finger began throbbing violently. A rose thorn had lodged in it two days before, as I pruned my roses. It was now turning septic. I straight away applied tea tree oil neat to the finger. By the time I arrived in Bangalore the swelling had almost gone and the throbbing had stopped.

Other oils have the power to comfort. Just before my guru, Marguerite Maury, died, she gave me a personal formulation of different oils which she asked me to spread on her coffin. Their strong aromas, released in the confines of the small church in Switzerland, enveloped me and comforted me as Marguerite had so thoughtfully intended.

More recently, during the late nights spent writing this book the stimulating odiferous molecules of basil placed near my desk helped me overcome the physical tiredness I felt, and helped to keep me going.

Over the years plants, flowers and their essential oils have been my great companions, healers and fortifiers, and it is impossible to visualize a world without them.

Sadly, however, it is a false claim that the therapy is 100 per cent safe, and that the therapy is for everyone; there are actually some severe dangers in self-help aromatherapy.

It is for this reason that this book gave me as much pain as joy to write. On the one hand, I have enjoyed all the research, talking about the plants encountered on my travels, their therapeutic values and the method of treatments. But on the other I have had to use a critical eye and condemn certain essential oils and their curative values for safety reasons. The reader should also be aware that the demand for certain plant essences has contributed to the wrecking of forests and has added to the pollution of our planet. Further, for economic reasons some oils are often adulterated, and this of course affects their therapeutic value. Essential oils must be absolutely pure and of the very best quality for use in therapy.

This book has not been written to stop the public from using essential oils. On the contrary. But as demands for alternative therapies have increased in the last few years and aromatherapy has become more popular, it is time to make sure that the public takes serious precautions before embarking on self-treatment. Essential oils are drugs and should be considered as such.

As a result, no essential oils have been prescribed internally in this book. Many essential oils are very strong indeed, and have a corrosive action which could be a danger if used in this way. (If certain oils can perforate metal – for example clove oil – what can they do to the human body?) The methods used are external application and, my own preference, vapour inhalation. If the essential oil is well diluted in a chosen carrier oil or in water, it can give very good results, offer relief, and be very pleasurable, causing an immediated sense of well-being when inhaled. Essential oils are only used neat in special circumstances.

With the dangers of oils still in mind, I have also given alternative methods of treatment from the plant world. Instead of the oils, the plants themselves can be used in the form of tisanes or cooking, when you can still find and benefit from the essential oils in minute proportions. In fact, a dish without herbs is a dish without sense: the addition of herbs or spices to a dish enhances the subtle *fumet* (aroma) of the food and not only sharpens the appetite but facilitates the digestion – as well as, of course, pleasing the taste buds. Rosemary, for example, aids the functioning of the liver and promotes the body's digestion of fatty meats like lamb and pork.

I also show you how to make your own plant oils from bought or homegrown plants. The finished oils will contain tiny but beneficial proportions of essential oils, and will be absolutely safe to use.

This book is easy to read, giving over 80 plants with botanical and historical research on each, and their therapeutic values and uses. This is balanced by a section of over 100 symptoms and ailments, which will help you to select and chose the method of treatment and its application, after having had the condition carefully diagnosed.

I hope that you will enjoy using the book, but that you will also take care.

Danièle Ryman
London

Part One

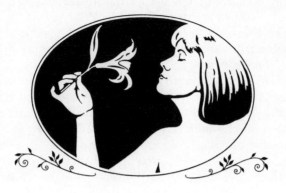

An Introduction
to Aromatherapy

THE OILS OF AROMATHERAPY

Aromatherapy consists of the use of natural aromatic essences or oils extracted from wild or cultivated plants. Wild plants are preferred as they yield the most active and best balanced product. Many plants under intensive cultivation lose some of their natural principles. The florist's rose, for instance, has lost its perfume and this was half the rose's attraction, certainly more than half its therapeutic value. Oils from cultivated plants are still good, though, if they are raised sympathetically and organically. It goes without saying that the therapeutic value of an oil distilled from a plant which has been sprayed with chemical pesticides, will be quite altered, if not destroyed completely. A plant which has been polluted in other ways – such as by heavy industrial pollution or, more horrifyingly, by fallout from Chernobyl – is rendered useless to the therapy.

These essential oils can come from many plants, and from many *parts* of plants. A great number of aromatherapy's essential oils come from culinary herbal plants like angelica, basil, marjoram and mint but these oils can vary in location: the roots of angelica, the flowers of lavender, and the leaves of rosemary. Oils come from culinary spices too – from the seeds of anise and caraway, the flower buds and leaves of the clove tree, the bark of cinnamon tree, the rhizomes that are ginger. Fruit and vegetables also produce essential oils – lemon, mandarin, carrot and celery among them. The orange is an aromatherapist's dispensary in itself: bergamot oil is distilled from the rind of the bergamot orange; neroli oil from the flowers of the bigarade orange; orange oil from the peel of sweet orange; and petitgrain oil from the leaves and tiny unripe fruit of the bigarade orange.

Flower essences are perhaps the most familiar to many who are not completely conversant with aromatherapy – and these include rose, geranium and ylang ylang. But that the resins and leaves of trees are used is probably not so well known: oils distilled from resins include benzoin, gaiac, pine and baume de Tolu; oils from tree leaves include eucalyptus, patchouli and bay. (This is not the culinary bay, but a West Indian tree leaf that was distilled with rum to make the Victorian men's hair dressing, bay rum. It is still used in aromatherapy as a hair remedy.) Aromatic grasses yield oils too, and these include lemongrass, palmarosa and vetiver.

Essential oils may have been developed by the plant to keep grazing animals away, or to attract pollinating insects, or may act internally as individual pesticides or fungicides. This is not known in any specific detail, but what is known from chemical analysis and from chromatography is that the oils are compounds. Each consists of very many organic constituents which unite in a delicate, complex balance to produce a wide range of therapeutic and olfactory qualities. Eucalyptus, for instance, contains no less than 250 different constituents; and in a 1978 chromatograph of Australian tea tree oil, prepared for the *Journal of Agriculture and Food Chemistry*, researchers identified 40 compounds. These included cineol, terpinene and cymene, as well as something called viridiflorene which had not previously been reported as occurring in nature.

Drugs Containing Natural Substances

Most of us are aware that plants contain chemical substances of various kinds many of which have been extracted and used for the benefit of mankind. The following are but a few of those used in conventional medicine.

- The simple **aspirin**, for instance, was originally derived from the willow tree, *Salix*, thus its chemical name, salicylic acid.
- **Quinine**, still used in the treatment of malaria, was originally derived from the bark of a South American tree, *Cinchona*.
- **Morphine** and **codeine**, used for pain control, are both derived from the milky juice of the unripe fruit capsules of the opium poppy (*Papaver somniferum*). This is thought to be the oldest medicine of all.
- One of the commonest ingredients of many laxatives is derived from the dried pods and leaves of **senna**, a species of *Cassia* tree.
- **Digitalis**, a crude drug once prescribed for many cardiac ills, originally derived from the simple cottage-garden flower, the purple foxglove. The more sophisticated **Digitoxin** and **Digoxin** are yielded by the white foxglove.
- The contraceptive pill was originally derived from Mexican yams.

Despite the development of the synthetic drug industry where drugs have been refined in the laboratory from the basis of plant compounds, many pharmacologists and drug manufacturers are turning once again to the plant world. Some are disenchanted with the strong chemicals and side-effects of modern drugs, but many have rediscovered the potential of plants and are seeking cures proving elusive in the test-tube.

Feverfew and the evening primrose are but two of the plants which have come to recent prominence and which are now under proper scientific evaluation. Feverfew has long been considered a herbal cure for migraine and these properties are now being investigated by the drug industry. The acid in the oil from the evening primrose is proving useful in such varied areas as eczema, heart disease and pre-menstrual tension: it is being prescribed in National Health Service hospitals in Britain.

Another plant remedy which is receiving current scientific attention is the Madagascar periwinkle, which contains a cancer-fighting substance used in the treatment of leukaemia. Russian research is achieving success in treating skin cancer with cotton-seed oil.

Aromatherapy may be thought of by some as an alternative form of therapy – as merely a beauty massage treatment even – but this is not the case. It consists of the medicinal use of natural plant compounds, exactly as do the conventional medicines described earlier.

THE HISTORY OF AROMATHERAPY

The use of plants to cure disease is as old as the human race, perhaps even older. Animals, for instance, have always sought out particular herbs or grasses when they are unwell – domestic dogs and cats still eat grass when they feel off-colour. Man has always been dependent on the nutritional value of the plant world. It was inevitable, therefore, that an awareness of how he felt after eating a plant would develop, and that a knowledge of herbal medicine would evolve. At first it must have been a case of trial and error – for many plants *are* poisonous – but, according to archeologists, the paintings on the walls of the Lascaux caves in the Dordogne in France, dating back to 18,000BC, tell of the use of plants in medicine.

The earliest written herbal text can be claimed by the Chinese. The *Pen Tsao*, or Great Herbal (which is still in print) was compiled by Shen Nung, an emperor who lived some time between about 1000 and 700BC. In this, he listed over 350 medicinal plants – many of which are familiar today, such as poppy and cannabis – and remedies.

The Egyptians and Aromatherapy

Aromatic substances also played important roles in the medicinal practices of the Hebrew, Arabic and Indian civilizations. But for the ancient Egyptians aromatherapy was a way of life. At about the time that the Chinese were developing acupuncture, the Egyptians were using balsamic substances in both religious ritual and medicine. Records dating back to 4500BC tell of perfumed oils, scented barks and resins, of spices, aromatic vinegars, wines and beers all used in medicine, ritual, astrology and embalming. When Tutankhamun's tomb was opened in 1922, many pots were found containing substances such as myrrh and frankincense (both derived from tree resins): these were used as much for medicine as for perfume, the two being interchangeable at the time.

Translations of hieroglyphics inscribed on *papryi* and *steles* found in the temple of Edfu indicate that aromatic substances were blended to specific formulations by the high priests and alchemists to make perfumes and medicinal potions. In the temples, aromatic substances like crushed cedarwood bark, caraway seeds and angelica roots were steeped in wine or oil, or burned, to perfume the air. The priests knew of the power of certain smells to raise the spirits of their congregation, or to promote a state of tranquillity. A favourite perfume was the famous *kyphi*, a mixture of sixteen different essences – including myrrh and juniper – and this was inhaled to heighten the senses and spiritual awareness of the priests. The incense used in present-day religious ritual serves much the same purpose.

In the 1870s, the Ebers Papyrus – seventy-odd feet of medical scroll – was discovered. It dated back to *c*.1500BC and listed over 800, mainly herbal, prescriptions and remedies. A scroll discovered slightly earlier, and called the Edwin Smith, dealt with medicine as well. From these scrolls, we learn that the Egyptians treated hayfever with a mixture of antimony, aloes, myrrh and honey. (Myrrh is still used for throat problems and coughs, by the way.) And they knew the basics of contraception: a blend of acacia, coloquinte (the pulp of the bitter-apple), dates and honey would be inserted in the vagina where it would ferment to form lactic acid – which is now known to act as a spermicide.

Aromatherapeutic principles were employed also in the famous Egyptian art of the embalmer. He knew of the natural antiseptic and antibiotic properties of plants and how these could be utilized in the process of preserving human bodies. Traces of resins like galbanum, and spices such as clove, cinnamon and nutmeg, have been isolated from the bandages of mummies. Such preservatives were obviously remarkably effective. Fragments of intestine examined under the microscope have been found to be completely intact after thousands of years. The remarkably preserved bodies extant in mummies, revealed by modern x-ray techniques, are a testament to the art of the embalmers, those early aromatherapists.

Another aspect of the Egyptians' use of aromatherapeutic principles was in cookery. They showed an amazing knowledge of the culinary value of aromatic substances. They would add spices such as caraway, coriander and aniseed to their breads of millet and barley to make them easier to digest. (Many spices and their oils are digestive in action, in fact, but recent research on caraway, for instance, has shown that one of its constituents, carvone, is extremely powerful, stimulating and releasing the gastric juices.) Onions and garlic were eaten often, onion bulbs invariably being found in or beside the tomb of a mummy as accompaniment into the next world. (Onion, of course, possesses potent antibacterial properties, and eating it daily can keep colds and 'flu at bay.) Garlic's bactericidal properties were as well known then as now: from an inscription on the Pyramid of Cheops we learn that every morning the slaves building the pyramid would be given a clove of garlic each to provide them with strength and good health. Today, garlic is well known as a powerful natural detoxicant, protecting against bacterial and viral infections.

The Greek and Roman Discoveries

If the Ancient Egyptians perfected the art of using the essences of plants to control emotion, putrefaction and disease, new discoveries of the medicinal power of plants continued to be made. The Greeks, for instance, developed medicine from a part-superstition to a science. Hippocrates, popularly known as the Father of Medicine, was the first physician to base medical knowledge and treatment on accurate observation, and ever since, of course, doctors have adhered to his principles outlined in the Hippocratic Oath. One of his beliefs was that a daily aromatic bath and a scented massage were the way to health, very much a central principle of today's aromatherapy. He was aware of the antibacterial properties of certain plants and when an epidemic of plague broke out in Athens he urged the people to burn aromatic plants at the corners of the streets to protect themselves and prevent the plague spreading. At this time, too, botanical knowledge was expanding, reaching its peak in the *Historia Plantarum* of Theophrastus, the so-called Father of Botany.

At the height of the power of Rome, it was 'immigrant' Greek physicians and seekers after knowledge who dominated the medical world. One of these was Dioscorides, a Greek surgeon in Nero's army, who wrote *De Materia Medica*, a comprehensive textbook on the properties and uses of medicinal plants. It was he who recorded further details such as when a plant and its active principles might be at their most powerful. This indisputable fact of plant life – that the principles are not always the same, depending on time of day, time of year, and state of development – is utilized by the essential oil industry today, nearly 2,000 years later. For instance, the poppy's yield in the morning is four times greater than in the evening. Jasmine's perfume and therefore its oil's powers, are strongest in the evening; this is why jasmine flowers are still picked at night in India for their olfactory qualities. Dioscorides also first used a decoction of willow to cure pain such as that caused by gout (it is this decoction which has since become our most common analgesic, aspirin).

The Romans, although more interested in the culinary than the medical properties of plants, were botanically enormously influential. As the legions advanced over Europe, the soldiers took with them seeds of the plants they needed or could not live without, to cultivate in the countries they occupied. Many herbal plants in England – parsley,

6

fennel and lovage, for instance – were introduced by the Romans. Many still grow in the greatest profusion in the wild along the routes taken by the soliders, seeds having dropped by the roadside, or around old Roman settlements.

Towards the Renaissance

Although rational medicine declined in Europe after these early beginnings, it still continued in China and India. The Arabs, whose civilization advanced from the fourth century AD, were also keeping the scientific spirit alive. An Arab was one of the founders of the famous medical school at Salerno, near Naples, and the Arabian physician Avicenna's book, *Canon of Medicine*, published in the eleventh century, remained a standard work until the mid-sixteenth century. Avicenna was also thought to be responsible for the invention of distillation as a means of extracting essences from plants, and many of his principles are still in use today. Great explorers and colonisers, the Arabs spread their knowledge throughout the known world. They were also great traders, and to a large extent were responsible for introducing many new plants from the East – spices in particular – which were used both in cooking and medicine.

The Middle Ages in Europe, stretching from roughly the sixth century to the Renaissance in the fourteenth century, was not an inspired time in terms of medical advance. A few lone voices were heard, though – one of them was that of the thirteenth-century Abbess of Bingen, St Hildegarde, who wrote four treatises on medicinal plants. The works are still referred to today.

The Black Death, which hit Europe in the early fourteenth century, destroyed between a third and a half of Europe's population, contemporary medicine offering no more advice than to carry aromatic herbal pomanders, or burn aromatics in houses and at the corners of streets. This was aromatherapeutic in theory, of course, but it was too little and too late.

With the Renaissance came the years of the great explorations. Christopher Columbus, unusually for his time, believed the world was round, and that he could reach the East – and its wealth of spices – by sailing to the West. He landed in 1492 in what he thought were the East Indies – in reality the Bahamas. It was from the opening up of America that many new plant species were introduced to Europe. The stimulant coca leaves chewed by the Incas were introduced from South America; and other plants used medicinally by the natives and the North American Indians, such as the balsams or *baumes* (of Canada and Peru), entered the European pharmacopoeiae.

The European Herbalists

The sixteenth and seventeenth centuries were the times of the great herbals in Europe, the British ones including those of Gerard, Parkinson and Culpeper. With the outbreak of plague again in 1665, methods of dealing with the disease had not advanced much from those employed 300 years before. Thereafter, though, knowledge grew in leaps and bounds, with the founding of the Royal Society in Britain, the plant classifications of Linnaeus, the explorations of Cook, and with many amazing medical discoveries such as digitalis, vaccination for smallpox, quinine and anaesthesia – the latter given the ultimate and Royal Seal of Approval by Victoria in 1853: 'We are having this baby, and we are having chloroform.'

Alongside the growth of the scientific approach to medicine, though, belief in aromatherapeutic principles still co-existed, and by the end of the eighteenth century, essential oils were still widely used in medicine. But, as chemistry began to flourish as a discipline, and plant cures could be synthesized in the laboratory – cures which were stronger and faster in action – aromatherapy and its oils began to lose their place in the pharmacopoeiae and the whole subject began to be thought of as rather cranky.

Aromatherapy in the Twentieth Century

It was not until the beginning of this century that a French chemist and scholar, Dr R M Gattefossé, rekindled interest in aromatherapy – a term he actually coined and about which he wrote several books. He explained at length the properties of essential oils and their methods of application, with examples of their antiseptic, bactericidal, anti-viral and anti-inflammatory properties. He related how, after burning his hand in the laboratory, he plunged the hand into the nearest receptacle which happen-ed to contain essential oil of lavender; he was astonished at how quickly the pain ceased and the skin healed. He continued to experiment with essential oils, using as his subjects men in military hospitals during the First World War. Essential oils such as thyme, clove, chamomile and lemon were used, with astounding results. Later the work was carried on by Dr J Valnet. Up until the Second World War essential oils of clove, lemon, thyme and chamomile were used as natural disinfectants and antiseptics to fumigate hospital wards and sterilise instruments used in surgery and dentistry.

Doctors used the oils throughout the war, and managed to prevent gangrene, cure burns and heal wounds in record time. This work was later translated into modern terms by Marguerite Maury, the French biochemist who trained me. She extended the research, bringing aromatherapy into the world of cosmetology, allying medicine, health and beauty. Aromatherapy is now widely practised by doctors on the continent – in conjunction with Phytotherapy (Herbalism) – and is referred to in France as *medicine douce*, or soft medicine, a significant appellation.

Around the same time that Dr R M Gattefossé wrote his first book on aromatherapy, Sir Alexander Fleming discovered the antibiotic penicillin. This was a 'natural' cure as well, being isolated from a culture of mould. Today, of course, natural penicillin is no longer used, for its constituents were identified long ago and it is now synthesized in the laboratory. Perhaps that is the reason why so many people have allergic reactions to penicillin, resulting in eczema and swelling: the artificial variety is considerably stronger than its natural counterpart.

And it is for this reason, I believe, that medicine is now turning once again to *natural* remedies. Using a strong synthetic drug to kill harmful bacteria is rather like cracking a nut with a sledgehammer, for not only do the drugs kill the harmful bacteria, they also destroy the beneficial ones present in the body. Natural remedies like using essential oils, on the other hand, may act more slowly in an antibiotic sense, but while killing off the bacteria or virus, they do not destroy anything else. In fact, they actually stimulate the body's immune system to strengthen its resistance to further attack.

Unfortunately, we have come to expect instant cures and think that the only medicines of value are made synthetically and come in pill form. Thus many find it hard to believe that the essential oils from plants are actually just as effective, if not more so. They may take longer to show results, but then illnesses do not develop overnight. There are no miracle cures, and a more valid option has to be the softer approach of something like aromatherapy.

THE COMPOSITION OF ESSENTIAL OILS

Each essential oil is made up of numerous different organic molecules. What gives every essential oil its uniqueness is not just one of its constituents, but the whole, delicate and complex admixture. The individual perfume of each oil depends on this balance; the therapeutic value of each oil depends on it too. It is the number of constituents of an oil which make it almost impossible to reproduce exactly with synthetic ingredients. The reaction between these constituents and their component molecules gives the oil its therapeutic value, which is why man-made imitations never have the same power to heal as their natural counterparts. In Part Two I give the principal constituents of each oil.

This balance of and reaction between constituents is also what makes one oil more or less toxic than another. The proportion of a toxic constituent in one oil may be balanced by other constituents which make the potential toxin less significant and allow the oil to be useful in therapy. In this way, aromatherapy is not unlike homoeopathy which also treats ailments with substances that are poisonous (belladonna and arsenic, for instance). The proportions are tiny, though, and when administered in correct proportions, even a poison can have a beneficial and dynamizing effect.

An experienced aromatherapist will also know how to combine essential oils so that these further admixtures can balance each other, with an alkaline constituent in one, say, being balanced by an acid constituent in another. This is chemistry in practice. There is no way in which knowledge like this can be gained in a short aromatherapy course (see page 29).

EXTRACTION OF THE OILS

The only methods of extracting *essential* oils are through steam distillation and expression. Methods of extracting plant oils include use of volatile solvents and dissolving. The choice of method is important for it will influence the ultimate quality and therapeutic value of the oil. Indeed, each method of extraction gives a different product, as each process extracts different constituents from the plant. I am concerned that as extraction methods become more sophisticated and mechanized, so new constituents which might alter the therapeutic balance of the oil may be extracted. They may be beneficial, but they may not: there is a huge amount of research that needs to be done into the vast subject of essential oils.

Whichever method is chosen, extraction is a painstaking process as the amount of oil present in plants is minute. So, huge quantities of plants are needed for viable amounts of oil: 200 kg (440 lb) of fresh lavender flowers, between 2 and 5 metric tonnes of rose petals and 3,000 lemons are needed to produce 1 kg (2¼ lb) of essential oils of lavender, rose and lemon respectively. This is what makes the essential oils so expensive, and why some producers are turning to more economical methods of extraction using volatile solvents. – and thereby cutting into the heart of the therapy. As oils extracted this way are in effect adulterated and not the pure essential oils, they should not be used for aromatherapy. Oils extracted by volatile solvents are intended for the fragrance industries, which carry their own restrictions.

Steam Distillation

This has been used as a method of extracting essential oils from plant material for thousands of years. The Ancient Egyptians are known to have placed their raw material and some water in a large clay pot. Heat was applied and the steam that formed had to pass through layers of cotton or linen cloth placed in the neck before escaping. The essential oils were trapped in this material, and all that had to be done to obtain them was to squeeze out the cloth occasionally. This is the basic method still used today, although a little more refined.

In the distillation of Australian tea tree oil, for instance, a common bush-still consists of a 1,600-litre (115-gallon) capacity tank with a removeable or hinged lid capable of being sealed to make the container steam-tight. A grid is fitted in the tank about 30 cm (1 ft) above the bottom to support the closely packed leaf (called the charge) and allow an even passage of steam through it. If steam is generated in the still itself (sometimes it is supplied by a separate boiler or steam generator), a constant level of water is maintained in the bottom and a fire built underneath it. An outlet at the top of the still carries the mixture of steam and oil vapour to the condenser, where the steam condenses back to water, and the oil vapour condenses as well. Because they are not water soluble, the oils separate and collect on the surface of the water when cool, and can be collected quite easily. That 1,600-litre tank holds half a metric tonne of fresh leaves, takes two to three hours to distill, and yields 7 – 10 kg (15 – 22 lb) of oil.

Extraction by Volatile Solvents

The process is similar to steam distillation, with the basic material placed in racks in a huge tank like a pressure cooker. Volatile solvents are heated and allowed to flow through the racks. The solvents, when saturated with the plant essentials, are evaporated off, leaving certain odiferous molecules and constituents behind, together with some chemical residue. It is a process which many producers and the perfume industry favour because its return in terms of fragrance is so very much higher than that of steam distillation, and with rose, for example, the fragrance obtained is actually stronger. The product extracted by this method is not essential oil, but what is known as a concrete. A concrete should never be used in therapy, since it not only contains chemical residue from the solvents, but because the balance of constituents extracted by the solvents is different to those extracted by steam distillation.

Benzene used to be one of the solvents used in the extraction of oils to obtain a concrete, but it is now used less and less as it leaves a residue behind that is known to cause allergies. Legislation has actually recommended that the traces left should be under 10 parts per 1,000. There are also formal restrictions for its use in the perfume industry due to its toxicity for the workers that handle it. The effects of its toxicity have been recognized by distilleries in Grasse as an industrial illness.

Hexane and chlorure of methylene are other extraction solvents which are even more volatile than benzene. It is estimated that 700 tonnes of chemicals per year disperse in the air around Grasse alone (see page 32).

Dissolving

To obtain an absolute from the concrete, the concrete is treated with a strong alcohol in which certain constituents dissolve. The alcohol is evaporated off completely, leaving behind the absolute. The absolute has a different balance of constituents to the concrete and the essential oil.

Dissolving can also be used for extracting gums and resins of plants and trees such as galbanum, frankincense and myrrh. The gums and resins are immersed in alcohol in which they dissolve. The alcohol is then evaporated off completely. What is left behind is called a resinoid and it is a heavy sticky substance. This process is cheaper than steam distillation and is widely used in the cosmetic industry. For aromatherapeutic use it is preferable to obtain oils that have been steam distilled.

Expression

This is the technique employed for obtaining the oils from the rinds and peels of fruits like oranges, mandarins and lemons. The rinds are pressed or grated, then the oils from the torn cells are collected in a sponge and squeezed out. It was once done by hand, but now it is performed by machine. It used to be the case that workers who handled the sponges full of essential oil for any length of time suffered allergies and problems on their hands. However, as mechanization has taken over, there are fewer problems of this kind.

USING ESSENTIAL OILS AND PLANTS

Essential oils can be massaged into the skin, added to warm bath water, inhaled or added to plant poultices or compresses. None can be taken internally, but many oils can be of internal benefit by eating the oil-containing plant itself (see pages 25 – 6).

Although I give warnings about particular oils throughout the book, it is appropriate to repeat here that one should always be very careful when using essential oils. This is particularly important in the case of pregnant women (see page 28) and children. Any treatment offered to a child should be used in half strength or less.

Before using *any* oil in any remedy, first do a skin test (see opposite).

Everyone is individual and has a different way of reacting to different oils. Age, size and sex all make a difference too.

In addition, when choosing which oil to use – for many have the same properties – for preference choose one from a plant which grows in approximately the same geographical area as that in which you live. If you are British, try lavender as a calmant before you try frankincense, for instance. And don't be surprised to see that many oils have apparently conflicting properties – *i.e.* stimulant *and* relaxant – depending on the proportions used. Lavender, for example, has stimulating properties when used in larger quantities, but in smaller amounts it is a relaxant. The concept can be likened to taking a drink of wine – one glass may act as a stimulant, whereas three or more might send you to sleep.

I do not advocate anyone to carry out continued use of essential oils, but to use them only when there is a problem requiring a remedy. Remember that they are a type of drug and just as you would not take an aspirin every day unless medically prescribed, so you should not use essential oils for prolonged periods of time without a reason or without first checking with your doctor or aromatherapist. Respect them and use them when they are genuinely needed.

You can, however, keep aromatherapy in your daily life in other ways, by using the plants rather than the essential oils, whether in decoctions, tisanes, cooking or other ideas suggested throughout this book.

Skin test

Everyone should carry out a skin test before using an essential oil, but it is particularly important if you suffer from hayfever or allergies of any kind, and should always be done before using the oils in treatments for children and the elderly.

Put one drop of the oil on a cotton bud and use it to just touch the inside of the elbow, the back of the wrist or under the arm. Cover the area with a plaster and leave unwashed for 24 hours. If there is itching, redness or any other type of reaction, don't use that oil on that person.

Base or Carrier Oils

Few essential oils are used neat, but are mixed into a fixed plant oil base like almond, soya or wheatgerm. (Fixed oils do not evaporate quickly on exposure to the air like essential or volatile ones.) These base or carrier oils contain certain benefits themselves, not least their contents of iodine and vitamin E. They also act as a balancing and stabilizing agent. A carrier or base oil should be pure, and preferably cold pressed when it retains its essential vitamin content better. It should have little or no smell of its own, and it should be penetrative. The quantities of essential oil to base oil will vary a little from oil to oil, but unless otherwise stated you should use 2-3 drops essential oil to 5 ml (1 tsp) base oil for use on the body, and 1 drop essential oil to 5ml (1 tsp) base oil for the face.

Almond oil

The plant: The almond tree (*Prunus amygdalus*, Rosaceae) is a native of the eastern Mediterranean, but is now established in other warm countries. It was introduced to Britain during Roman times, and its nuts were a common ingredient in medieval cooking.

The oil: The fixed oils of almond are extracted from two types of almond tree, the bitter almond (*P. amygdalus* var. *amara*) and the sweet almond (*P. amygdalus* var. *dulcis*). Only the latter is used in therapy. The nuts contain about 50 – 60 per cent oil, which is also used in baking and confectionery.

The oil is a lovely clear pale yellow, more or less odourless with a slight nutty note. Olein is its principal constituent, with a tiny proportion of glyceride and linoleic acid. It has a definite action on the skin as a softening agent, being a good lubricant, nourishing and revitalizing. Shop-bought oils are often adulterated, so beware.

Its uses: An almond remedy is wonderful for dry, wrinkled hands, but is also very beneficial for eczema and skin irritations of any kind. Warm some almond oil gently in a bain-marie then dissolve in it the same amount of cocoa butter. Remove from the heat, mix until paste-like and apply to the hands. Put on some cotton gloves and allow the oil to penetrate for at least an hour (or overnight).

Castor oil

The plant: Castor oil comes from a tall, quick-growing, perennial woody shrub or small tree (*Ricinus communis*, Euphorbiaceae) native to India, but is now seen in many warm countries. It is often grown as an ornamental, but it is also of value as a windbreak and a shade tree. It bears seed profusely and it is these that are pressed for the oil. This was known to the Greeks and Romans as a purgative or laxative, which is still a major role of the oil today; lots of common laxatives contain a proportion of castor oil.

The oil: It has a very viscid consistency, is colourless, has a slight fragrance, and is disagreeable to taste. The major constituents are palmatic and other fatty acids, ricinoleic acid and glycerine.

Its uses: The Ancient Egyptians called the oil *kiki*, using it as an unguent for skin rashes, and in embalming. It is still useful for numerous skin complaints, ranging from eczema to dryness of the skin. For very dry eczema, mix 30 ml (2 tbsp) of castor oil with 15 ml (1 tbsp) of almond oil and 2 drops of wheatgerm oil, and apply gently to the affected part.

Because the oil is so viscid, it is a good idea to mix it with another carrier oil to help its penetration.

When in India I drove past field upon field of the plant. My skin was so dry from the heat and dust that I asked the driver to stop so I could rub my hands and face with the leaves and berries of the plant. Indian women also do this to keep their skin young looking and supple.

Grapeseed oil

The oil: Grape seeds contain between 6 and 20 per cent oil. The oil is pale greeny yellow in colour and is very pure, high in polyunsaturates, and extremely light – it is almost as thin as water. This means that it is easily absorbed by the skin, which is very useful in aromatherapy because the essentials can penetrate very quickly.

It uses: The seeds and leaves of grapes are rather astringent, so I tend to use the oil for conditions like acne.

Soya oil

The plant: This comes from the soy or soya bean plant (*Glycine hispida* or *soja*, Leguminosae), an erect annual sometimes reaching 1 – 1.75 m (4 – 6 ft) in height, which is native to China and Japan. Although used in the East for the last 4,000 years, it did not appear in Europe until the end of the seventeenth century, nor in Britain until the beginning of the twentieth century. It is high in polyunsaturates, and one of the most popular of cooking oils. The bean itself is one of the world's major and most nourishing foodstuffs (it is the only plant source containing complete protein).

The oil: There is approximately 12 – 25 per cent oil in the beans, and this contains many acids (oleic, linoleic, stearic, palmitic, etc) and traces of chlorophyll. It is a very nourishing oil of a very pale colour with a tinge of yellow; it is a good carrier oil as it is quickly absorbed when applied to the skin. It must be of the best quality, though. I use it a lot in preparations for acne – as you will see in this book.

Its uses: The French value soya oil for its medicinal properties: the linoleic acid content helps lower cholesterol levels. Take some every day in your salad dressings, on top of freshly cooked vegetables, or with rice dishes.

Wheatgerm oil

The plant: Wheatgerm, the germ of the wheat grain, is a highly nutritious food, rich in proteins (one of the few plant sources which provide near complete proteins), and vitamins B and E.

The oil: Wheatgerm oil contains a very high proportion of vitamin E, which is said to be the skin vitamin.

15

It uses: Because of its high proportion of vitamin E, it is very effective in contributing to the treatment of skin problems when used as a carrier oil.

Another benefit of using wheatgerm oil is that as it is an antioxidant it stabilizes essential oils and makes them last longer. Add a drop or two of wheatgerm oil to any remedy.

Massage

That essential oils can pass through the skin is indisputable. After all, the skin eliminates, so it can just as easily absorb. Modern scientific research has shown that many more substances pass through the skin than was previously thought possible, and some of the best scientific units in the world are investigating the medical potential of this. It is known, for example, that steroid creams held in place underneath occlusive dressings can contribute to a dangerous build-up of steroids in the body as they are passing through the skin. A simple test for the sceptical is to rub the soles of the feet with a cut garlic clove; in a few hours the smell of the garlic will be detected on the breath.

One effective way to treat ailments with essential oils is by massage. This could be as professional or as perfunctory as you like, but the rubbing action will activate the nerve endings and stimulate the circulation of blood to the surface of the skin – and thereby ease the entry of the oils.

Even if correctly applied, essential oils will only be taken up by the skin for a period of about seven to ten minutes, and will not be absorbed well if applied when the body is eliminating – when sweating through anxiety or heat, for instance, or after exercise. And their efficiency in penetrating the skin and reaching the other organs also depends very much on the individual. A large amount of subcutaneous fat will impede their passage, as will water retention and poor circulation.

The oils can be massaged into the face, back, chest, top of the hands, soles of the feet – or relevant part of the body in the case of rheumatic pain, say – and this in itself is relaxing. Even if you don't have time for a proper massage, apply an appropriate essential oil mix on the top of your hands, back of the neck, temples, the third eye (between the eyes), under the nose, and behind the ears; this activates the circulation, and the relevant oil will help you regain vitality. The hands are particularly useful because the skin on top is very thin, and there are many visible main veins.

On the face

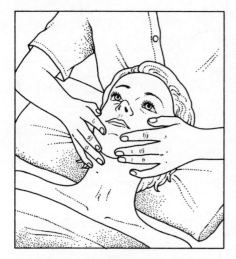

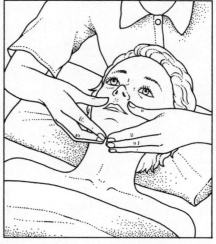

Having applied the appropriate massage oil to face and neck, use the fingers to apply pressure at several points along the jawline. Work from the chin to the ears.

Apply pressure with the thumbs to the hollows at the side of the nose, then work at intervals along nose-to-mouth lines to the centre of the chin.

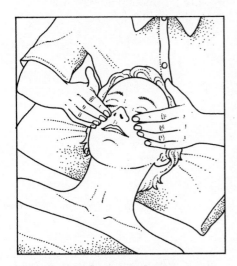

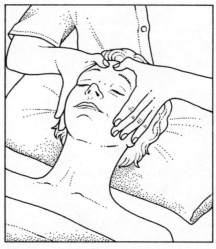

Use all your fingers to apply pressure under cheekbones, working from the side of the nose out to the ears.

Working in parallel lines from the eyebrows upwards to the hairline, use the thumbs to apply pressure at several points along the lines. (This is good for headaches, catarrh and general puffiness.)

17

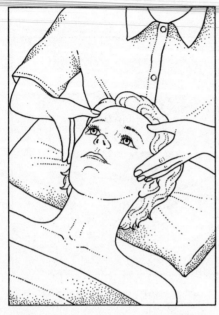

Work with your thumbs in smooth, sweeping movements to trace a line from the centre of the forehead to the temples.

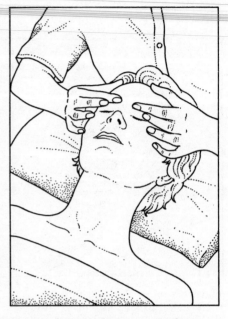

Use your index fingers to apply pressure to the tearduct at the inner corner of each eye. Disperse the pressure by smoothing outwards under the eyebrows.

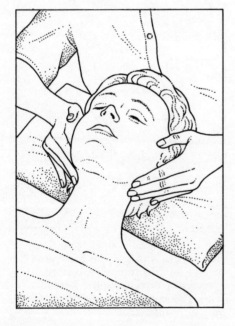

Press the hands gently against the outer ears. Massage the whole ear from back to front, using a circular motion, but without rubbing the skin. Massage the other ear at the same time in the same way.

On the back and shoulders

Obviously you have to do this to someone else or get someone else to do it to you! The recipient should be lying on his/her stomach on a table or firm bed, head on arms. Clothes should be removed to the waist, and a towel can be used for warmth.

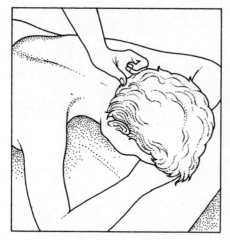

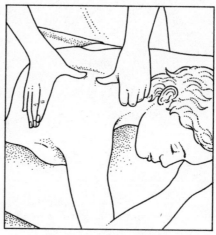

Start the massage by applying oil to the back of the neck and down the back. Then, using one thumb, work down the neck, one side at a time, applying pressure at equal intervals.

Using both thumbs together on the same side of the spine, work down the spine from the base of the neck.

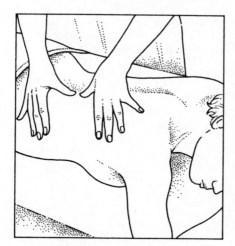

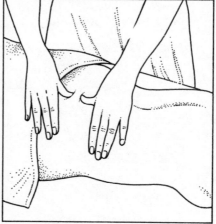

As you work down the back, apply the pressure about 1 cm (½ in) from the spine). Use a fast movement for a stimulating effect and a slow movement for a relaxing one.

Finish this first stage at the coccyx. Then work down the other side of the spine as you did before, trying to keep the pressure points parallel.

19

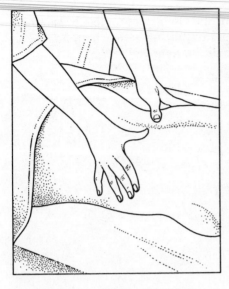

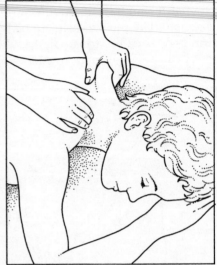

With thumbs on either side of the spine, work up the back using small upward and outward movements. Start at the base of the spine, and finish at the base of the neck. The idea is to slowly disperse energy from the pressure points.

Massage the shoulders with a kneading motion. Your aim is to relieve the knots of tension that build up there.

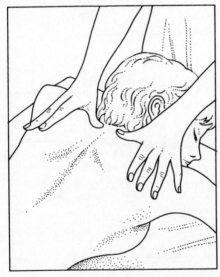

With thumbs on either side of the spine, work down the spine with gently downward movements about 1 cm (½ in) from the spine. Start at the base of the neck and finish at the coccyx as before.

If there is no one available to give you a full back massage, apply the oil to the sacrum area (the lower part of the back) and massage in well.

On the legs and feet

To give a leg massage to someone else, ask him/her to lie down and apply oil to the legs, working up from the feet and squeezing gently. Always work towards the heart.

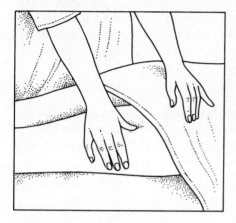

Apply pressure with your thumb to the back of the thigh (to improve circulation).

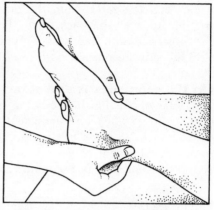

Using your thumb, apply pressure to the inside back of the ankle (this relieves poor circulation, fluid retention and bladder problems).

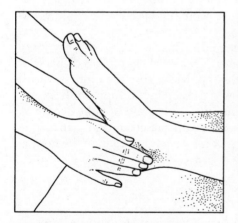

Using the fingers of both hands, massage the back of the ankles on the inside and outside of the leg simultaneously (this relieves strain in the back).

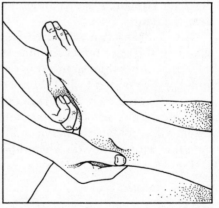

Using the knuckles of one hand, press firmly in one even movement from the arch of the foot to the heel (again to promote good circulation).

Or simply sit on the floor, and massage an appropriate oil into the soles and tops of the feet and between each toe. You can do this while watching television and, along with a scalp massage, it is a wonderful way to spend ten minutes before you go to bed which will help you to sleep.

On the scalp

This is particularly good for tiredness, loss of hair and ageing. Start at the back of the head, on the dip at the back of the neck, and work upwards towards the crown of the head. Press from the left towards the centre of the neck with the thumb of your left hand, all round the back of the neck, then the same from the other side using the other hand. Then friction up over the back of the head, and all over the cranium using the fingers of both hands as if giving yourself a very vigorous shampoo. Feel the skin becoming loose.

On the solar plexus and stomach

The solar plexus lies between the ribs, and you should simply press the oiled palm of one hand against it and rub in a clockwise direction (it doesn't seem to work in the opposite direction). Do the same with the stomach. The heat of your hands will help the absorption of the oils. Avoid this massage in pregnancy.

In the Bath

Another effective way of treating with essential oils is to use them in the bath. Recent scientific research using radio-active isotopes has provided proof that essential oils added to bath water *are* absorbed through the skin. So when Hippocrates recommended an aromatic bath every day, he was near the truth.

Mix 3 drops (unless otherwise stated) with a capful of very mild shampoo and pour under running water. This will help the oils disperse in the water rather than sit in a film on the top. Make sure the room is warm, and that the door and windows are closed to keep in the vapours. Immerse your body completely for at least ten minutes, relax and breathe deeply. A certain quantity of odoriferous molecules will penetrate the skin, while others will stimulate the nerve endings of the olfactory organ in the nose in the same way as they do when inhaled as a vapour.

Facial Saunas

For deep-cleansing the skin, have a facial sauna once or twice a week. Have ready a bowl, the chosen oil(s), and a towel. Boil a kettle of water and wait until it has cooled to hand-hot temperature (about 38 °C ® 100 °F⅜), not scalding. Put in a few drops (or as many drops as specified) of essential oil. Put the towel over your head and lean over the bowl so that the towel encloses both head and bowl. Do not get much closer than about 30 cm (12 in).

The essential oils in the steam will get to work on the skin. The effect is twofold as the essences in vapour form are absorbed through the delicate membranes of the nasal passages as well. Their action is thus internal as well as external.

Inhalations

Inhalation, which is most obviously useful for congestive ailments like catarrh and colds, uses the same principle as a facial sauna. It also operates on the same principle as traditional home or chemist-shop remedies for the blocked noses of colds and 'flu: these involve a simple towel-over-head inhalation of friar's balsam (derived from benzoin essential oil), or eucalyptus or wintergreen (essential oils of Australian and North American trees respectively).

You can buy inhalers from specialist chemists, or use your own 'built-in' inhaler: put 1 drop of the chosen oil on your hands, rub together to warm, then cup together over your nose, making sure the hands are firmly closed. Inhale deeply several times, and the benefits of the oils will be very quickly absorbed.

Poultices

Poultices are an age-old way of drawing impurities out through the skin to soothe irritation, or to relieve congestion or pain. Their history goes back many thousands of years, indeed, they were among the first forms of medicine developed by man. What they consist of is a raw or mashed herb, which is sometimes applied in this state directly to the body, or is moistened first before its application (see individual plant descriptions). Sometimes, too, the contents of the poultice are left exposed to the air; otherwise the ingredients are wrapped in a cloth and then applied.

Traditionally the poultices in most frequent use were made of linseed or mustard; they were particularly popular when dealing with chest complaints and skin ailments – and still are.

Linseed

The seeds are those of the plant *Linum usitatissimum* (Linaceae), which also yields the fibre flax. Linseed oil is used occasionally as a base oil in aromatherapy, but its main commercial value is in paints and varnishes (and in conditioning the willow of cricket bats). The seeds contain 30 – 40 per cent fixed oil, which is viscid and yellow, containing linolene and palmotine. The oil is reputedly good for constipation; in Switzerland they sell it to mix with muesli.

The seeds form a good base for a poultice as they crush easily, swell up in liquid, and hold heat for a long time; they are also very lubricant because of the oil content of the seeds.

Depending on the area to be covered, use from 3 tablespoons up to about 100 g (4 oz) seeds. Crush them in a mortar or a coffee mill. Place in a saucepan and pour in enough boiling water to make a smooth paste. Add the essential oil – from 2 to 5 drops, depending on the amount of linseed used (see also individual recommendations) – and mix. Spread on an appropriately sized piece of gauze or muslin, and cover with a second piece. Fold the ends over and apply while still hot (but not scalding). Leave for at least ten minutes, or until cool.

Apply an oil afterwards to reinforce the action of the poultice and lubricate the skin (see individual recommendations). If used on the face, the poultice can leave the skin feeling a bit sticky (although it gives a wonderful glow and an amazingly supple feeling). Use a flower water, like rose, orange or witch hazel, to remove this stickiness.

Mustard seeds

A poultice of mustard should not be used on the face: it is most effective, though, on the chest and back for a number of ailments.

You can either use crushed seeds (use a mortar or coffee mill, but wash them well afterwards!) or mustard powder. A mustard seed poultice is made in the same way as a linseed poultice, using boiling purified water (available from chemists) or still mineral water; but as the seeds are less bulky than linseed, add some linseed as well. If using mustard powder, add it to linseed or oatmeal.

Apply the poultice warm, not hot. A mustard seed poultice will make the skin red and hot (a sign it is having the desired reaction) so after removing apply talcum powder, to absorb the heat, and wash your hands. Do not leave for longer than ten minutes as it can make the skin swell.

Mustard poultices can be bought ready-made in France.

Oatmeal

Like linseed, organic oats swell up, retain heat and are easy to spread on gauze. Oatmeal contains a significant amount of vitamin E, too. Use as for linseed, but these poultices are a little too sticky to be used on the face.

In Clay Masks

Some clay is included as a base in many commercial mask formulas as it helps absorb excess oil from greasy skin, and lifts dirt out of the pores. Clay masks should not be used on a dry or sensitive skin.

Powdered clay (green especially) is available in selected chemists. Mix with just enough purified water (or still mineral water or chamomile or rose water) to make a paste, then add the relevant essential oil. Apply to the face and leave to dry. Wash off with water or a flower infusion like chamomile (see opposite).

As Compresses

These are used externally on the eyes in particular, and are either hot or cold depending on the effect required.

To make compresses soak pieces of lint (or thin pieces of *real* cotton wool) in an appropriate infusion, decoction or maceration and hold over the affected area (or bandage in place). When a cold compress warms through contact with the skin, replace with another cold one; when a hot compress becomes cold, replace that as well.

Infusions

Pour boiling water on to fresh bruised herbs or dried herbs, and leave for six to ten minutes. Strain. To bruise herbs use a mortar and pestle. For large quantities roll the herbs in a clean tea-towel and walk on them.

Decoctions

Used for harder stems, roots and seeds. Bruise the plant material using a hammer, then bring to the boil in water for one to two minutes. Cover, and leave to infuse for 15 minutes. Strain.

Macerations

Bring the material to the boil in water, remove from the heat, and leave to infuse, covered, for several hours. This becomes very potent and has a strong effect. Strain.

None of these preparations lasts very long, so store them in a fridge and use within two days.

In Diet

A sensible diet is vital for maintaining body health, and this I have emphasised in almost every entry in Part Three, the ailment section. A sensible diet should include plants – vegetables, fruit, herbs and spices – many of which actually contain oils which are extracted for use in aromatherapy.

That the principles of aromatherapy have a natural place in the kitchen is easily understandable, not least because one of the major properties of many plant oils is digestive: the smell of a food reaches the nose, nerve stimuli are sent to the brain, and this in turn triggers the secretion of saliva and gastric juices. This means the digestive process can start before any food is actually placed in the mouth. And this, along with the oils in the food, will naturally help facilitate complete digestion once the food is actually in the body. To use aromatic plants in cooking is virtually to be a do-it-yourself doctor!

The body requires many basic nutrients – proteins, fats, carbohydrates, fibre, vitamins, minerals, trace elements and fluid – and to utilize as much as possible of these it is best to eat the food raw for many nutrients are destroyed by heat. Salads, for instance, are delicious, filling, and can contain very many healthy ingredients. Some people, however, cannot digest raw food, such as cucumber and green pepper, properly which is why digestive herbs should be taken in combination with them. Very many herbs, leaves and flowers, can be scattered into salads, for their digestive properties. Lemon juice, too, because of its antiseptic effect, is good in dressings for salads.

Even with cooked food, aromatherapeutic principles can still apply. The orange in the traditional sauce for duck helps the body assimilate the fat content of the bird's flesh; savory and other herbs help the digestion of difficult foods such as pulses. The time to add herbs and spices (even salt and pepper) to food is at the last moment.

To dress your salads and to cook with, use pure cold-pressed oils such as olive, safflower and soya. If cold-pressed, they retain more of their own essential nutrients. Or make your own herbal oils (see page 27) and use these.

A healthy liquid intake is an equally important part of a balanced diet. Man can survive for many days without food but only a few without water, which has a vital role in the proper functioning of the kidneys. The liquid drunk should preferably be mineral water and for complete health, tea, coffee and alcohol should be drunk in moderation, or replaced with herbal teas and tisanes.

Herbal Teas and Tisanes

These are the aromatherapeutic answer to the liquid requirements of the diet. Everyone could benefit from drinking tisanes. A rosehip tea with some honey is popular with children and it is rich in vitamin C. A herb tea could replace tea or coffee at home or in the office. All you need to do is make room in your kitchen for a range of herbs and spices. You can buy herbs in teabag form in health food shops, or you can grow and dry your own. When buying spices, buy whole rather than ground.

To use herbal teabags, infuse in boiling water in a cup covered with a saucer for 3 – 5 minutes. For herbs, use a dessertspoon of chopped fresh herbs or ½ dessertspoon dried herbs per person, in a warmed teapot. Add boiling water and infuse for about 7 minutes. Spices may need longer to infuse in boiling water, and you will want to experiment with quantities to suit your taste. To all, add a little honey to sweeten if preferred. Drink throughout the day – gradually replacing tea or coffee completely – and taking a last calming cup at night is a lovely way to finish the day.

MAKING YOUR OWN PLANT OILS AND VINEGARS

Making your own plant oils and vinegars is one way to be certain of the quality, especially if you use homegrown or organic plants. The oils will not be as strong as bought essential oils but they will still be effective, while being safer to use. What is more they won't need diluting in a carrier oil so they are actually easier to use. They can also be used in cooking and make delicious marinades and salad dressings. Good herbs to try are lavender flowers, thyme, marjoram, rosemary, sage or chamomile, but it's fun to experiment with your own favourite herbs.

Herb Oils

You will need 250g (8 oz) fresh herbs or 100g (4 oz) dried to every 600 ml (1 pint) grapeseed or soya oil.

First wash and dry the fresh herbs quickly and carefully. Place the fresh or dried herbs in a clear glass bottle. Cover completely with the oil, seal and stand on a sunny windowsill for two to three weeks. Remove the herbs from the oil and decant into dark bottles. The oil is now ready for using.

Herb Vinegars

Use 250 g (8 oz) fresh herbs or 100 g (4 oz) dried for every 600 ml (1 pint) cider vinegar. Quickly wash and dry the fresh herbs before using. Place the fresh or dried herbs in dark glass bottles and place the bottles in the dark. Shake them every two or three days. The herbs should be left in the vinegar for at least 10 days, after which time the vinegar is ready for using.

Mint and raspberry vinegar skin freshener
This is a wonderful skin freshener to cool the skin in summer, or to use as a daily rinse after cleansing. Use 50 g (2 oz) fresh mint and 100–200g (4–7 oz) fresh raspberries to 600 ml (1 pint) cider vinegar and make as above.

THE TOXICITY OF ESSENTIAL OILS

Certain constituents of essential oils are very toxic, particularly to vulnerable people like the old, the very young, and pregnant women (see page 28). On the whole, this toxicity applies to an oil when taken internally, which is something I am passionately against. Certain of these toxins in certain oils *can* be dangerous when applied externally (or inhaled), and I have given clear warnings where necessary throughout the book. In many cases, though, because of a balance of constituents in the oil, or because of a balance of more than one essential oil in a remedy (or even just because of the calming influence of a certain carrier oil), the oil can still be used safely. It is usually only when potentially dangerous oils are used in too large quantities that the dangers become a reality and for this reason the proportions of essential oils recommended must be respected. One must remember that *one* little drop of an essential oil represents between 25 and 35 g (1 and 1 ¼ oz) of the plant itself. Proportion is the key to everything.

The International Fragrance Association (IFRA), has issued a list of oils whose use is restricted in the industries which use fragrancies in their products, for example cosmetics and household products. IFRA gives these oils strict proportion controls and of those used in aromatherapy they include angelica root, *baume de Pérou*, bergamot, cassia, cinnamon, cumin, sassafras and verbena. IFRA has no international legal powers, but most fragrance companies worldwide do follow their guidelines.

In addition to those oils restricted by IFRA, I consider the following to be worthy of close and careful attention: anise, aspic, basil, clove, coriander, hyssop and sage. These worries mostly concern constituents such as anethol, estragol (methyl-chavicol) and thujone, but I'm also careful about those containing eugenol (which can corrode metal).

Toxic reactions can be felt immediately, and range from dizziness and nausea to exhaustion, epilepsy and even death. Some toxins cause allergy: the tansy flower, used in perfumery (and now restricted in the industry by the French Ministry of Health), has caused terrible eczema on the hands of the pickers.

Pregnancy

I don't advise anyone who is pregnant to use any essential oils. Not only does the skin become more sensitive during pregnancy, but some women find that smells they once had no problems with now make them feel nauseous or irritable. More alarmingly, certain essential oils, particularly those containing apiol and myristicine, have abortive powers and cause miscarriage or have other undesirable effects on the womb. Parsley, for example, in very large doses was once used as an abortive. In France apiol was used in contraception before the advent of the pill, and in South America it is still used today.

Instead of using the essential oils, try very weak herbal teas, in small quantities, and bring aromatherapy into your life in other ways – for instance by bringing flowers into your home, by using the relevant herbs in cooking, or using weak infusions of the plants themselves.

If you think you may be pregnant, do stop using essential oils immediately, and of course always consult your doctor.

THE FUTURE OF AROMATHERAPY

Sadly, in the ten years or so that aromatherapy has regained popularity in Britain, a country more wedded than my native France to traditional medicine, the therapy's true origins and values have been eroded. Anyone can now take a brief course, invest a few thousand pounds in oils, and set up as an aromatherapist. This is an appalling situation showing a disrespect for the therapy and is an insult to those who want to believe in its efficacy.

How can anyone just beginning in the therapy possibly diagnose a condition, know how to treat it, and which essential oils to use? Diagnosing and treating a condition require considerable expertise, knowledge and practice, and the short courses given are grossly inadequate. I have received many letters from young women who have gained 'diplomas' in aromatherapy, but who want to learn more because they feel they know so little. Some top nurses in the Churchill Hospital, Oxford, use essential oils in their treatments, but even they, with all their medical knowledge, are very careful in their usage, and are extremely worried about some claims made for the therapy in the last few years. It is actually dangerous, too, for many of the oils are very strong, poisonous even, and can have powerful effects in the wrong – or uninformed – hands; the results could be disastrous to vulnerable people – children, the old, or pregnant women (see page 28).

Aromatherapy was once a proper therapy because the oils were pure and natural essential oils, having been water distilled from plants grown especially for the therapy. Today there are many methods of gaining essences from plants (see page 10), most being steam-distilled. Through the demands of commerce though, many distillers are now using volatile solvents rather than water to extract the oils (see page 11). These modern methods produce far more oil and oil with a stronger fragrance, which is beneficial to the perfume industry – the largest client of the distillers. But, as even the tiniest trace of the solvent remaining in the essential oil changes the balance of its constituents, the oil cannot therefore be used as safely and therapeutically as before. Many inexperienced aromatherapists do, however, use these oils, not questioning or caring about the method of extraction and the purity of the oil. Unfortunately, as the therapy accounts for such a tiny percentage of the oils sold, we have little or no say in how they are extracted.

Essential oils for aromatherapy were once produced from plants raised naturally – and, indeed, many still are – but most, again through the demands of commerce, are now being 'helped along' by modern agricultural methods, using pesticides and fertilizers. These affect the essential constituents of the plant and therefore the essential oil. Traces of agricultural nitrates, for instance, show up in chromatographs ('x-rays' of plant oils), and as a result a lot of research is being done to evaluate the dangers of this in therapy. These pesticides are normally used by those who have huge acreages of plants; most distillers of essential oils for therapy are smaller and are more careful.

Another worrying aspect is the aftermath of the nuclear disaster at Chernobyl. The fallout has probably affected the whole world, but European plants in particular have suffered and, in turn, so have the plants' oils (as can be seen when the oils are tested for radioactivity). I now import a lot of my oils – particularly thyme, which seems to 'fix' pollutants more than other herbs – from Israel, ie. as far as possible from Kiev and the path of the fallout.

Distillers and bottlers have a great responsibility in ensuring the future of the therapy. There are many who distil by steam, bottle pure oils and are honest, but others cut corners. If the clary sage crop has not been good enough, they might top up with sage and sell the oil as that of pure clary sage. Sage oil is a very strong oil, and can have disastrous effects on vulnerable or sensitive people. This practice is very common indeed now, so what are practitioners, let alone members of the public, to do?

Checking Quality

It is not always easy to check on the quality of oils, even if you have in your hand all the right answers such as the chromatography and the marks of quality. One has to depend entirely on one's nose to make the ultimate check, and experience in this comes only after many years of smelling different qualities of essential oils. For instance, lavender, lavandin and aspic all smell the same to an inexpert nose, and lavandin and aspic are taken for lavender in most cases. (There are huge differences therapeutically and in cost.)

An expert nose should also be able to detect adulteration of the product. This is not easy and only comes with time. Many years ago the agent and importer of essential oils with whom I dealt died. His business was bought by someone who had very little knowledge. Shortly afterwards I purchased some essential oil of rose from Morocco, and when I opened the bottle I immediately recognized that the smell was different – it had an added note – also the colour had changed and the consistency was more fluid. My suspicions raised I rang the new agent but was told that the quality was the same as I had purchased in the past. I sent a sample to my laboratory in France for analysis, and I was right. The oil had been adulterated in two ways: first by diluting it with a vegetable oil, and second, by adding geranium. Was the new agent dishonest or had the distillers taken advantage of his lack of expertise? As one depends on total honesty from the distiller and supplier, where does this leave the practitioner? One must always be on the alert.

I am now actively campaigning to have the provenance of essential oils recorded on their labels by the distiller. This will be difficult because of the very many countries which produce oils, but it is a step in the right direction. I also want to have the dates of the distillation recorded on these labels, for oils deteriorate very quickly if not kept properly, and lose their therapeutic properties if too old. Some can actually cause allergic reactions. Two clients reacted badly to lavender that they bought in shops; it is a gentle oil, but it had been stored for far too long.

Storing essential oils
Essential oils should always be stored in dark bottles (glass or metal) to protect them from light, and preferably kept in a dark, cool place (not under the bright lights of a shop interior). Stoppers have to be very carefully and properly sealed, for air can also have a deleterious effect on the oil. (And the oils can, of course, dissolve certain types of stoppers and seals.) Certain oils, clove for example, can also corrode metal. Because it may be impossible for you to check the quality of essential oils, where relevant I have given remedies using the plants themselves. Alternatively you could make your own plant oils (see page 27) and use these in therapy. Don't forget that they won't need diluting.

The Effects of the Perfume and Food Industries

Commerce is also responsible for yet another blow to the future of aromatherapy. The largest market for most essential oils is the perfumery industry. This industry is so powerful that it can actually specify to growers around the world what is to be grown. We need rose this year, they might say, not geranium, so distil that. The growers will, of course, agree, thereby cutting down the availability of certain oils which, although very valuable in therapy, are not so valued in perfumery. Certain houses in the perfumery industry, for instance, have recently monopolized almost the entire world market in sandalwood oil. As a result, that oil, of great value therapeutically, particularily for Ayurvedic medicine in India, will not be readily available for aromatherapy for years to come, to say nothing of the effect that the perfumery industry's demands are having on the destruction of forests (see page 195).

The food industry, too, uses a huge proportion of essential oils for flavouring all manner of foods and drink. About a teaspoon of an oil like sage could kill a child, and indeed seven cases of 'food poisoning' were recently registered in France where the sufferers had eaten sausages flavoured with sage oil instead of fresh sage. What effects, therefore, are the inclusion of oils like nutmeg in food having on the rest of us? Hyperactivity in children, now believed to be related to additives in food, could be one result.

A Look to the Future

All in all, the therapy is no longer what it once was, and in the wrong hands, can be positively dangerous rather than beneficial to health. The future and the success of the therapy are dependent on a whole chain of people doing the right thing at the right time and in the right way: growing the plant organically, cutting the plant at the right time, distilling the plant in the most natural way, bottling the oil honestly, and storing the oil sensibly. I believe that this essential 'trust' is diminishing all the time. An expensive 'rose oil' could have been solvent extracted from chemically fertilized plants then adulterated with geranium or gaiac oil.

The city of Grasse in the south of France, once so famed for its fields of flowers and its mild winters, illustrates these points all too well. Very few plants are now cultivated there for distillation and many small factories have been closed down in the last few decades, leaving the big factories to deal with most of the trade. The intensive labour cost, the cost of land and the pressures and demands of certain plants, have been the main factors leading to this demise, and the growers have turned to new sources of income. Some of them have lost all their money and have had to sell their land to developers. Now tall buildings, blocks of flats and houses have replaced the endless fields of aromatic flowers which once composed the unique landscape in and around Grasse.

Neither can its reputation as *the* 'climatic' city of France be applied any more. Nominated this because of its flowers, altitude and proximity to the sea, this lovely city has become one of the most polluted in France. Some 700 tonnes of solvent escape into the air above it each year because Grasse is still one of the world centres of the perfume industry, but chemically so. In the last two decades the chemical syntheses for perfumery have taken great strides forward resulting in the stability in pricing, the lower cost, the good synthetic reproduction of natural smells, and the continuity of colour of products.

There are not enough plants to supply the world demand for perfume, which is why chemical equivalents are being produced. As a result, some flower distillations have completely ceased: some of the flowers which used to make the great perfumes of the past – gardenia, lilac, lily of the valley – are all now recreated in the laboratory, but for me the synthetic smell will never compare with the subtlety of the natural. Such synthetic equivalents, although they can't be used in aromatherapy, can't be totally condemned as rather this than that the earth should be further wrecked and deprived of its flora and vegetation, and forests destroyed (see Bois de rose and Sandalwood).

If the future looks gloomy, it remains that the basic principles of aromatherapy still hold good. I do use essential oils in my prescriptions, and I have recommended using many in the remedies throughout this book. However, these are used in very careful dilutions to ensure safety, and I give warnings about those which have even the smallest doubt attached to them. Instead, the majority of my remedies utilize the actual plants themselves, which of course contain the essential oils in smaller but safer quantities. This is a sensible path to choose.

Always consult your doctor for a proper diagnosis of any symptoms, particularly as they may be indicative of a more serious underlying cause.

Aromatherapy has been, and always should be, effective, with a part to play in modern medicine, health, beauty and life – but I do urge you to take care.

Part Two

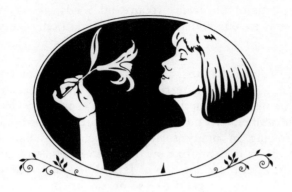

A-Z OF AROMATHERAPEUTIC PLANTS & OILS

Illnesses marked in bold appear in Part Three, the A-Z of Ailments, where more detailed information will be found.

ANGELICA *(Angelica archangelica/officinalis – Umbelliferae)*

'The whole plants, both leafe, roote and seeds, is of an excellent comfortable sent, savour and taste.' (John Parkinson, *Theatre of Plants*, 1640)

An old legend claims that the benefits of angelica were revealed to a monk by an angel during a terrible plague – thus the common and horticultural names, and another local one, 'root of the Holy Ghost'. Angelica is an umbellifer and is native to northern Europe and Syria, commonly growing in many sorts of habitat. Various varieties are known: the *norvegica* in Scandinavia, the *sativa* in Holland and northern France, and the *refracta* and *japonica* in Japan; *sylvestris* is the wild British variety, but this is not so good to use or eat as the *officinalis* which is generally seen in the wild as a kitchen garden escapee.

The plant can reach a height of 1.5 – 2 m (5 – 6½ ft), and the seeds, stems, leaves and roots are all aromatic. The stems are hollow and ridged, the leaves bright green and large, divided into toothed leaflets. Small yellow-green flower groups in large umbels bloom from early summer.

All parts of the plant have been used over the centuries for many purposes. A third-century Chinese physician wrote that 'when I tell the common people that ... angelica and peony can cure colic ... they doubt or deny it and prefer to believe in wizardry.' John Gerard, herbalist to James I, attributed many virtues to angelica, and during the plague of 1660, angelica stems were chewed as a preventative against infection, and seeds and roots burned to purify the air. The same measures had been prescribed by Paracelsus some 150 years earlier during an epidemic in Milan.

Angelica is cultivated and used in many European countries, as well as China, for its medicinal properties. The seeds (best gathered on a dry day after the sun has dried the dew) are used along with the leaves, in teas and tisanes. The stems and roots are used too: the former should be cut in late spring/early summer; the latter should be dried as quickly as possible so that they retain their medicinal properties, and stored in hermetically sealed brown glass jars. Dried roots are wrinkled and brown and have a very pleasant aromatic odour of benzoin, pepper and musk.

The leaves, seeds, roots and stems possess carminative, diaphoretic, stimulant, stomachic, expectorant and tonic properties. John Gerard prescribed angelica as a preventative against viral infections. Two well-known seventeenth-century French herbalists, Nicolas Lemery and Jean-Baptiste Chomel, described angelica as being sudorific, tonic, depurative and an expectorant. Dr Leclerc prescribed it for anorexia as it stimulates the nervous and digestive systems.

THE ESSENTIAL OIL

Description: *There are two angelica essential oils, one distilled from the seeds, one from the roots. Sometimes they are combined. As an essence, angelica has been distilled only recently in Europe. At first it is colourless, but with age it turns yellow and then dark brown. It must not be used when dark brown. It is quite thick, but still fluid. The seeds contain more essential oil than the roots, but the root oil is much stronger and more concentrated.*

The principal constituents: *Seeds – these are dependent on the variety but include angelic acid, sugar, valeric acid, volatile oil, bitter principle and a resin called angelicin. The essential oil is extracted from the roots when the plant is approximately one year old and it contains angelicin, bergaptene, two furocoumarines, phellandrenic compounds and terebangelene and other terpenes (limonene).*

Danger: *Exposure to sunlight or ultra-violet light after use may cause dermatitis.*

ITS USES

In illness

In general, angelica can be used for **rheumatic conditions**, virus infections, a smoker's cough, for **indigestion, flatulence, colic** and urinary infections or complaints. It is also an emmenagogue, a blood cleanser, and can help the symptoms of **PMT** and the **menopause**.

It is a remarkable healer for scars, wounds and **bruises**. Mix about 5 drops of angelica essential oil with 10 ml (2 tsp) of a vegetable oil like almond, and apply three times a day at first, then once every day until cured. Patience is necessary. *Caution:* Don't expose yourself to the sun or ultra-violet light straight after use.

Two drops of angelica seed oil added to 20 ml (4 tsp) base oil together with a few drops of eucalyptus, niaouli or cajuput oil is good for **coughs** and **colds**, either warmed and rubbed on the torso every morning, or added sparingly to the bath. (See *Caution* above.) Slices of dried roots chewed twice a day for six months builds up a resistence to viruses. Stems chewed after meals prevent **flatulence** and **indigestion** – or you could steep some stems for a fortnight in some brandy, and drink a little before or after meals.

Vin d'Angelique

This is very useful in convalescence as a fortifier, and you should take a large spoonful three times a day before meals. It can also help the symptoms of **PMT, menopause,** and is wonderful after meals for **flatulence**.

> *1 litre (1 ¾ pints) Malaga wine*
> *30 g (1 ¼ oz) angelic roots*
> *20 g (¾ oz) angelica seeds*
> *10 g (½ oz) cinnamon*

Mix together and stand for ten days in a hermetically sealed glass container. Strain into a bottle.

(*See also* **cuts and wounds** *and* **fatigue**)

In beauty
Many writers, ancient and modern, recommend angelica eye and face washes. Use a mild decoction of the seeds. Angelica was also a major constituent of one of the earliest perfumes, Carmelite water, first distilled in the Middle Ages.

In cookery
The best known culinary use of angelica is as the green candied stem used in confectionery and cakes. Chunks of the sugar-preserved and dried stems can also add flavour to preserves, jams and marmalades. To make your own is very simple, and it will have a better flavour and more health-giving benefit than shop-bought. The Elizabethans used angelica leaves on their salads, and both leaves and roots can be used for flavouring fish and soft cheese dishes, and for sweetening stewed fruit. During times of famine, the dried roots – which can weigh up to 1.4 kg (3 lb) – were once ground and used as bread flour.

   Angelica plays an important part in the history of alcohol: it flavours many spirits such as gin and absinthe, as well as Chartreuse and vermouths.

Other uses
The roots and seeds can be burned on the fire for a wonderful and purifying fragrance, and both leaves and roots can be part of a pot-pourri.

ANISE/ANISEED (*Pimpinella anisum – Umbelliferae*)

Anise or aniseed is a tender annual, growing to about 60 cm (2 ft) high, belonging to the same family as parsley and fennel. It is sometimes known as sweet cumin. Its leaves are feathery, rather like coriander, and its yellowish-white flowers set to pale brown, ribbed and hairy fruit seeds which taste like liquorice. The plant originates from the Orient but, like most herbs, grows both in the wild and cultivated state around the Mediterranean and especially in Egypt and the Middle East. It is cultivated in Spain, France and Russia. It can be cultivated further north, but it rarely sets seed.

It was introduced to northern Europe by the Romans, and early settlers took it to North America. It was used by the Romans as a digestive – in a cake eaten after meals containing other digestive seeds such as cumin and fennel – and by the Ancient Egyptians to help digestion of their millet and barley breads. Pliny claimed it helped insomnia, and Pythagoras considered aniseed bread a great delicacy. Dr Leclerc recommended an anise herbal tea for **asthmatic conditions** and for **menstrual problems**.

THE ESSENTIAL OIL

Description: *The oil is distilled from the seed fruits. It smells sweet and very characteristic, a little like fennel. It is colourless or a very pale yellow.*

The principal constituents: *Anethole forms 80 – 90 per cent of the oil shared with a little aldehyde, anisic acid and methyl chavicol (see page 28). In commerce it is often found falsified by essential oils of fennel or caraway.*

Dangers: *The essential oil is very toxic and dangerous, a real poison for the nervous system, causing a muscular numbness followed by paralysis. Since 1959, it has been under strict controls from the Ministry of Health in France. It can be more dangerous than pure alcohol, and should never be left where children might find it. The high proportion of anethol, plus the tiny amount of methyl chavicol could be extremely toxic, so the oil should not be used in therapy nor sold to the public.*

In commerce, a synthetic anethole is found, but this too is very toxic. The annual production of the authentic oil in 1987 was 40 – 50 tonnes. It is said that the consumption has slowed down since the appearance of the synthetic anethol as the price of this is very low in comparison to the pure oil.

ITS USES

In illness

Anise can be very successful in treating **PMT** and **menopausal symptoms**, particularly in counteracting retention of fluid. Make a tisane by boiling 10 ml (2 tsp) anise seeds in 600 ml (1 pint) water for 3 minutes then infusing for 5 minutes. Drink this slowly at difficult times, and stop all other stimulants until symptoms have ceased.

The main property of anise is digestive, as has been appreciated for so long, especially in Indian and Chinese medicine. The tisane helps **indigestion** due to anxiety and nervousness, and nervous **palpitations**, relieving breathing and promoting relaxation after a meal. Drinking the tisane – or chewing seeds very slowly, as they do in India – can prevent hiccoughs and **flatulence**. A few deep breaths and a few minutes' relaxation help as well.

(*See also* **appetite, loss of, colic,** *and* **dysmenorrhoea.**)

In cookery

Anise seeds can be cooked in breads, cakes and biscuits, in fish dishes, soups and curries, and some European dessert and fruit dishes. They flavour confectionery such as dragees in France, and a solitary seed was once the centre of the much-loved aniseed ball.

Anise seeds and their oil are used mostly to flavour various alcoholic spirits and liqueurs such as the *pastis* of France – Pernod, Ricard, *anisette* – the *ouzo* of Greece, *raki* of Turkey, and the *arrak* of other eastern Mediterranean countries. Sometimes, particularly in the case of Pernod, the majority of the anise flavour comes from the Chinese star anise (see below). However, that anise oil is added to these drinks as well is fairly certain; but the oil is not now allowed to be sold to the public for making their own *pastis*-type drinks. Often the flavour of aniseed can be given to a dish by adding the spirit or liqueur rather than the seeds, and in France there are many specialities named 'Ricard', for instance.

The leaves of anise may be used in salads, with vegetables like carrots, and in fish soups.

Other uses

The French use the oil, under strict control, to scent pharmaceutical products such as toothpastes, mouth washes and syrups. In veterinary practice, seeds have been fed to cows as this apparently helps the production of milk (which has a faint aniseed flavour). Seeds, crushed or whole, can scent pot-pourris, and other household pomanders.

ANISE, CHINESE OR STAR (*Illicium verum* – *Magnoliaceae*)

This spice, also known as Badian anise, is the star-shaped fruit of a small evergreen tree belonging to the magnolia family. It is native to China and Vietnam, and has not been successfully cultivated elsewhere.

THE ESSENTIAL OIL

Description: *Star anise oil is extracted from the dried fruits, and is very similar to, though rather coarser than, that distilled from anise seeds.*
The principal constituents: *Like oil from anise seeds, star anise contains a high proportion of anethole but, despite that, is used in the drinks industry. It should not be used in therapy.*

ITS USES

In cookery
Not surprisingly, it is much used in Chinese cookery, and, together with cassia or cinnamon, cloves, fennel and Sichuan peppercorns is one of the Chinese five spices. It is particularly good in duck and pork recipes, flavouring the best Chinese spare ribs.

ASPIC (*Lavandula spica – Labiatae*)

Aspic oil comes from a variety of lavender, known once as sticadore, spike lavender or Old English lavender. Like true lavender, the plants grow around the Mediterranean, but at a lower altitude, around 700 (2,300 ft). The bush grows up to 1 m (3 ft) in height, with larger leaves and more intensely coloured flowers than true lavender. Aspic plants have been hybridized with *L. angustifolia* and others to produce lavandin.

(*See also* **lavandin** *and* **lavender**.)

THE ESSENTIAL OIL

Description: *The plant is largely cultivated for its essential oils, chiefly in Spain, and a major proportion is used in perfumery and toiletries. The*

41

essential oil is pale yellow in colour and very fluid; when badly stored or left in the air, it becomes dark yellow and thickens so do not buy or use when like this. The smell is very camphory and lavender-like (like the flowers), with a note of rosemary.

The principal constituents: *Borneol, camphor, cineol, geraniol, linalool, pinene and terpineol. It is often falsified with rosemary and turpentine.*

Dangers: *Never use aspic in too large a quantity – in the bath for example – as it can be toxic. Instead of the correct reaction, you could end up with headaches, nervousness and exhaustion. Please respect the dosages.*

ITS USES

In illness
Doctors R M Gattefossé and Leclerc considered aspic to be a diuretic and sudorific, and found it to be effective for **fevers** and virus infections.

Externally, like its close relative lavender, aspic can be used for **bruises**, aches and pains, chapped hands, allergies caused by too much sun, and **burns**.

As it is a very active antibiotic, it is very successful in the treatment of **acne**, and to heal wounds. It is more efficient, though, if used in conjunction with another labiate oil such as true lavender. To reinforce its action, I like to add chamomile or geranium. Mix 5 ml (1 tsp) soya oil, a few drops of wheatgerm, 3 drops aspic and 1 drop chamomile or geranium, and apply two to three times a day to very bad acne.

(*See also* **backache, dermatitis, frostbite, oedema** *and* **pediculosis**.)

Other uses
Aspic is used a great deal in veterinary medicine in France. After long races, horses' legs and backs are rubbed with an aspic oil. It is also rubbed on the paws and sore legs of old dogs and cats suffering from rheumatic conditions.

BASIL (*Ocimum* spp – *Labiatae*)

There are more than 100 varieties of the herb basil, and they come in different sizes, shapes, colours and scents (some lemony, some tarragon- or clove-like). The common variety has dark green leaves which, if bruised, yield a very aromatic scent. The plant grows to a height of about 20 – 50 cm (8 – 20 in), and the flowers are white, arranged on the stem in several crowded, bristly whorls at the point from which the leaft stalks grow. Basil originates from India, but is now cultivated in many countries – around the Mediterranean, in Java, the Seychelles, Réunion, in Florida and Morocco. It is thought to have reached Europe in the sixteenth century.

The botanical name of basil is derived from the Greek *okimon* meaning quick, because the plant grows so rapidly. The name *basilicum*, that of the commonest culinary herb, derives from the Latin for royal, thus the plant is often known as the royal herb.

In Europe basil is considered by many to be a symbol of fertility; others associate it with death or evil (in Crete especially). The Greeks believed that when the plant was sown, words of abuse should be said or sung or the plant would not flourish; a belief echoed in the French phrase, '*semer* (to sow) *le basilic*', to slander someone.

Basil was recommended by Pliny against jaundice and epilepsy, and as a diuretic. It was also known as an aphrodisiac, so no wonder the Romans used it in so many culinary recipes! In the Middle Ages it was prescribed for melancholy and depression.

THE ESSENTIAL OIL

Description: *This is obtained by steam distillation of the flower tops or young shoots and the leaves. The oil is yellow, and it is very aromatic, similar in many ways to the essential oil of tarragon, but warmer and more camphory. It has been distilled in France since the sixteenth century, mentioned at that time by Jerome Brunschwig in one of his treatises on distillation.*

The principal constituents: *The essence is rich in camphor, cineol, estragol (or methyl chavicol), eugenol, linalool and pinene but all vary in proportion according to the plant and to its provenance.*

Dangers: *Following scares about the effects of estragol (or methyl chavicol) which can cause adverse reactions in sensitive subjects, and may even cause cancer in high doses, the essential oil industry is looking at types of basil which contain little or none. These include* O. canum *(Sims), camphor type, also known as* O. Americanum *(Linn), which comes from India and Russia, and has a very high proportion of camphor;* O. canum *(Sims), linalool-type, introduced from Kenya, which obviously has a high linalool content; and* O. gratissimum *(Linn) which is indigenous to India and Sudan, and has a high phenol content.*

ITS USES

In illness

Basil's properties are known to be carminative, galactogenic, stomachic, acts as a tonic and is antispasmodic. Dr Jean Valnet, a contemporary leading French aromatherapist, says it also helps normalize the menstrual cycle. An oil with basil in is useful as a rub on the tummy and solar plexus during **menopause**: use 3 drops in 20 ml (4 tsp) grapeseed oil. You could also add 5 drops to the bath water. You might not like the smell of the oil – more a 'cooking' smell to many people – so add a little of another essential oil to the bath water: orange, for instance, or, if you're feeling rich, some rose.

Basil is also a good fortifier of the nervous system, and is valuable for nervous fatigue, **nervous insomnia**, and mental and physical tiredness. A simple remedy for anxiety or **stress** is a mixture of 5 ml (1 tsp) soya oil, a drop of marjoram and 2 drops of basil oil. Rub all over the body.

Basil is particularly effective as a **migraine** remedy (see page 297). It is also valuable when used for **colds**, and a loss of the sense of smell, due to colds, **hayfever** or virus infections. Put 1 drop of basil oil in a bowl of hot water, and inhale for a few minutes two to three times a day until the symptoms improve.

Basil leaves can be eaten after garlic consumption to sweeten the breath. Basil is also a very good natural antiseptic: add a few drops to the water you wash the kitchen floor with, or the water for washing a sick pet's basket. A few drops on a piece of cotton wool left on top of a radiator will purify the atmosphere.

(*See also* **abscesses and boils, anosmia, depression, dyspepsia, fatigue, headaches, insomnia, oedema, palpitations, pre-menstrual tension, sexual problems** *and* **stings and bites**.)

Basil aphrodisiac

This is a very old family recipe from Cahors, my birthplace. For its aphrodisiac effect, drink a glass before meals with your loved one. It is also effective for impotence, depression, mental fatigue and melancholy; likewise drink a glass before meals.

1 litre (1¾ pints) red wine of Cahors
50 g (2 oz) fresh basil leaves

Uncork the bottle, push in the basil leaves, and replace the cork. Leave to mature for two days in the dark, shaking the bottle from time to time.

In cookery

Needless to say, eating fresh basil or using it in cooking, will give many of the above benefits, especially the digestive ones. Add the fresh flower heads and leaves to salads just before serving and, if to be cooked, add just moments before the cooking time is up. It goes well with fish, chicken and eggs, with peppers, aubergines and tomatoes.

To preserve the flavour and medicinal benefits of basil, macerate it in olive oil; dried, it tastes and smells rather musty and curry-like. Grow it in Britain on a sunny inside windowsill; on the Continent, it flourishes outside.

Other uses

These are legion. Basil was used as a strewing herb, in pot-pourris and herb bags, and the oil is still used in soaps and perfumery. In Spain and Greece, the plant is used to keep flies away, but the oil used neat, or crushed leaves, can soothe wasp stings.

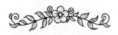

BAUME DE CANADA/Canada Balsam
(Abies balsameae – Pinaceae)

All the silver, or true, firs smell aromatic and yield resin to a greater or lesser degree. For this reason, the fir trees in North America have been called balsams for many years. Firs are evergreen conifers with single needles and flowers of both sexes on the same tree. The topmost branches bear the solid cylindrical cones. The balsam fir of Canada and the Lake States grows to a medium height, reaching a maximum of 18 m (60 ft), although in gardens it usually reaches about 7.5 m (25 ft).

The first mention of the therapeutic properties of the oil was in the 1606 journal of Marc Lescarbot after he had visited Canada. He related how the Indians used the oil for medicinal as well as domestic purposes: as a very strong antiseptic on wounds and ulcers, in the form of liniment; in veterinary practice on animals; and on their bows to lubricate the wood. It was only much later, in the eighteenth century, that the oil appeared in the European pharmacopoeiae.

THE ESSENTIAL OIL

Description: *The resin is collected by tapping the trees in July and August, when the resin is at its peak. It is then steam distilled. The essential oil is very* *similar to that of the pine trees which yield oil of turpentine. It is very aromatic with a pleasant scent, reminiscent of a mixture of caraway and juniper. It has a bitter taste.*

The principal constituents: *Camphene, pinene and resinic acid.*

Dangers: *The oil should, preferably, be prescribed only by reputable practitioners and should not be used for self treatment.*

ITS USES

In illness

The properties of *baume de Canada* are antirheumatic, expectorant, and antiseptic. It is a valuable remedy in diseases of the reproductive organs and urinary systems, and of the **mucous and respiratory systems**.

(*See also* **coughing, pneumonia** *and* **sinusitis.**)

Other uses

A considerable North American industry has grown up around the balsam firs. The needles are used to give their inimitable fragrance to soaps and other cosmetics.

If you are lucky enough to find some resin, you could use it to buff old furniture, so lubricating it and helping protect it against woodworm.

BAUME DE PÉROU/Balsam of Peru

(*Myroxylon balsamum* var. *pereirae* – *Leguminosae*)

Myroxylon pereirae is a large spreading tree of tropical America, closely related to the tree which yields *baume de Tolu* (*M. toluiferum*) (see page 47). It grows in Guatemala, San Salvador and Honduras, but, funnily enough, not in Peru. The name stems from the fact that the tree and its resin were sent from Peru by the Spanish Conquistadors.

THE ESSENTIAL OIL

Description: *This comes from the oleoresin, which is obtained by removing the bark at the foot of the tree and burning it with a flame to make the resin* *exude. Sometimes solvents such as ethylic ether, petroleum ether and sulphuric carbon are used for extraction. The colour of the oil I recommend for therapeutic use is browny red; it is thick and can be soluble in alcohol. It smells quite unique, flowery and sweet but not sweet at the same time, slightly medicinal like wintergreen, with notes of pine or cedar.*

The principal constituents: *The oil is sometimes called cinnameine as it is essentially composed of cinnamic acid, with benzoic acid, farnesol, nerolidol, peruviol and vanillin.*

Dangers: *As it can provoke skin reactions and unpleasant side effects in some people, it should only be prescribed by a reputable practitioner, and is on the list of restricted oils prepared by IFRA.*

ITS USES

In illness
Chomel and Lemery have prescribed and recommended its usage for **asthmatics** and for those with weak constitutions or weak chests after illness. At one time it was dissolved in alcohol and taken internally. *Baume de Pérou* is classifed as balsamic, a pectoral antiseptic, a skin bactericide, and as being calming and beneficial for **coughs** (bronchial or smoker's), **'flu** and **asthma**. It is still included in many pharmacological products in France for chest and skin problems.

Its bactericidal properties make it very effective for **burns, cuts, frost-bite** and many **skin problems** such as ulcers, **abscesses** and **eczema**.

Other uses
Baume de Pérou is used in perfumery as a fixative. In veterinary practice, many domestic animals respond well to it.

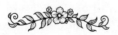

BAUME DE TOLU/Balsam of Tolu
(*Myroxylon toluiferum – Leguminosae*)

The balsam tree, *Myroxylon balsamum*, is a large evergreen of tropical America, which can reach a height of 20 m (about 66 ft). It has small, pinnate, dark green leaves, and a fruit which appears in June and

December consisting of a lance-shaped, one-seeded pod. *M.toluiferum* is a similar tree, but it yields the fragrant gum resin known usually by its French name, *baume de Tolu*. This is obtained by tapping – making an incision in the bark from which the resin exudes.

Baume de Tolu has been used in medicine for centuries, and was first mentioned by the Spanish naturalists, Hernandes and Monardes, in their book *Nova Plantarum* (1574). In the seventeenth century, it was included in the European pharmacopoeiae. The resin has always been used by the natives of South America and Mexico for its balsamic and expectorant values.

THE ESSENTIAL OIL

Description: *After collecting the resin it is steamed to separate out the oil. Fresh, the oil is of a grey colour, but matures to a reddish brown. The smell is sweet, pleasant and aromatic; when warmed, it has notes of benzoin, vanilla and even of hyacinth.*

The principal constituents: *Benzoic acid (up to 15 per cent), plus benzoate, cinnamate, cinnamic acid, nerolidol, and vanillin. Its properties are very similar to* baume de Canada *and* baume de Pérou *(see pages 45 and 46).*

ITS USES

In illness

The oil is an expectorant and is **bechic**, and is a good natural antiseptic. In the Second World War, Japanese troops were issued with bandages imbued with *baume de Tolu* to use on their injuries to avoid **tetanus**, the vaccination not then being practised in Japan. *Baume de Tolu* is particularly valuable for problems of the skin (see page 278 for a **frostbite** and **cracked skin** remedy) and of the urinary and **respiratory systems**. I have also found it useful for aches and pains such as those caused by **rheumatic conditions, fever,** or **pre-menstrual.**

Always use the oil in combination with other essential oils. It can be added, for instance, to juniper, rosemary or Siberian pine to reinforce the actions of those essences.

Chest infection remedy

This is good for colds which end up on the chest. Warm up the *baume de Tolu* by placing the bottle under a hot tap.

10 ml (2 tsp) soya oil
3 drops baume de Tolu
2 drops eucalyptus
1 drop myrrh

Mix together, and keep in a well-corked bottle. Rub on the chest vigorously twice a day, then wear a woolly vest and dress warmly.

(*See also* **bunions, coughing, dermatitis** *and* **sinusitis**.)

BAY (*Pimenta acris – Myrtaceae*)

The bay or bayberry tree originated in South America, but is now cultivated in the Antilles, Mexico, Venezuela, Barbados and Jamaica. This is not the culinary bay, which is a laurel; neither is it the bayberry shrub, wax myrtle or *Myrica pensylvanica*, from which early American settlers made candles. It is, however, closely related to *Pimenta officinalis*, the tree which produces allspice berries, also known as whole-spice, Pimento and Jamaica pepper. The tree is is small and erect – 7.5 – 9 m (25 – 30 ft) in height – and has a smooth greyish bark, and oval, aromatic, green leaves. It, too, bears berries. Another relation, the *P. acris*, var. *citrifolia*, has lemon-scented leaves.

THE ESSENTIAL OIL

Description: *This is distilled from the dried leaves and the berries, and the most esteemed oil comes from St Thomas in the Virgin Islands. The oil is amber to brown and has quite a strong smell, similar to clove. It is difficult to find the best quality as the oil is so often adulterated with turpentine or pimento, or even with clove and there is little distinction in smell between the pure and the adulterated oils.*
The principal constituents: *As much as 65 – 70 per cent of the oil comprises phenols (chavicol, eugenol, methyl eugenol); other constituents are myrcene and phellandrene, with some citral.*
Danger: *Eugenol can corrode metal, so use the oil with care.*

ITS USES

In illness
The properties of the essential oil are much the same as those of clove or laurel (see pages 83 and 121). In addition, because of the high proportion of phenols, the oil is a good antiseptic for the respiratory system, for the nose, throat and lungs, recently confirmed in research done in 1930 by Ridéal and Walker. It is also a good tonic.

In beauty
The major use of bay oil is as a remedy for **hair loss**. The bay rum used as a hair-wash and hair-dressing by men in Victorian times was a liquid obtained from distilling the leaves in rum. Many hair recipes and shampoos contain the essential oil, most of the cultivated (and wild) leaves going to America for that purpose. A great deal of the oil is used locally, so if you ever travel to South America or the Carribean, do buy some. Use it to make a remedy for hair loss, for greasy hair or a flaky scalp, or to give vigour and lustre to fragile hair. Mix 100 ml (4 fl oz) alcohol of 40–60 degree proof with 25 ml (1 fl oz) purified or mineral water and 3 ml (a scant tsp) oil of bay. Massage into the scalp before shampooing. Alternatively make a strong decoction of the leaves by boiling 10–12 leaves in 600 ml (1 pint) water for 5–10 minutes. Cool, add 20 ml (4 tsp) white or dark rum and store in the fridge. Use as a scalp rub.

Other uses
The essential oil, with its good masculine smell, is used to perfume shaving soaps, which will be antiseptic as well. It has always been one of my favourite oils, and is a constituent of a toilet soap I formulated for a major London hotel. It is so smooth that many male guests use it as a shaving cream.

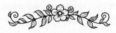

BENZOIN (*Styrax benzoin – Styraceae*)

Styrax benzoin is a tree which originated in Laos and Vietnam, but now grows in and around Malaysia, Java and Sumatra. It grows to a height of about 20 m (66 ft). The leaves are oval and hairy, the flowers are fleshy, greenish yellow in colour and slightly balsamic. Benzoin is the gum resin which exudes from the bark after tapping and the trees can apparently produce resin in this way for about 15 to 20 years.

Benzoin was first known in English as *benjoin* (recorded in the six-teenth century), which was popularly corrupted to *benjamin*. This is an adaptation of the same word in French, Spanish and Portuguese which derived from the Arab *luban-jawi*, 'incense from Sumatra (Java)'. In old recipes, benzoin is variously called gum benzoin, gum benjamin, benjamin, benzoin, oil of ben, even storax (which is a sweet-smelling gum resin extracted from the tree *Styrax officinalis*).

The Ancient Greeks and Romans knew benzoin, although they called it by quite different names – 'Silphion' to the Greeks, and 'Laserpitium' to the Romans. They would include the powdered resin in pot-pourris because of its very powerful fixative properties. Benzoin was highly valued by all. In 1461, for instance, the Sultan of Egypt, Melech Elmazda, sent the Doge of Venice a gift of two Persian carpets and 30 *rotoli* (100 *rotoli* is the equivalent of 80kg/177 lb) of benzoin. The Queen of Cyprus received a similarly sumptuous present from the Sultan in 1476, 15 *rotoli* of benzoin. The Portuguese navigator, Barboza, is thought to have introduced the precious resin to Europe. Later, in 1623, the resin's properities were sufficiently valued for the British to set up a factory in Siam to produce and export it.

Nostradamus, famous for his prognostications, gave many recipes including benzoin in a 1556 book. It was classified as an antispasmodic and tonic for skin infections and eruptions. In France it was called '*baume pulmonaire*', pulmonary balsam, and the resin was burned near the ill person, the fumes inhaled. In France many proprietary medicines are based on benzoin: sweets called *pastilles de serail* are taken for colds and 'flu, and tablets made that are bechic and anti-asthmatic. Its properties were not unknown in British medicine either, because friar's balsam, used as an inhalant and application for ulcers and wounds, is a tincture of benzoin compound.

THE ESSENTIAL OIL

Description: *As it exudes, the resin is yellowish, but when it thickens and hardens, it becomes brownish-red. It has a strong smell of vanilla, and is very aromatic; to taste, it is rather acrid. The resin is cleaned, and is available powdered, in two forms of tincture, simple and compound (the latter too strong for use on the skin), or as an essential oil.*

The principal constitutents: *70–80 per cent resin, 20–25 per cent cinnamic acid, a small quantity of vanillin (thus the smell), coniferyl benzoate, benzoic acid, phenylethylene and phenylpropylic alcohol.*

Danger: *Benzoin can cause allergic reactions, so do a skin test (see page 13) before use.*

51

ITS USES

In illness

Benzoin is particularly useful for **eczema** and **psoriasis**, using powdered clay (green if possible). Place 25 ml (1 ½ tbsp) clay in a small dish, add 3 drops benzoin, and enough distilled water to make a smooth paste. Apply immediately to the affected areas, leave for a minimum of 20 minutes, then rinse off with a chamomile infusion (put 3 heads of the dried flowers in a cup of boiling water, infuse for 10 minutes, then strain and cool). The eczema and psoriasis should look much better, much less angry and irritated, as the paste is very soothing. Repeat a few times per day when the condition is acute.

For psoriasis of the scalp, add 5 drops benzoin oil to a very mild shampoo and shake well before use. Rinse the hair finally with cold mineral water. (If your shampoo is too strong, add a proportion of distilled water to dilute it.)

Many other skin complaints can benefit from the use of the balsamic resin – **frostbite, bed sores, wounds, burns** and **skin ulcerations**. Mix 10 ml (2 tsp) almond oil, 2 drops wheatgerm oil and 6 drops benzoin oil. Apply on affected areas.

For **catarrh** and **chest infections**, put 3 drops benzoin oil in a bowl of hot water and place the bowl beside your bed at night. During the day, add 4 drops benzoin oil and 1 drop eucalyptus to a bowl of hot water, cover your head with a towel and breathe in the fumes for as long as you can. Several times during the day, rub your chest, torso and sinus areas with the following oil: mix 10 ml (2 tsp) soya oil with 1 drop wheatgerm, 8 drops benzoin oil and 2 drops eucalyptus.

(*See also* **impetigo, melanosis** *and* **sinusitis**.)

In beauty

Benzoin is useful for brown marks on the face, decolletage and hands, particularly in association with lemon oil. Mix 10 ml (2 tsp) almond oil with 2 drops lemon, 2 drops wheatgerm and 4 drops benzoin oil. The simple benzoin tincture could be diluted with distilled water to make an effective skin toner.

Other uses

Benzoin is one of the most favoured of perfume fixatives and is widely used in the perfumery industry and in pot-pourri mixtures, old and new. It can also be used in herb pillows or in sweet bags to perfume linen. Benzoin was once burned as incense in churches, and the gum could be burned to perfume the air at home.

Benzoic acid was discovered in gum benzoin in 1608; it has been used as a food preservative.

BERGAMOT *(Citrus aurantium bergamia – Rutaceae)*

Bergamot is the oil produced from the rind of a bitter orange tree said to have been exported by Christopher Columbus from the Canary Islands to the New World. It is now cultivated exclusively for its oil in and around Calabria in southern Italy and in Sicily; smaller producing areas are in Africa, especially along the Ivory Coast. The trees are much smaller than other members of the *Citrus* family, growing up to only 4.5 m (15 ft), and are thought to be an orange cross. The small, yellowish fruits are pear-shaped, and are harvested from December to February. There once were pears known as bergamot pears, and this is possibly where the name originated – from the Turkish *beg-armûdī*, 'bey's pear'. The bergamot orange should not be confused with red bergamot (bee balm, Oswego tea, *Monarda didyma*) which is an herbaceous perennial. The herb's name, however, is probably derived from the orange, as the scent of the herb flowers is very similar to that of the orange and its oil.

Essence of bergamot has been used since the sixteenth century in France, and is mentioned in many old manuscripts and herbals.

(See also neroli, orange *and* petitgrain.)

THE ESSENTIAL OIL

Description: *The oil is extracted, like that of orange, by pressing the peel, or grating the rind without touching the white albedo, or pith. The essence runs from the torn cells into a sponge which is then squeezed out over a container. In his book* Tropical Planting and Gardening *(1935), H F Macmillan says that 'about 1,000 peels are required to produce 30 oz of the oil which is usually valued at 35 – 50s per lb, according to purity'.*

The essence is a lovely emerald-green colour, with a subtle, spicy lemon scent.

The principal constituents: *A good essence contains up to 50 per cent of linalyl acetate; other constituents are bergamotine, bergaptene, d-limonene and linalool.*

Dangers: *Because of the bergaptene and bergamotine, the essential oil needs to be used with care when applied externally. These two furocoumarines increase the melanin-producing properties of the skin, and thus bergamot is often used in proprietary suntan preparations. But the furocoumarines are very often responsible for an over-pigmentation of the skin when exposed to the sun (or even just light in some circumstances), and can provoke abnormalities which can degenerate. Bergamot therefore is a very dangerous oil to use in any suntan preparation, particularly in these days of increased skin melonomas and cancers. I have always been very careful about using it on all skins, especially very fair skins, or those with large moles.*

ITS USES

In illness
Bergamot is mainly used in aromatherapy because of its antiseptic properties, and research by many therapists has proved it to be as effective as lavender. I don't recommend it as an external treatment for the skin (because of the problems outlined above), but its antiseptic properties – and its wonderful smell – can be used as a vapour in the home. Put hot water in a bowl with a few drops of the essential oil, or put some oil on a tissue near the radiator in a warm room. Replace every few hours.

(*See also* **oedema**.)

In cookery
The fruit is not used for eating but the peel is dried and used in cooking and in the drinks industry (*see* neroli); and it is also candied and used in pâtisserie. The essential oil is more famously used to flavour Earl Greay tea.

Other uses
Bergamot oil is used a great deal in the cosmetic industry in soaps, in perfumes and aftershaves. However, even at this dilution, it can provoke over-pigmentation of the skin.

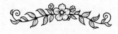

BOIS DE ROSE (*Aniba rosaeodora*)

Bois de rose – literally 'wood of rose' – is given the French name to prevent confusion with actual rosewood. The tree from which the essential oil is distilled originates from tropical Africa and Brazil (where the oil is known as '*oleo de Pau-Rosa*'). It grows wild and in abundance in the Amazon forests. A similar tree is found in Guyana (where the oil is known as 'Cayenne'.)

The distilleries in Brazil are situated in and around Manaus, and the huge quantities of oil produced in the past – once as much as 150 – 300 tonnes annually, principally for the American and European markets – have resulted in the deforestation of millions of hectares. The oil is distilled from the bark of the tree, but to obtain it, the whole tree is felled. Despite a drop in the exportation of the oil in recent years, the environment and climate have been irrevocably changed, and I feel that the oil should be completely banned, and its usage stopped. Many aromatherapists, however, still sell products containing it.

THE ESSENTIAL OIL

Description: *The smell of* bois de rose *is valued above all. It is woody, mossy, flowery, quite rose-like. It is also a good base, a natural fixative, thicker and more viscous than other essences and is greatly used in perfumery.*

The principal constituent: *Between 70 and 80 per cent of the oil is linalool and this has been much valued by perfumers for many decades. However, linalool can now be reproduced synthetically so there is no excuse to continue the usage of* bois de rose. *Obviously, the therapeutic properties of a synthetic will not be the same, nor is the smell, but it is better than continued pointless destruction. There are other sources of linalool too: the leaves of a plant from Taiwan (called* Ho *or* Shiu) *yield an oil with 80 – 90 per cent linalool. Equally, other essential oils are rich in linalool: aspic, basil, bergamot, coriander, lavender, lemon, thyme and ylang-ylang. Although the therapeutic properties won't be identical, they can happily serve as a substitute.*

ITS USES

In illness and beauty

The Amazon natives used the bark in therapy for its medicinal properties and, indeed, it has a remarkable action on the **skin**, helping wrinkles, stretch marks and **scars**. It is a great toner, and can be used for ageing skin (with rose, it could rejuvenate), and for skin that has lost its tone or has become flabby after illness or weight loss.

Galbanum and rose would be the oils possessing the properties closest to those of *bois de rose*.

CADE (*Juniperus oxycedrus – Cupressaceae*)

Juniperus oxycedrus is the Mediterranean equivalent of the common juniper. Known as prickly juniper, it is a hardy spreading plant, which can vary in size from a low shrub (very typical of the Mediterranean *maquis* and *garrigue*), to a tree of about 6 m (20 ft). The leaves are tiny, narrow and prickly, and have little surface from which moisture can escape during summer droughts; they are white and green above, dark green beneath. The cones are yellow and rounded, and the fruits are berry-like, growing in clusters, and black when ripe. (*See also* juniper.)

Cade oil was introduced into French medicine in the middle of the nineteenth century to treat skin irritation. It was listed as having antiseptic, vulnerary and anti-parasitic properties, and was used in the treatment of dermatitis, eczema, psoriasis, scalp infections with hair loss, herpes, all skin eruptions and chronic rhinitis. (It was also used in veterinary practice, externally on horses and other animals, to treat ulcers, scabies, worms and parasites.)

THE ESSENTIAL OIL

Description: *The oil is distilled from the young twigs and wood of more mature plants. The oil is resinous, a darkish brown colour, and has a strange waxy smell which is even caustic and tar-like (not surprisingly, as creosol forms the main constituent of creosote).*
The principal constituents: *Phenols (creosol, guaiacol), sesquiterpenes (cadinene) and terpenes.*
Dangers: *Unfortunately, cade is often adulterated with pine, birch, petrol and tar, so the benefits this oil can offer to the skin are limited (the name 'creosote' comes from the Greek words meaning flesh-saving, referring to the powerful antiseptic action on the skin). In fact the false oil can provoke terrible skin reactions so, to check, hold the oil up to a light: if it is blackish-brown instead of reddish and dark, it may have been adulterated.*

ITS USES

In illness
The unadulterated oil is one of the best remedies for **hair loss, dandruff,** hair weakened by dyeing and bleaching, and **skin eruptions.**

Dandruff remedy

This makes enough for only a few applications.

> *5 ml (1 tsp) castor oil*
> *2 drops wheatgerm oil*
> *3 ml (a good ½ tsp) soya oil*
> *10 drops cade oil*

Mix all the ingredients together well, and place in a dark bottle. To use, rub gently into scalp, massage for a few moments, then leave for a couple of hours. Wash off with a mild shampoo. Use twice a week.

I would advise consulting a practitioner concerning any other hair problems, as they can be caused by diet or other conditions, and will need expert or specialist treatment.

CAJUPUT *(Melaleuca leucadendron – Myrtaceae)*

Cajuput oil comes from a tree thought to have originated in the Moluccas, but which is now found in the East Indies, Malaysia and tropical Australia. The name of the oil is derived from the Malay *Kayu-Puti* or *Caju-Puti* meaning white tree, as the trunk with its irregular ascending branches has a whitish bark. This is remarkably fibrous, loose and scaly and may be pulled off in large strips. There are more than a dozen varieties of *Melaleuca* from which essential oil is distilled: among them *M. hypericifolia*, *M. veridifolia* (niaouli), *M. decussata*, *M. erucifolia* and *M. alternifolia* (the Australian tea tree). It is the young twigs, leaves and buds which are fermented before distillation.

The oil only seems to have made an appearance in the early seventeenth century in Europe, while in Malaysia and other Indonesian islands it had long been known for its therapeutic properties. It was considered particularly valuable for colds, 'flu and chronic rheumatism, and was prescribed for cholera as well, because it is sudorific. The bark was also used by native doctors. Until the Dutch gained territory in the Moluccas, it remained a very rare and expensive remedy in Europe.

One of the first French mentions of the therapeutic properties of the tree was in *The Natural History of Simple Drugs* by Dr G Guibourt in 1876. In a long study of *Melaleuca*, he described its properties as antiseptic for intestinal problems, dysentery, enteritis, urinary complaints, cystitis and infections of the urethra. They were also considered good for the respiratory system and for virus infections like 'flu. These researches were much later confirmed by the 1963 work of Dr Costet.

THE ESSENTIAL OIL

Description: *The oil distilled from young twigs, leaves and buds is colourless and limpid, with a very strong aroma reminiscent of camphor and spicy pepper, hot followed by a feeling of cold.*

The principal constituents: *Cineol (45 – 70 per cent), followed by several aldehydes such as benzoic, butyric, valeric, pinene and terpineol.*

Dangers: *Couvreur, a pharmacist writing in 1939, warns the practitioner to be on guard against the oil being taken internally: he said that vomiting followed by internal bleeding could occur. It can be a very dangerous remedy, so must always be used externally only, and for complete safety store it out of the reach of small children.*

The essential oil is often adulterated with other essential oils such as rosemary, turpentine and camphor, and with colorant. If this is the case, the oil will have none of its natural therapeutic properties and, in skin conditions, could cause further blistering and eruptions.

Only use cajuput oil if you are absolutely sure of its purity, and on the recommendation of a practitioner.

ITS USES

In illness

I have had good results in many cases of **rheumatism** and **stiff joints**. Mix 10 ml (2 tsp) soya oil with a few drops of wheatgerm and 10 drops cajuput. Rub gently on the affected parts, repeating several times a day whenever pain is felt.

Cajuput is also a valuable treatment for **cystitis**: add 3 drops to a warm bath. Niaouli, cajuput's close relative, (see page 156) is even more effective.

(*See also* **bursitis, chest infections, colds, coughing, hayfever, headaches, pneumonia, psoriasis, sinusitis** *and* **throat, sore.**)

In beauty

Cajuput is good for any **skin** eruptions. Mix 5 ml (1 tsp) each of almond oil and castor oil with 2 drops wheatgerm and 5 drops cajuput. Apply gently on the skin eruption, and repeat a few times until better. This acts as a mild counter-irritant.

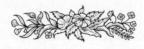

CALENDULA/MARIGOLD
(Calendula officinalis – Compositae)

Calendula oil is distilled from the petals of the pot marigold, a species of flower native to southern Europe, but which grows well further north in even the poorest of soils. It grows to a height of 60 cm (2 ft), has light green leaves, and daisy-like flowers which vary in colour from bright orange to yellow, and can bloom from May until the first frosts. The Latin name is derived from the fact that it blooms on the calends, or the first, of most months. The name marigold is a corruption of the Anglo-Saxon *merso-meargealla*, or marsh marigold. The flower was also later associated with the Virgin Mary and then with Queen Mary in the seventeenth century.

There is a considerable amount of folklore pertaining to calendula: if cut when the sun is at its highest calendula flowers are said to act as a heart tonic and fortifier. Old French sources claim that by merely looking at the flowers for a few minutes each day, this will strengthen weak eyes. Garlands of calendula were once attached to door handles to keep evil, particularly contagion, out of the house.

The therapeutic values of the flowers in treating skin problems have long been known. Marigold poultices were used to heal and obliterate the scars of smallpox, for instance. Marigold skin remedies are very highly regarded in today's homoeopathy and herbal or holistic medicine.

THE ESSENTIAL OIL

Description: *This is distilled from the flower tops, and it is quite sticky, and viscous. It smells very strange – musky, woody, rotten even, rather like the flowers themselves. This smell does not appeal to many people, even when it is used in a remedy.*
The principal constituents: *Flavinoids, saponosene, triterpenic alcohol and a bitter principle.*

ITS USES

In illness
The properties attributed to the oil are tonic, sudorific, emmenagogic and antispasmodic, but it is mainly used dermatologically. It is useful for very **sensitive skin**, and to help heal the scars of those who

have had very bad **acne**. It is very calming, even in the smallest proportions, mixed with other oils. I also use if for **burns**, mixing a little into a calming lotion. Very little oil is needed in any preparation.

Dried marigold infusions make good **toners**, and good calmers for the itchy eyes of **hayfever**. A tisane could help **PMT**. Some oil in a parsley compress (see page 241) is good for **broken capillaries**. A drop of oil in a bath is good for **psoriasis**.

(*See also* **abdominal pain, bruises, cold sores, cuts and wounds, dermatitis, dysmenorrhoea, ear problems, frostbite** *and* **impetigo.**)

In cookery

Marigold petals have been used as the poor man's saffron to colour cheeses, butters and dishes since the Middle Ages. The Elizabethans would use both petals and leaves in salads (although the latter are very strong). The petals flavour soups and stews, and they can be crystallized.

Other uses

Marigold has long been used as a dye, and the dried petals can be included in pot-pourris.

CAMPHOR (*Cinnamomum camphora – Lauraceae*)

The crystalline substance commonly known as camphor (the one which was used for moth balls) comes from a member of the laurel or bay family, *Cinnamomum camphora*, also known as *Camphora officinarum* and *Laurus camphora*, and it is related to the cinnamon and cassia trees. *C. camphora*, which can grow to over 30 m (100 ft) in height, is native to China, Taiwan and Japan, but is cultivated also in Sri Lanka and California. It is evergreen, often with growth right down to the ground, and can have an enormous trunk circumference (over 12 m [40 ft] has been recorded in China); it can also live, so the Chinese say, for up to 1,000 years.

THE ESSENTIAL OIL

Description: *The older the tree, the more oil it contains. The clippings, wood and roots are distilled for both the crystalline ketone camphor ($C_{10}H_{16}0$), and the oil.*

The principal constituents: *The composition of the oil is extremely complex and the constituents include azulene, borneol, cadinene, camphene, carvacrol, cineol, citronellol, cuminic alcohol, dipentene, eugenol, phellandrene, pinene, safrol and terpineol.*

Dangers: *Because it is a terpenic ketone, the essential oil can be highly toxic, particularly to those who are allergy prone or suffer from asthmatic conditions. The very hot and acid fumes should never be inhaled. I do not recommend camphor oil for therapeutic use.*

ITS USES

'Solid' camphor was once used as insecticide, but moth balls are now composed of naphthalene, a crystalline substance derived from coal tar or petroleum. Natural camphor is hardly produced today as it can be derived synthetically from oil of turpentine.

CAMPHOR OF BORNEO/BORNEOL
(Dryobalanops aromatica/camphora – Dipterocarpeae)

Dryobalanops camphora is native to the west coast of Sumatra and the north of Borneo, and produces a camphor oil which is known as Camphor of Borneo, Malaysia or Sumatra, or borneol (camphor).

Borneol camphor is the camphor which has been valued for many centuries in medicine. In the Indian Ayurvedic system it is mixed with other plants for eye injuries and infections, headaches and migraines, insect and snake bites, leucorrhoea and vaginitis; and it is considered as a tonic for the kidneys, a diuretic, and is a strong antiseptic. In Chinese medicine, it has been used for over 2,000 years. In Europe it was difficult to obtain, and its price at one time was higher than that of gold. Avicenna was one of the first to mention its use in medicine in the eleventh century.

In France, many researchers have investigated the therapeutic properties of borneol camphor. Dr Leclerc considered it a cardiac and general tonic, as well as a mild sexual stimulant; he also found it analgesic for rheumatic conditions, and highly antiseptic for many pulmonary infections.

THE ESSENTIAL OIL

Description: *As with the other camphor (page 60), the older the tree is, the more oil it will produce. Borneol exudes naturally from the cracks in the tree trunk, although an essential oil can be obtained by distilling twigs and wood fragments. Young trees produce a more liquid camphor, which is pale yellow and does not crystallize easily. This camphor is quite different from the* Cinnamomum camphora *camphor; it is borneol, an alcohol, which crystallizes in small grains or thin layers and it is white when it solidifies. It is also harder than the other camphor. Borneol is present in many other essential oils, among them aspic, ginger, lavender, marjoram, rosemary, sage and thyme. Although primarily smelling characteristically of camphor, the oil also has patchouli and amber notes.*

Dangers: *I have found it very difficult to obtain a good quality oil on which to absolutely rely. If you think you have found a source of borneol, buy very carefully, as the other camphor is so toxic.*

Never use borneol camphor if you are taking homoeopathic remedies – it will act against the remedy.

ITS USES

In illness

As it is so difficult to obtain good quality oil I use borneol camphor very rarely, choosing plant essentials containing borneol instead (see above) for treating joint stiffness, inflammations and **bursitis.**

(*See also* **stings and bites.**)

In Malaysia, camphor of Borneo is included in many analgesic preparations and balms for migraines, headaches and rheumatic pains.

CARAWAY *(Carum carvi – Umbelliferae)*

Caraway is a biennial plant, native to south-eastern Europe, and now grows in the wild and in cultivation all over Europe and temperate Asia. It is not native to Britain, and has become naturalized in the USA. It is an umbellifer, like cumin and coriander, and grows to about 60 cm (2 ft) in height. Its leaves are feathery, rather like carrot leaves (*Umbelliferae* is the carrot family), and umbels of white or pink small flowers are followed by the seed fruit. These are sickle-shaped and striped, the shape dictating the confusion with cumin (the tastes are essentially quite dissimilar). The plant self-seeds easily, and it is found wild in France in the Vosges, and in Alsace, near to Germany. It is cultivated for culinary use, particularly in Holland, Germany, Austria and Russia.

The name in English is thought to derive from the Arabic *al-karwiya* or *al-karawiya*, which became in Old Spanish *alcarahueya*. Because it is known as *carvi* in French, Lemery, a seventeenth-century botanist, decided that the name originated from the Carie province in Asia Minor where caraway was thought to originate (but that was probably cumin – the confusions are many). Another species exists, *C. copticum* or Ajowan, and this is used in Indian cooking and native medicine; the seeds are rich in thymol.

Fossilized caraway seeds have been found in Neolithic dwellings in Switzerland, and in Mesolithic sites, so it was in use up to 8,000 years ago. The Ancient Egyptians used the spice in religious ritual, and in cooking to make foods like bread and onions more digestible. Theophrastus recorded a recipe for oysters, eaten with caraway for the same reason; another culinary expert, Etimus, cooked lentils with caraway and thyme. The Romans ate the seeds after meals to sweeten their breath, and in cakes with other seeds to ease digestion. Caraway seeds are frequently offered after an Indian meal to sweeten the breath.

The School of Salerno and St Hildegarde considered caraway to be carminative, a stimulant, a diuretic, emmenagogic, galactagogic and stomachic.

THE ESSENTIAL OIL

Description: *The oil, distilled from the seeds, is colourless, sometimes with a tinge of yellow which darkens as the oil matures. The smell is more musky than cumin, more fruity and hot.*
The principal constituents: *50-60 per cent carvone; others are carvacol, carvene, and limonene. Researches have confirmed that this high proportion of carvone helps the digestion, stimulating and releasing gastric juices.*

ITS USES

In illness
Caraway is excellent for all digestive problems like flatulence, pain, dyspepsia, colic and colitis. The oil is also considered to be a mild antiseptic.

For difficult adult **digestion**, chew a few seeds slowly, drink a glass of warm water, and try to breathe deeply for a few minutes. Digestion should start, and the pain will be relieved. For a tisane for indigestion, steep 5 ml (1 tsp) lightly crushed seeds in 600 ml (1 pint) water for 10 minutes. Drink after meals. This is also good for **dysmenorrhoea**.

For children's nervous **colics**, mix together well 50 ml (2 fl oz) soya oil, 2 drops wheatgerm oil and 12 drops caraway. Put the bottle under a hot tap to warm the oil, then massage some gently into the child's stomach clockwise for a few minutes. Apply a warm poultice of linseed or oatmeal to the stomach (see pages 23 – 4), cover with a towel, and leave for 15 minutes. The pain should disappear.

(*See also* **dysmenorrhoea** *and* **dyspepsia**.)

In cookery
Caraway is used as a seasoning mostly in Central Europe. In Germany and Austria, particularly, the seeds are used in sausages, pâtés, in cheeses, rye and other breads, *sauerkraut* and fresh cabbage dishes, beetroot dishes, with meat (especially pork) and in some goulashes and other meat casseroles. Caraway seeds added to bread doughs and soft white cheese makes them both much more digestible. You could also add them to butter eaten with cheese for the same purpose. Mixed with aniseed and fennel seeds into butter and spread on wholemeal bread, they can help digestion of the latter.

Other uses

The oil is also used in perfumery and in the soap industry. Historically, the seeds have been used in bags to scent drawers and clothes, and to keep moths away. Napoleon is said to have used a soap scented with caraway. The oil of caraway is used in baked goods and confectionery.

Caraway, known as *Kümmel* in Germany, flavours (often along with some cumin) the liqueur also known as *Kümmel*. The earliest recorded caraway liqueur was that made by Lucas Bols in Amsterdam in 1575. The confusion between caraway and cumin exists even in the drinks industry, as reputedly the finest of all *Kümmels* is something called *Crème de Cumin*!

CARDAMOM (*Elettaria cardamomum – Zingiberaceae*)

There are several botanical varieties of cardamom, a tall herbaceous perennial native to India and Sri Lanka. *Elettaria* produces the small seed pods that are most commonly imported into Europe; two principal types are known as Mysore and Malabar. Other plants which produce seeds pods sold as cardamom are members of the *Amomum* family which includes *A. melegueta*, known as Grains of Paradise, Guinea grains, Guinea or Melegueta pepper. This was imported into Europe from the coast of West Africa – thus its name of Pepper Coast – and it was very popular in medieval and Tudor recipes.

Elettaria grows wild and in cultivation, preferring moist soil at a height of about 600 – 1,500 m (2,000 – 5,000 ft) above sea level. The leaves are long and lanceolate, and the flowering and fruiting stem grows from the base of the plant; those of Mysore are erect, those of Malabar trail on the ground. The flowers, which appear around May, are usually yellowish with a purple lip; the fruits, following around early October, are ovoid capsules of up to 2 cm (¾ inch) long, each divided into three sections which contain rows of dark brownish-red seeds. The plant has strong, creeping rhizomes which reveal its close relationship with ginger and turmeric. One of the main hazards of cultivating cardamom is said to be the loss of pods to gourmet lizards – they are partial to the seeds!

The pods must be gathered just before they are ripe: if fully ripe, the seeds would burst out of the pods during the drying process, and they would also have lost their essential oils and so their fragrance. The pods

65

are spread out in the sun on trays to dry and bleach, or in kilns. It was once customary to bleach the pods over sulphur fumes – the export market preferring white pods rather than the fresh pale green ones so valued in Indian cookery – but this practice is gradually decreasing.

The majority of Indian production is for local use, with less than 5 tonnes being exported annually. Other producers are Sri Lanka, Guatemala, Indochina and Thailand. Tanzania has recently attempted cardamom production too. Cardamoms are the third most expensive spice after saffron and vanilla.

Cardamom has been used in India as spice and medicament since the very earliest times: the Ayurveda, the Hindu system of medicine dating from at least 1,000 years before Christ, mentions it under the name of 'Ela'. In the first century the Greek philosopher Plutarch described how the Ancient Egyptians used it in their religious ceremonies and added it to their perfumes. It was introduced to Europe via the caravan routes of the Arabs, and was used mainly in Ancient Greek and Roman times in perfume. In fact the name is thought to be derived from the Arab 'Hehmama', itself derived from a Sanskrit word meaning something hot and penetrating. Hippocrates referred to it as 'kardamomon', and Dioscorides recorded that he preferred the kind that came from Armenia. Ovid and other poets sang the praises of cardamom's exquisite aroma.

Medicinally, the Ancients found it to be a diuretic, and effective against epilepsy, spasms, paralysis and rheumatic stiffness of joints. They added it to their wines to extract the therapeutic value of the seeds. The School of Salerno valued it in cases of cardiac disorders, and classified it as a good diuretic and stomachic. Chinese medicine, old and new, attributes a multitude of therapeutic values to cardamom, believing it a panacea for all intestinal illnesses.

Nearer our own time, Dr Leclerc attributed carminative and stomachic values to the seeds, considering them a good stimulant for all the digestive functions. Mme Maury considered them a wonderful pulmonary antiseptic, a good antispasmodic and a tonic for people with a weak heart condition due to emotional problems.

THE ESSENTIAL OIL

Description: *This is obtained by steam distillation of the aromatic, fragrant seeds. The essence is liquid and colourless, with a tinge of yellowish green. It has a lovely, warm, soft and spicy scent which is used a great deal in floral perfume compositions.*

The principal constituents: *Cineol and terpineol, with a little limonene* and traces of eucalyptol and zingiberene. Every variety of oil varies in its constituents, though, depending on the type of plant used, and indeed on variations in climate, soil etc.

There are few fragrances to compare with that of cardamom, and thus it is impossible to reproduce synthetically.

ITS USES

In illness
If the spice is used in cooking, cardamom can be a natural diuretic for fluid retention, and can help around the time of **periods** or during the **menopause**. A massage oil is useful for the same conditions. Mix together 20 ml (4 tsp) soya oil, 2 drops wheatgerm oil, 2 drops cypress oil and 8 drops cardamom oil. Rub clockwise on the stomach, solar plexus and thighs, preferably in the morning.

The seeds can be drunk in a decoction to help **digestion** and **flatulence**: boil a few seeds in 600 ml (1 pint) boiling water for 2 minutes, then add some fresh mint. Drink after meals with honey if desired.

In cookery
The small, greenish, unbleached pods (*choti elaichee*) are the most valued in Indian cooking; the large black pods sold as cardamom (*bari elaichee*) are very much less subtle, inferior, and cheaper to buy. The pods are used whole or lightly crushed in curries and *pilaus*; the ground seeds are a constituent of many curry powders and almost every *garam masala*. Always freshly grind the seeds; bought powder can be adulterated, and its loses its fragrance, as do all ground spices, very quickly. Cardamom also flavours sweets and sweet dishes in India, and the seeds are sugar coated for use at Hindu festivals and ceremonials.

In Sweden, cardamom is used as a flavouring for cakes, breads and pastries (reportedly taking a quarter of the Indian production) as it is in Germany, other Scandinavian countries and Russia. In Germany, cardamom often finds its way into meat dishes such as *Sauerbraten*, as well as pâtés, sausages and pickles. In France, cardamom is a little neglected, giving its subtle flavour happily to some *pains d'épices* and, less happily, to some *bouquets garnis* for fish. Cardamom can be used in punches and hot spiced or mulled wines such as the German *Glühwein*. Bedouin coffee is flavoured with cardamom pods stuffed into the spout of the coffee pot.

Other uses
The oil is added to toothpaste and used in a syrup for pulmonary problems in France. The seeds can be used, coarsely ground, in pot-pourris

and herb pillows. In India, the seeds are considered to be an aphrodisiac as well as a digestive aid; they are used in *paan*, the seed and spice mixture served after meals to help digestion and to freshen the breath, especially after eating garlic (this is also good for heavy smokers).

CARROT *(Daucus carota – Umbelliferae)*

Carrots have become one of the world's most important root vegetables, and are rich in nutritive and curative properties. They originated in Afghanistan, and were known to the Greeks and Romans. The wild variety spread all over Europe, and can still be found, mainly in chalky soils near the sea; the roots are whitish, small, hard and elongated, with an acrid pungent aroma. The cultivated variety – the familiar orange tubular shape, *D. carota* spp. *sativus* – was not developed until the seventeenth century, by the Dutch. The flesh is crisp, and has a sweet, pleasing aroma and taste. The leaves are finely divided and feathery. On the continent, carrots can also be found which are white, deep purple and red.

Carrots and parsnips are both umbellifers, and for centuries they shared the same name, together with anise, chervil, both types of fennel, parsley and rather more alarmingly, the poisonous hemlock. The wild flower, Queen Anne's lace, which grows so enthusiastically along roadsides in the New World, is the wild carrot, brought there by colonists from England. Carrots are hardy biennials, and are among the easiest of vegetables to grow at home.

In France in the sixteenth century, carrots were prescribed as a remedy because of their carminative, stomachic and hepatic properties. They were grated and used on ulcers, and have been thought of ever since as a blood cleanser, the panacea for liver and skin problems, all the pulmonary conditions, allergies, inflammation of the intestines, and as a tonic for the nervous system. They are said to be good for eyesight too: pilots in the Second World War were issued the vegetable to help their night vision.

THE ESSENTIAL OIL

Description: *It is the small hairy seeds that are crushed for the essential oil. Apart from in therapy, the oil from carrot seeds is used in perfumery.*

It is yellowish orange in colour, very fluid, and smells like a spicy, peppery carrot. Most of the oil used in therapy comes from Europe.
The principal constituents: *acetic acids, alephatic aldehyde, carotal, ß-carotene, cineol, formic acid, limonene, pinene and terpineol.*

ITS USES

In illness

The carrot, wild or cultivated, is one of the best possible vegetables to eat as it contains so many important vitamins and minerals: vitamin A and carotene, the B complex vitamins plus vitamins C, D, E and K; as well as copper, iron, magnesium, manganese, phosphorus, potassium and sulphur. It also contains easily digested sugar, levulose and dextrose.

Carrots are rich in carotene (the precursor of vitamin A) and, according to the work of Dr Leclerc and that of Artault de Vevey (at the end of the last century), this reinforces the body's immune (or defensive) system. They should be eaten every day because of their many therapeutic properties – at least 150–200 g (5–7 oz). Carrots eaten during lactation help to stimulate a good flow of milk. Carrots are good for liver problems, **diarrhoea, constipation** (they are rich in fibre), **anaemia** and **rheumatism**.

A carrot and fennel water can soothe a **colicky baby**: boil 2 carrots in 300 ml (½ pint) water with a few fennel fronds, for 10–15 minutes, strain, cool and add a drop of honey. Nothing is better for the **teething baby** than a chunk of carrot on which to chew: the natural oils help soothe the inflamed gums (under no circumstances rub the essential oil on the baby's gums).

(*See also* **broken veins and capillaries, burns, coughing, impetigo** *and* **mouth ulcers.**)

In beauty

Eating carrots is also good for the **skin**; its known blood-cleansing properties will help clear up spots and blemishes. For ageing of the skin, wrinkles and a bad colour, mix 10 ml (2 tsp) almond oil and 4 drops essential oil of carrot (*see also* **burns**). Use twice a year, for one month only each time, applying twice a day, and your skin will regain elasticity and firmness, and will acquire a good colour. The smell of the oil is not to everyone's liking, so for a face oil you could also add a drop of rose oil.

Carrots are very useful in preparing the skin for the sun, particularly extra sensitive skins. They help prevent dryness, burns, and the very early stages of skin cancer. For two months before going on a sunshine holiday, drink some carrot juice every day. (Use the pulp from the juiced carrots as a mask once a week on any skin that needs moisturizing.) Every night massage in a little of the above carrot oil blend. Hazelnut is a good oil to use instead of almond, as it actively helps a tan.

Another trick is to apply some carrot juice to the face and decolletage: this makes the skin look slightly more tanned, and is particularly effective if you are going out for the evening, as it covers up any little blemishes.

(*See also* **ageing skin** *and* **dermatitis**.)

In cookery

Carrots really need no words to describe their place in cookery. They have become a foundation vegetable rather like onions, forming the basis for stews, casseroles and braises, to which they contribute flavour, colour and texture. Carrots make a delicious soup, and they are also lightly cooked as an accompaniment vegetable – older roots cut into chunks or sticks, and young ones whole – and Carottes Vichy, roots cooked in water from the spa, used to be prescribed to cure eating excesses and digestive problems. The nutritive properties of carrots, though, are best when ingested uncooked, and carrots can be eaten raw as a snack, grated in salads, or in chunks as a crudité with a dip. Carrot juice is now freely available in good supermarkets, and juicers can be bought.

An important point. The flavour and goodness of carrots is in or near the skin, so they should never be peeled or scraped, only scrubbed.

CARROT QUICHE   *Serves 4 – 8*

Carrots are rich in vitamin A and they make a delicious quiche which is good for the skin and all respiratory problems. You could decorate it before baking with little circles of raw carrot.

225g (8 oz) shortcrust pastry

FILLING
1 kg (2¼ lb) carrots, scrubbed and chopped
1 onion, peeled and chopped
15 g (½ oz) butter

2 sprigs thyme
150 ml (5 fl oz) buttermilk
1 medium egg, beaten
30 ml (2 tbsp) chopped fresh parsley
salt, freshly ground pepper and freshly grated nutmeg
30 ml (2 tbsp) grated Gruyère or Emmenthal cheese

Roll the pastry and use to line an 18 – 20cm (7 – 8 inch) flan tin. Chill.

Boil the carrots until soft, then mash. Meanwhile sweat the onion in the butter until soft. Mix the onion and carrot together, then mix in the thyme, buttermilk, egg and parsley. Season with salt, pepper and nutmeg. Pour into the prepared pastry case and place in an oven preheated to 180 °C (350 °F) Gas 4. Bake for 40 minutes, sprinkling with the cheese after 10 minutes.

Other uses

The reddish juice of wild carrots was once used as a food colouring; a tincture of carrot seed oil was sometimes used in French liqueurs, and roasted carrot roots were used in times of hardship as a substitute for coffee. Carrots are also used in France to colour natural cosmetics.

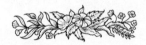

CEDARWOOD *(Cedrus atlantica Manetti – Pinaceae)*

Cedrus, or true cedar, is a genus of four species of evergreen coniferous, hardy and long-lived trees. *C. atlantica*, the Atlantic or Atlas cedar, is native to the Atlas Mountains of Morocco; *C. libani*, the cedar of Lebanon, is native to Syria and south-east Turkey; *C. libani* var. *brevifolia* comes from Cyprus; and *C. deodora*, the deodar, comes from the western Himalayas. The needles of the true cedars form in bunches; yellow male flowers appear in early summer, the females appearing as the males shed pollen. Cones take up to two years to ripen and disintegrate on the tree, after releasing seed. The wood is very balsamic and a reddish-brown.

Because cedars are reputed to be very long lived, they have been grown in churchyards. An enormous grove of cedars of Lebanon – from which King Solomon is said to have built his temple – exists still on the slopes of Mount Lebanon. The first cedar of Lebanon planted in Britain was

71

in the Thames valley in 1646 – and it is still alive and healthy. The first Atlas cedar in Britain was planted on the Welsh borders in 1845 and is also still alive. A forest of Atlas cedars, planted in 1862, stands on Mount Ventoux in Provence in the south of France.

Cedars are the trees most mentioned in the Bible, symbolizing everything that was fertile and abundant. The wood and its oil were used in embalming by the Ancient Egyptians. Later, Dioscorides and Galen in the first and second centuries mentioned a species of tree which they called *cedrium*, whose resin preserved the body from putrefaction. In 1698, Nicolas Lemery mentioned the therapeutic nature of the resinous matter, describing it as a urinary and pulmonary antiseptic. Later research confirmed the therapeutic properties of the oil, and doctors Michel and Gilbert in France recorded in 1925 the good results obtained in cases of chronic bronchitis, and its tonic and stimulant properties.

THE ESSENTIAL OIL

Description: *For therapeutic use, the only recognized oil of cedar is that from the Atlantic, or Atlas, cedar which grows in Morocco. The Moroccans produced some 6 – 7 metric tonnes of oil per year in the late 1980s.*

The oil is steam-distilled from the wood itself, and it is like syrup, yellowish and very balsamic; it has a turpentine scent, but one which is sweeter and more agreeable, similar in some ways to sandalwood.

The principal constituents: *Terpenic hydrocarbons, a little cedrol (which crystallizes when isolated) and sesquiterpenes, especially cadinene.*

Dangers: *Other varities of 'cedarwood oil' that are quite different to the Moroccan oil are on sale, so beware. The cedarwood oil from the USA is obtained from junipers,* J. *flaccida, mexicano and* virginiana. *The essential oils of these trees are rich in cedrol. The latter is high in thujone, and is used to falsify sage oil (itself very dangerous, see page 192). These American essences are used primarily in perfumery as they give a nice woody base to scents, eau de toilettes and soaps. For therapeutic use, insist on the oil from the true cedar, that from Morocco.*

Cedarwood has been prescribed internally in the past, but stomach problems with intense burning sensations, thirst and nausea were recorded. Never take the oil internally. Externally, it can sometimes be used neat or diluted, depending on need.

ITS USES

In illness
Over the last 100 years, cedarwood's beneficial effect on **eczema, skin eruptions and disease** has been noted, and it is highly valued in dermatology. For eczema and rashes, add 8 drops of the oil to 20 ml (4 tsp) wheatgerm oil. Apply three to four times daily.

As a stimulant, cedarwood can be added to your body oil, or to men's products. Add 4–5 drops to a cold cream, and apply after shaving.

As the oil is also considered a **sexual stimulant**, it could be used for men's body preparations. The oil on its own, though, is rather dull, and needs to be mixed with oils with livelier notes like lavender or rosemary.

(*See also* **cystitis, dermatitis, oedema** *and* **pneumonia**.)

In beauty
Cedarwood has a very therapeutic action on the scalp in cases of **alopecia, falling hair** and **dandruff**. In France, it is included in commercial shampoos and hair lotions for alopecia. For any loss of hair – for both men and women, whether after illness, or during stress or pregnancy – cedarwood can be very helpful. Mix 35 ml (a good 2 tbsp) grapeseed oil, 5 ml (1 tsp) first pressing virgin olive oil, 5 drops of wheatgerm oil and 20 drops of cedarwood. Rub this gently into the scalp a few hours before shampooing. Add 15 drops of cedarwood to an average sized bottle of mild shampoo.

If you have fair hair, use cedarwood with discretion. The oil has a tendency to darken the hair colour.

Other uses
Cedarwood essences, wood, wood shavings or powders were used in early pot-pourris and anti-moth bags. Many expensive fish are smoked over cedarwood.

CELERY (*Apium graveolens – Umbelliferae*)

Also known as 'smallage' and 'ache', *Apium graveolens* is a wild celery native to European salt marshes; *A.g. dulce* is the cultivated variety, first recorded in France in 1623, but was probably developed by the Italians rather earlier. The wild plant has a ridged stalk, the familiar toothed leaves and an extremely pungent flavour and smell; its domestication aimed to soften the pungency and thicken the stalk and ribs. Garden celery, as we know it, only really became popular in Europe and the US in the nineteenth century. It is a hardy biennial vegetable, grown for its crisp, long, crescent-shaped stalks. There are green and white varieties, some blanched by earthing-up during cultivation.

Wild celery was familiar to and esteemed by the Greeks and Romans. Pliny ate it as a vegetable rather than using it just as a seasoning, and the Romans, ever wary of drunkenness and hangovers, would wreath the leaves around their heads to avoid both! The Greeks called it *selinon*, moon plant, and at this time the vegetable was said to have an action on the nervous system, and to be a strong tonic. Hippocrates and Dioscorides thought of it as a strong diuretic, echoed later by St Hildegarde. All the properties attributed to celery by the Ancients were confirmed nearer our own time by Dr Leclerc, who recorded its effects on some of his patients.

THE ESSENTIAL OIL

Description: *All parts of the plant yield oil, but the most esteemed is that from the seeds which produce 2 – 3 per cent essential oil. This is pale yellow and very fluid, with a strong celery aroma.*
The principal constituents: *Lactone sedanolide, palminic acid and terpenic hydrocarbons (limonene, selinene).*

ITS USES

In illness
Celery has a number of diverse uses, both as a vegetable, raw or cooked, and as an oil. The vegetable should be eaten often, the best kind being those heads that are loose and perhaps with some soil still clinging to them – better than those already washed and wrapped in polythene. It is particularly good for **diabetics** who suffer from hypoglycaemia as it can be eaten freely.

Celery is a remarkable remedy for **chilblains**. Boil a large head of celery, root and leaves as well, in 2 litres (3½ pints) water for about 15 minutes, then strain into a large receptacle. Place hands or feet into the hot water and leave for 15 minutes. Repeat three times a day, reheating the celery water each time. A celery water could also be drunk as a cure for a liver deficiency. Cook the celery in the same way.

A head of celery can be juiced to make a liquid that is valuable for a number of complaints. Celery is a diuretic, so before and during a period if you retain fluid, or during menopause, the juice can help. For the same reason, it is also useful in a diet for weight loss. Drink several times a day, perhaps with a little lemon juice added. I have found this excellent, especially after heavy festivities such as Christmas and New Year. Sufferers from **cystitis** can also benefit from celery juice. The vegetable can be liquidized raw and eaten, or juiced and drunk: I think the latter is better.

As a gargle for voice loss caused by nervousness or a chill, put 1 drop of the essential oil in a mug of boiled warm water, plus a little sea salt. Gargle for a few moments, and repeat three or four times per day.

When suffering from nervous fatigue, take a warm bath with 8 drops of celery essential oil in it. Rest for 10 minutes afterwards. I always do this when I come back tired from the office, and feel very much better the next day.

(*See also* **throat, sore.**)

Celery aphrodisiac

This is an old family recipe, and was always given to the bride or bridegroom – one glass per day – for one week before the wedding! Not only does it have aphrodisiac properties, but it is a wonderful diuretic as well. It is said in the family that it is a recipe for long life, and as my two great-grandmothers lived well into their eighties it may indeed be because of their celery elixir!

> *1 large head celery (about 600 g/1¼ lb)*
> *1 litre (1¾ pints) good French white wine*
> *100 g (4 oz) fructose*

Clean and cut the celery into small pieces and put into a food processor with the wine and fructose (better than sugar, you can find it in health shops). Blend well, then filter into a bottle, cork firmly and leave in the dark for 48 hours. Filter again thoroughly, re-bottle, and drink one glass per day.

In cookery

Celery has little nutritional value, but its flavour and crisp texture enhance many dishes. Raw, the stalks are eaten dipped into salt (only really by the British), eaten with cheese, chopped to use in salads, or as crudités or containers for canapés. Celery can also be braised with a good sauce as a vegetable accompaniment, or used as a 'foundation vegetable' like onion and carrot in casseroles and stews. The leaves, which are mildly pungent, can be dried, and they are useful in *bouquets garnis*. The seeds are quite bitter, but can also be used to flavour; they are particularly good pounded with sea salt for a home-made celery salt.

CHAMOMILE
(Chamaemelum nobile; Matricaria chamomilla/recutita – Compositae)

There are many species of chamomile growing in temperate climates. All have attractive, finely divided leaves, and daisy-like flowers. The sweet, common or Roman chamomile (*Chamaemelum nobile*, once known as *Anthemis nobilis*) is very highly valued as a herb; so is the wild or German chamomile (*Matricaria chamomilla* or *recutita*, known also as the scented mayweed). *Chamaemelum* comes from the Greek for 'apples on the ground' because the plant is low and mat-forming, and leaves and flowers have an apple fragrance; *matricaria* comes from the Latin *matrix*, womb, because chamomile was and still is effective in treating menstrual problems. The sweet variety flowers from June to August, the wild from May to August; the former reach a height of about 15 – 23 cm (6 – 9 in), the latter up to 1 m (3 ft).

Chamomile was apparently sacred to the Ancient Egyptians, according to Hippocrates who 'dedicated it to the Sun because it cured agues'. By the seventeenth century, chamomile was well established in monastery and domestic herb gardens as a medicine and beauty herb – it had been taken to the New World by the Pilgrim Fathers – and in the late nineteenth century, the herb was commercially grown in Mitcham, Surrey, alongside the famous lavender, for medicinal purposes.

THE ESSENTIAL OIL

Description: *Distilled from the freshly dried flowers, the oil of sweet chamomile is pastel bluish, and later turns greenish yellow. The oil from the wild chamomile is a deeper colour, and makes a stronger, less acrid oil.*
The principal constituents: *The most important part is azulene, a fatty aromatic substance which is anti-inflammatory and promotes rapid healing of skin problems and wounds. This substance is not present in the flower, but is formed during the distillation of the oil.*

ITS USES

In illness
The oil's main properties are tonic, digestive, sedative, anti-allergic and antiseptic. Indeed, chamomile oil and a few others were commonly used until the Second World War as natural **disinfectants**

and **antiseptics** in hospitals and surgeries. The antiseptic power of the plant and its oil is said to be 120 times that of sea or salt water.

Many of the claims for chamomile made by the great herbalists still hold good. In his 1656 *Earthly Paradise*, Parkinson wrote that in bathing, it could be used to 'comfort and strengthen the sound and to ease pains in the diseased'. A few drops of the essential oil can be added to a warm bath to remove weariness and ease pain in any part of the body. Such a fragrant bath could also be a tonic for children and old people who have been ill. For general aches and pains, rub in a mixture of 10 ml (2 tsp) grapeseed oil, 2 drops camphor oil and 4 drops chamomile oil after a chamomile bath. A simpler massage oil made with 10 ml (2 tsp) soya and 3 drops chamomile can be massaged into the spine of a weary child after a warm chamomile bath. Chamomile is one of the gentlest essential oils, and so is ideal for use with children: a drop of the essential oil mixed with a dessert spoon of grapeseed oil and put on an index finger can safely be massaged into the gums of a fretful teething baby for relief.

Dried flower tisanes and inhalations would also relieve the pains of **headache, migraine, 'flu, coughs, facial neuralgia** and **sinusitis**. For the latter, mix 5 ml (1 tsp) soya oil and 4 drops chamomile, and massage for a few minutes around the sinus area and eyes from the nose to the temples: there should be immediate relief. For general irritability or an intermittent nervous **fever**, massage clockwise on the solar plexus, and bottom of the spine once or twice a day: use 5 drops chamomile to 5 ml (1 tsp) soya.

Chamomile is good for allergies like **hayfever**, too. Put a few drops in a bowl of hot water beside your bed, or on a clean handkerchief left near the pillow. This would also help relieve the symptoms of asthma, catarrh, bronchitis and pneumonia.

Chamomile is still extremely useful in the treatment of many women's problems such as **amenorrhoea, dysmenorrhoea, PMT** and **cystitis**. Chamomile baths, rubs and tisanes can help avoid the build-up of fluids before a period and any dropsical complaints.

A major property of chamomile is digestive, and infusions are excellent in cases of **indigestion, colic, loss of appetite, gout,** and can stop summer **diarrhoea** in children.

A simple tea taken before going to bed is not only digestive, but can also relax you for sleep and prevent nightmares.

(*See also* **abdominal pain, abscesses, amenorrhoea, anosmia, bedsores, broken veins and capillaries, catarrh, cold sores, colitis, cramp, cuts and wounds, ear problems, eye problems, fatigue, frostbite, halitosis, impetigo, menopause, oedema** *and* **teething pains**.)

In beauty

I have found chamomile most useful in treating skin complaints such as **dermatitis, acne** and **eczema**. Thanks to the properties of azulene, **abscesses and boils** can also be cured very quickly: steep some chamomile flowers in hot water and make into a poultice to apply directly (or use a steeped chamomile tea bag). You could also apply some oil neat. A steeped chamomile tea bag will help reduce facial puffiness suffered by some women pre-menstrually or during attacks of allergies such as hayfever. Chamomile oil can be mixed with others to make facial oils for many types of skin, and chamomile infusions make a good tonic cleanser for dry skin. Chamomile facial saunas are good too for many skin problems.

Chamomile is most famed for its use in hair preparations. It is used commercially in shampoos for fair hair, and it can lighten hair colour. Use an infusion as a final rinse for fair hair.

(*See also* **dandruff, hair problems** *and* **psoriasis**.)

In cookery

Chamomile is not much used in cooking, although it contains traces of calcium, the mineral which is so vital for healthy teeth and bones (and which accounts for the herb's natural tranquillizing properties). To benefit from fresh or dried chamomile, though, drink it as a tea, or add tiny sprigs of leaves to salads, sauces, omelettes or bread doughs.

Other uses

Chamomile can be used in pot-pourris and in tussie-mussies; it was listed by Tusser as a strewing herb, and as a clothes freshener in Edward III's household accounts. The Elizabethans smoked chamomile to prevent insomnia before the advent of tobacco. A related plant – *Anthemis tinctoria*, dyer's or ox-eye chamomile – yields an orange-brown dye.

A principal use of chamomile is, not unnaturally, in the garden. It was cultivated for herb seats along with thyme in Elizabethan times, and also for tough, fragrant lawns. Strong infusions of chamomile are said to be good as an activator for the compost heap, and also as a tonic spray for young plants. Many modern scientific gardeners weed chamomile out ruthlessly because they claim it takes so much goodness out of the ground: but old-fashioned gardeners and many herbal experts say it is the best of all 'plant doctors', reviving any sickly plant nearby. In France, the herb is particularly valued for its effect on roses; one French gardener I talked to had saved a favourite bush by planting some chamomile around it.

CINNAMON/CASSIA
(Cinnamomum zeylanicum/Cinnamomum cassia – Lauraceae)

Cinnamon and cassia come from the bark of trees or bushes belonging to the laurel family. These are evergreen, and the trees can grow to a height of 18 m (60 ft), more commonly 6 – 9 m (20 – 30 ft). The leaves are shiny and ovoid, and the yellow cluster flowers are tiny, as are the fruit. The whole tree – flowers, fruits, leaves, roots and bark – exudes a spicy aroma.

Cassia is thought to have originated in Burma or China (thus its name in many countries, *canelle de Chine*, for example). Cinnamon was native to Ceylon, but is now cultivated in other tropical countries such as India, the Seychelles and Mauritius.

This most ancient of spices – probably cassia, but cinnamon and cassia have long been historically confused – was mentioned in the treatise of the Emperor Shen Nung (2700BC) under the name of *'kwei'*, and in the *Pen T'Sao* (the first compendium of *materia medica*) under the name *'ten-chu-kwei'* meaning 'cinnamon of India'. Very few prescriptions seem to have been issued in China without the inclusion of the spice, and it was registered as a tranquillizer, tonic, stomachic, and as being good for depression and a weak heart. The spice is mentioned in the Bible under the name of 'quesiah'. In Exodus, God told Moses to take myrrh, cinnamon, olive oil and bulrushes with him from Egypt. The Ancient Egyptians were known to have used it to keep epidemics at bay, and in embalming.

The Arab traders supplied the spice to the Greeks and Romans, trying to keep its origins secret, but the quest for the coveted cinnamon was pursued so enthusiastically that it was the principal incentive of the Portuguese in discovering the route around the Cape to India and Ceylon in the sixteenth century. The Dutch, who took possession of Ceylon – now Sri Lanka – in the mid-seventeenth century, monopolized the cinnamon trade for some 150 years, but it was also they who began its systematic cultivation (as late as 1770). Thereafter, the spice became more widely available, and its use more affordable, in the West.

THE ESSENTIAL OIL

Description: *When the trees are six to eight years old, the bark is removed in long strips and left to dry in the hot sun. These strips roll up into tubes, the 'quills' familiar as the culinary spice. An inner corky layer is stripped* *for cinnamon, but is left in place with cassia, which is redder in colour, often chipped, and more coarsely pungent than cinnamon. To give the bark time to grow again, it is removed about every two years, and it is said that a good tree can produce for almost 200 years.*

The essential oil of cinnamon is obtained by steam distillation of the bark and leaves; that of cassia – which is not easy to find – from the leaves, barks and young twigs. The consistency of cassia is thicker, and it is less subtle and aromatic.

The principal constituents: *Cinnamon – cinnamic aldehyde (60 – 65 per cent), caryophyllene, cymene, eugenol, linalool, methylamine ketone which gives the characteristic aroma, phellandrene, pinene and many others. Cassia contains a higher proportion of cinnamic aldehyde, as much as 80 – 85 per cent.*

Dangers: *The oils should never be self-administered, but always used by a reputable practitioner. They can be toxic for many people, and they always have to be well diluted in a base oil and used in combination with other essential oils. If used pure in a bath or on the skin, they could cause terrible blisters and burns. The high eugenol content of cinnamon oil means it could corrode metal. Both cinnamon and cassia oils are restricted on the list issued by IFRA.*

ITS USES

In illness

The properties are antiseptic, digestive and anti-rheumatic. As cinnamon leaves contain such a high proportion of phenols (5 – 10 per cent eugenol), it has been classified as one of the strongest antiseptics and antivirals in nature. One source states that the essential oil destroyed a culture of the typhoid bacillus in less than half an hour. Such strength should, understandably, be used only by practitioners.

For safety, I recommend that it is used at home in bark or ground form only, when it can help the symptoms of 'flu or **colds**, and act as a stimulant for the **digestive system**. A sugary, cinnamon-scented drink – milk or brandy and milk, for instance – can ease a cough or sore throat.

CINNAMON CURE-ALL

60 g (2 oz) cinnamon sticks
30 g (1 oz) vanilla pods
30 g (1 oz) ginseng

20 g (¾ oz) rhubarb, chopped
7.5 g (¼ oz) root ginger, peeled and grated
1 litre (1¾ pints) Malaga wine

Mix the ingredients together and leave to rest in the dark for four weeks, shaking the bottle from time to time. Drink one small liqueur glass per day before meals as a preventative when 'flu is around, as a pick-me-up after a bad illnes or for a sluggish digestive system. A little, one to two liqueur glasses, can also be added to puddings such as compôte of fruits, fruit salads and crème caramel.

Cinnamon, ground or sticks, can be used in mouthwashes, and simply chewing a stick is an instant breath freshener.

(*See also* **coughing, pneumonia** *and* **throat, sore.**)

In cookery
Cinnamon and cassia for culinary use can be bought in stick or chip form; cinnamon can also be bought ground (it is difficult to grind at home), but buy sparingly, as the flavour quickly goes. In the West, ground cinnamon is generally used in desserts, cakes, pastries and biscuits; the sticks can give their flavour to syrups, creams and aromatic or mulled wines. Simply using cinnamon as a swizzle stick for hot drinks like cocoa or chocolate can significantly flavour and benefit.

Elsewhere, cinnamon and cassia, particularly the latter, are used in Arab and Indian meat dishes: because of the phenol content, this serves the practical purpose of destroying or discouraging the bacteria responsible for putrefaction. Dried cassia leaves, which are as aromatic as the bark, are much used in India: they are *tej-put*, the Indian 'bay'. Cassia buds, which are clove-like, are also used in meat dishes.

Cassia is, not surprisingly, one of the spices in the famous Chinese five-spice mixture, and cinnamon is found in many *garam masalas*.

Other uses
Cinnamon or cassia bark was often burned as incense in the past, and a fat obtained from the fruit was once used to make church candles. The powerful fragrance of either spice can be used in pot-pourris, in herb pillows and herb bags to keep moths away. Cinnamon is also one of the ingredients of Carmelite water. Pliny used cinnamon in a perfume recipe for men in his *Natural History*, and many sources recommend it as a spice with which to perfume linen – but beware, the Book of Proverbs warns against the woman who perfumes her bed with enticements such as these!

Cinnamon is now popular in many soaps and men's cosmetic preparations.

CITRONELLA *(Cymbopogon nardus − Gramineae)*

Citronella belongs to the same family of aromatic, oil-rich tropical grasses as lemongrass and palmarosa. These were once known by the generic name of *Andropogon*, but are now included in the genus *Cymbopogon*. There are a few varieties, but all are large, coarse and robust, growing to about 1.2 − 1.5 m (4 − 5 ft); they can grow wild at height, but are cultivated largely near the sea. They are propagated by root division, and the leaves are ready for cutting about eight months from planting, and thereafter about every four months, subject to weather. Replanting is necessary every four to five years.

The most esteemed of varieties come from Java, Sri Lanka, the Seychelles, New Guinea and Guyana. In 1933, it was estimated that 30,000 acres of Sri Lanka were given over to citronella production; in 1987, 100 − 120 tonnes of oil were exported; but since then cultivation and production have diminished.

THE ESSENTIAL OIL

Description: *This is distilled from the leaves, and is yellow to dark brown with a very strong aromatic lemony smell. The production of oil varies from season to season.*

The principal constituents: *These vary depending on the origins of the oil. That from Java, for instance, is high in citronellol (30 − 50 per cent) and geraniol, with traces of citral, methyl-eugenol and various terpenes. The oil from Sri Lanka contains less citronellol (only 8 − 18 per cent), with some geraniol, 5 − 8 per cent eugenol, and traces of borneol, citral, and various terpenes.*

Dangers: *Because citronella oil is quite cheap, it has been used, along with sandalwood, to imitate geranium oil; with lemongrass and geranium to imitate rose (which contains geraniol and citronellol); and to imitate verbena.*

ITS USES

In illness

For bites and to use as an insecticide, take a small bottle of citronella oil with you on holiday. Put a few drops on your bedding and next to your pillow. Apply to mosquito and other insect bites a few times a day: this will stop the itching and will act as an **antiseptic** as well. For children under eight years old, dilute the oil (10 drops in 25 ml/1 fl oz almond oil).

If you have **rheumatic problems** or other aches and pains, mix 50 ml (2 fl oz) soya or other vegetable oil and 20 drops of citronella. Rub on the affected parts.

(*See also* **stings and bites**.)

Other uses
The oil is hardly used in therapy but because of its highly antiseptic and deodorizing properties, it is used a great deal in commercial preparations – soaps, cleaning products and insecticides. The citral content is utilized for the base of industrial menthol.

CLOVE (*Eugenia caryophyllata – Myrtaceae*)

The evergreen clove tree originated in the Moluccas, the 'Spice Islands', but has now been introduced into most tropical countries and Madagascar, Zanzibar and Tanzania dominate the world trade. Cloves grow best near the sea, thus the preponderance of island cultivation. The trees are fairly small, growing naturally up to 9 m (30 ft), but usually kept at a more accessible height, 5 – 6 m (16 ½ – 20 ft), for cropping. They are conical, looking a little like laurels, but the leaves are longer than laurel, brighter green and although as shiny, they have visible dots containing the aromatic substances. These are released if you bruise or crush the leaves. The trunk, covered with a smooth greyish bark, divides quite low into large branches, at the end of which the crimson flowers grow – or would, if they were allowed to reach that stage. The cloves are the unopened, long, yellowish-green flower buds which appear at the end of the rainy season. When these turn pink, just before opening, they are picked by hand or beaten from the tree. The flowers are then dried in the sun, or gently over heat, for a few days until they are the familiar dark brown colour of the spice.

The tree does not produce the spice until aged about five years, and can carry on increasing its yield until it is about 20 years old. The yield of a mature tree is generally around 3 – 4 kg (6 ½ – 8 ¾ lb) fresh buds. When these are dried, the weight reduces to about 1 kg (2 ¼ lb), and in turn this yields about 15 – 20 per cent essential oil. The contents of one little 150 ml (¼ pint) bottle represents the output of one tree – a very small quantity for all the work involved!

In the middle of the rainy season, the hot humid atmosphere disperses the fragrance of the clove trees all over the islands where they grow. The lack of epidemics on Penang was attributed to the medicinal scents from the tree (clove is a very strong antiseptic). Significantly, after the Dutch destroyed the clove trees in the early seventeenth century island inhabitants began to suffer from disease, and many died.

The Greeks called the tree '*caryophyllum*', meaning 'leaf of walnut tree' and this derived through Arabic to '*girofle*', part of the French name for the spice, *clou de girofle*. *Clou* is the French for nail, deriving from the Latin *clavus*, which is also the origin of the English word (the dried buds look like little nails). Cloves were also known to the Ancient Egyptians, Greeks and Romans.

Pliny praised cloves, as did the great Roman doctor, Alexander Trallianus. St Hildegarde, in her book *Morborum Causae et Curae*, wrote that cloves were included in treatments for headaches, migraines, deafness after a cold, and dropsy. She advised that cloves would warm people feeling the cold, and cool down those who felt hot. During the Renaissance, pomanders were made with cloves to keep epidemics and plague at bay.

THE ESSENTIAL OIL

Description: *Clove oil is distilled from the leaves and unripe fruit. Some salt is added to the water to raise the boiling temperature, and the clove buds must be distilled over and over again to extract all the essential oil. This is colourless with a little tinge of yellow when freshly distilled: as it matures it turns a dark brown. It has a spicy vanilla scent, peppery with a little note of carnation.*

The principal constituents: *The largest part are the phenols (70 – 80 per cent), particularly eugenol. This was only isolated by Bonastre in 1827, and is one of the most antiseptic of the phenol family, three to four times stronger than any other. Further constituents are acetyleugenol (which gives the specific fragrance), benzoic acid, benzyl benzoate, furfurol, sesquiterpene (β-caryophyllene) and vanillin.*

Dangers: *Clove oil is often adulterated with a vegetable oil (usually palm) and oil of pimento berries and leaves. Sometimes the adulterant is copaiba, an oil made from the gum resin of a Brazilian balsam tree, Copaifera* officinalis. *This is a great pity, as the therapeutic values are only present in the absolutely pure essential oil. Because of the eugenol content the oil can corrode metal.*

ITS USES

In illness

The old texts all seem to agree on the many therapeutic properties of clove – it is a stimulant and has stomachic, expectorant, sedative, carminative, antispasmodic and digestive qualities. It helps **flatulence, stimulates digestion** and **restores appetite**, so is good for convalescence. It is a general tonic for both physical and intellectual weakness; and for those suffering from frigidity. Its principal therapeutic value, though, is antiseptic because of the high proportion of eugenol. This is used for intestinal parasites, and for prevention of virus infections. It is good for the immune system, and particularly effective in **mouth and tooth infections.**

When I am under physical or mental strain, or simply tired, I suck a clove several times a day. It has an agreeable taste, and acts as a relaxant. Sucking cloves is a particularly good idea for those trying to give up smoking.

The **dental value** of cloves is well known. They are antiseptic, but have sedative and minor anaesthetic properties too (a sucked clove will slightly numb your tongue). If you have a toothache, either suck a clove on the side of the sore tooth, or apply a cotton bud with a drop of the essential oil to the tooth. This will give you relief until you get to the dentist, and also helps to keep the mouth clean because of the antiseptic effect. Never use *too* much of the oil, and don't leave it *on* the tooth (on a piece of cotton wool, say) as your gums could begin to flake. A good mouthwash can be made for **halitosis**: boil a few cloves in a little water for 5 minutes, let it cool down, then add a few mint leaves and rinse and gargle with the strained liquid.

For **rheumatic pains**, mix together 25 ml (1 fl oz) castor oil, 5 drops each of juniper and wheatgerm oils, and 5 drops clove oil in a brown bottle. Rub on the affected parts and keep warm.

In popular medicine, an infusion of cloves was given to **activate labour** after the first pains were felt. This could also ease the pains.

(*See also* **bronchitis, colds, dental abscess, fever, gum disease, pneumonia** *and* **throat, sore.**)

In cookery

Cloves can be used in cooking for their therapeutic values in a variety of ways, although always with care as they can dominate. A single clove can be stuck into an onion to flavour a stock or bread sauce, or added to a meat or chicken dish to strengthen and enrich its flavour. A boiled meat dish should always have a few cloves in the cooking water, and a clove plus a clove of garlic inserted into the end of a leg of lamb before roasting greatly adds to the flavour. Meat marinades should include cloves as well. Onions cooked with cloves become sweeter and the clove aroma blends very interestingly with the onion. Clove also perfumes the classic German *sauerkraut*. Cloves are a constituent of many *garam masalas*, and flavour curries and rice dishes; they are also one of the Chinese five spices.

The flavour of cloves goes particularly well with apples: sweet apple pies, or the apple sauce to accompany pork.

Many drinks benefit from cloves, particularly spicy, hot mulled wines. Many local liqueurs use cloves: that from Grenobles called 'Nossolio' or 'Merisat', and the 'Tafia' of Martinique and Guadaloupe.

CLOVE SOUP   *Serves 4*

This 'soup' should be taken when minor discomforts start to appear at the beginning of winter – colds, sore throats or snuffles. As soon as any symptoms are felt, make and drink this concoction.

600 ml (1 pint) beef stock
2 onions, peeled and thinly sliced
1 bay leaf
6 cloves
salt to taste

Put all the ingredients in a pan, bring to the boil, then simmer for 30 minutes. Remove the cloves and bay leaf, and serve hot.

Other uses
The classic way to use cloves is to stick them into an orange for a pomander to sweeten the wardrobe and keep moths away. This is an interpretation of the anti-plague properties utilized in the Middle Ages. Whole or ground cloves can be included in pot-pourris. The oil is used a great deal in perfumery – to recreate the smell of carnations – and in soaps and bath salts. In the Indonesian islands – reputedly the consumers of half the world's output – tobacco and cigarettes are perfumed with cloves.

It is said that courtiers at the Han court in China in the second century BC would suck cloves to sweeten their breath when appearing before the emperor. If not in deference to Chinese emperors, eugenol, the principal constituent of clove oil, is still used in some brands of mouthwash.

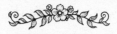

CORIANDER (*Coriandrum sativum – Umbelliferae*)

The name coriander comes from the Greek *koris*, meaning bug, because there is supposedly a connection between the smell of the young leaves and that of bed bugs. Indigenous to Southern Europe, India, North Africa, South America and the USSR, coriander is an umbelliferous plant; its leaves are a bright green, deeply indented at the base of the plant like Continental parsley, and feathery at the top. The plant bears umbels of mauve flowers which later set to seed. Both leaves and seeds are used.

Coriander, both spice and herb, can be traced back over many centuries, and it could be one of the oldest flavourings in the world. It was cultivated in Ancient Egypt where its seeds were bruised to mix into bread, and an essential oil obtained from the seeds was used in religious ceremony. It was one of the bitter herbs designated in the Bible to be eaten at Passover, and in India it was used for magic incantations to the gods, and was – and is – added to many dishes. Coriander was also said to be an aphrodisiac.

The Greeks and Romans believed coriander had stimulant, digestive and carminative properties. Dioscorides claimed it was a calmant and Galen lauded it as a tonic. Some considered it a poison, a suspicion echoed in the warnings to apothecaries by Renaissance doctors that they should sell it with enormous caution. Others swore by its therapeutic properties. A major usage at one time was in obstetrics: a few seeds placed at the top of a woman's thigh while in labour would facilitate birth and ease pain; and by taking seeds regularly, a woman could cease menstruating and quickly become pregnant.

THE ESSENTIAL OIL

Description: *The essential oil distilled from the seeds is slightly yellow and has a musky, aromatic and pleasant smell. Approximately 100 kg (about 222 lb) are needed to obtain 2 – 3 kg (4 – 6 lb) of essential oil.*
The principal constituents: *An alcohol (coriandrol, 60 – 65 per cent), geraniol and pinene, with traces of borneol, cymene, dipentene, phellandrene*

87

and terpinene. The provenance of coriander oil must be 100 per cent, as it is easily simulated with orange and turpentine essential oils.

Dangers: *The oil should not be used internally by any but the most experienced practitioner: if the wrong dosage is taken the effect could be fatal.*

ITS USES

In illness

In more modern aromatherapeutic practice, Dr Leclerc believed coriander combated fatigue, and Mme Maury prescribed it externally for **rheumatic conditions** and **fevers**.

Externally, coriander is useful in alleviating **facial neuralgia, toothache, nervous facial cramps**, and the facial pain associated with **shingles**. It is also effective when used after 'flu, and for **solar plexus cramps**; a few drops in almond oil can be massaged in daily, in a clockwise direction. This also helps to regulate the breathing.

(*See also* **headaches**.)

In cookery

Coriander is used to good effect in many of the world's cuisines: the Chinese claim it as their own, calling it Chinese parsley; in Mexico, where it flourishes, it is frequently used; Moroccan *souks* are heady with its scent; and it is also popular in the Middle East, Africa, Asia and southern Spain. The seeds are a major ingredient in curry powder – they are also used to halt the putrefaction of meat – and the leaves are an essential in many types of curry. Coriander also lends a superb flavour, used sparingly, to mushroom dishes, meatballs, lamb stews, and lamb or pork kebabs.

When baking bread, ground seeds mixed into the dough give an interesting flavour and help the digestion of the starch.

CORIANDER SOUP   *Serves 4*

This is a good therapeutic soup when one is under stress, as it has carminative, warming and diuretic properties. It is recommended for helping to alleviate the symptoms of PMT and the menopause, and to prevent retention of fluid and cellulite.

1.8 litres (3 pints) water
a little sea salt
1 tsp virgin olive oil

225 g (8 oz) coriander leaves
2 potatoes, peeled and diced
1 large onion, peeled and diced
a little lemon juice
1 bay leaf
10 ml (2 tsp) coriander seeds, freshly ground
a little goat's milk or soured cream (optional)

Bring the water to the boil with the salt and olive oil. Add the coriander, keeping aside 2 sprigs of leaves, along with the potato, onion, lemon juice and bay leaf. Simmer for 15–20 minutes until the potatoes are tender, then liquidize.

Add the ground coriander seeds at the last moment, along with a little goat's milk or soured cream if desired. Finely chop the remaining coriander leaves and sprinkle them on the top of the soup just before serving.

A CAUTIONARY TALE

A large container in a herb distillery was knocked over and 50 litres coriander oil (from 5,000 kg of crushed coriander seed) were spilled on to the cement floor. Eight workers came to clean up the mess, but it was too late: the essential oil had found its way everywhere, having penetrated every crack and hole in the large room. The workers continued trying to save as much as they could, but the atmosphere became unbearable. During the next half hour they all started laughing and giggling and telling jokes, and seemed to be quite unconcerned about the disaster, and quite unaware of the effect the fumes were having on them. After a while they became aggressive, and loud voices could be heard in different parts of the distillery. When the chief chemist came to investigate, he found two workers fighting in the intoxicating atmosphere. Two others had extreme nausea, and all of them had to be sent home for a few days to get over the extreme fatigue which followed. (Schmoller & Bompard, Grasse, 1973.)

CUBEB (*Piper cubeba* – *Piperaceae*)

Cubebs are the fruit of a vine belonging to the same family as that which produces the familiar black, white and green peppercorns (*Piper nigrum*). *P. cubeba* is a climbing perennial shrub with dioecious flowers, and spherical fruit containing a kernel. The fruits grow on strings like black pepper, but on separate little stalks which account for one of the common names, tail pepper (in French, *poivre à queue*). The fruits look very similar to black pepper, but are rather larger. They are less perfumed too than black pepper; they taste peppery and aromatic, pungent and bitter.

Cubeb pepper is native to the East Indian 'Spice Islands', to Java, Borneo and Sumatra, and is also grown in India, Sri Lanka and Réunion.

Cubeb pepper has been used since ancient times in China and India as a spice, and in Indian Ayurvedic practice as a medicine. The Arabs used it, too, for medicinal purposes, the name *kubeba* appearing for over four centuries in Arab manuscripts. St Hildegarde thought highly of cubeb as a remedy, considering it a great tonic of the nervous system, a good antiseptic and vulnerary. (She recommended it for warming the stomach and brain, for the weak, and for those with no colour in their cheeks!) In India, it was used to help gonorrhoea (a venereal disease with excessive mucus discharge), and it was from there and for that purpose that it was introduced to Europe at the beginning of the nineteenth century. The essential oil was listed in the French pharmacopoeia until 1937 for the above properties, but was deleted after the advent of chemical antibiotics.

THE ESSENTIAL OIL

Description: *This is viscous, thick and of a pale green or bluish colour, with a very characteristic scent of pepper plus a note of camphor.*

The principal constituents: *Cubeb is similar to pepper (see page 172) in its constituents, but has a high percentage of cubebine (40 – 55 per cent); others are amorphous cubebic acid, azulene, camphor, cubebin, dipentene, lineol, pinene and an alcohol which crystallizes when cold.*

Dangers: *Cubeb oil is often used to adulterate other essentials, and it in turn is often falsified with other oils. This, of course, completely destroys the therapeutic properties. It would be nice to revitalize the interests in cubeb oil, but it would mean that distillers would have to produce an absolutely pure oil. For a long time I have been unable to find a supply on which I can rely 100 per cent. There are, in fact, several cubeb distilleries in India, but the oil is not exported because there is no current demand in the West.*

ITS USES

In illness
Cubeb is well worth using on **skin rashes and inflammations**: combine 50 ml (2 fl oz) almond, 2 drops wheatgerm and 5 drops cubeb. It is also useful for laryngitis, sore throat and other **throat infections**. Add 3 drops cubeb to a bowl of hot water for use as an inhalation, or cool this down for an antiseptic gargle.

Other uses
Cubeb is not used much as a spice, although in medieval times it was combined with other weird and wonderful sounding spices such as galangale and grains of paradise. It was one of the spices used in the wine cordial called Hippocras.

CUMIN *(Cuminus cyminum – Umbelliferae)*

Cumin is a delicate annual plant thought to originate from Egypt, but grown in the Mediterranean area for many years BC and now naturalized in hot countries all over the world – the North African coast, Malta, the Middle East and America. It has a slender and fragile stem, leaves that are divided into narrow strips, and tiny part-umbels of flowers which are white to pinkish purple. The plant later sets the narrow-ridged seed-fruit that are the spice, and the only part of the plant used. These seeds look rather like those of caraway, and indeed they are often confused in Europe: caraway is called *cumin des prés* in France; *cumino holandese* (Dutch cumin) in Spain. There is no real resemblance in flavour. The name comes from the Hebrew *kammon* or Arabic *kammun*, and later became *kuminon* in Greek.

There are two types of cumin spice, which are most clearly defined in Indian culinary terminology. *Kala* or *shah zeera* is the 'true' or black cumin, and this is quite rare and expensive. White cumin, *safeid zeera*, is the seed more commonly available in ethnic shops and better supermarkets.

Cumin seeds were found in the tombs of the Pharaohs in Egypt. The plant was cultivated by both Ancient Egyptians and Hebrews, much as it is today. It was mentioned in both Old and New Testaments, and the Hebrews also used it in their ceremony of circumcision as an antiseptic.

To the Greeks, cumin was a symbol of selfishness, and they referred to people so avaricious that they would divide everything, even their cumin seeds. Dioscorides thought of it as one of the best aromatics to help with flatulence, and recognized it as a stimulant for the digestive system. The Romans used cumin a great deal in their cooking: to spice their olive oil, to sauce their shellfish and grilled fish, to keep their meat fresh, to spread on bread, and to substitute for pepper. Cumin seeds were also used in digestive cakes at the end of a meal, along with caraway, dill and fennel. Cumin apparently helped congested people regain their normal pale colour, so it was popular with over-eaters and heavy drinkers; Pliny even suggested that this 'whitening' property was utilized by scholars wishing to impress their teachers that they were working harder than they actually were!

Pierre Pomet, in his book *History of Drugs* (1694), recommended cumin for rheumatic conditions in the essential oil form. Nearer our own time, Dr Leclerc classified it as a general tonic for the heart and nervous system. Eugene Perrot, in his 1940s and 1970s researches, found it a tonic and aphrodisiac.

THE ESSENTIAL OIL

Description: *The oil is distilled from the seeds and it is colourless, sometimes with a tinge of yellow which, with age, becomes a deeper yellow. The aroma of the oil is very pungent, reminiscent of anise, but with a very spicy, musky note.*

The principal constituents: *Cuminol, or cuminic aldehyde, of between 35 and 50 per cent; others are cymene, pinene and terpineol.*

Dangers: *The oil is on the restricted list issued by IFRA, and may cause dermatitis if there is exposure to sunlight or ultra-violet light after use.*

ITS USES

In illness

Cumin is a good general tonic, antiseptic and bactericide.

A decoction of the seeds is good for the deafness that often comes after a bad virus 'flu infection. Boil a good 15 ml (1 heaped tbsp) of the seeds in 600 ml (1 pint) water for 15 minutes. Leave to cool, then strain. Insert a little of the liquid in the ear and repeat a few times a day. Massage behind the ear and on the neck with a mixture of 5 ml (1 tsp) wheatgerm oil and 4 drops cumin oil.

Cumin is most successful for **cellulite**. For a tisane, crush 5 – 10 ml (1 – 2 tsp) cumin seeds slightly, and infuse in 600 ml (1 pint) boiling water for 5 minutes. Drink warm after meals, adding honey if desired.

Cellulite body oil
The only disadvantage of cumin is the smell, which many people dislike, but the addition of orange or lemon oil helps enormously. Do a skin test with this body oil before use (see page 13) and never expose yourself to sunlight or a sun bed after use.

15 ml (1 tbsp) almond oil
2 drops wheatgerm oil
8 drops cumin oil
2 – 3 drops orange or lemon oil

Mix together and use to massage legs, thighs, and tummy area. This oil is also good for before menstruation. Rub on the tummy, and blot after use.

In cookery
Cumin is not much used in European cookery but it is most appreciated in Indian, North African and Middle Eastern cuisines.

Cumin can be bought whole or ground; buy the latter in small portions as the aromatic essential oils fade quickly. To bring out the flavour of the seeds and make them more nutty, toast them quickly in a hot dry pan – this is a common appetizer and digestive in the Middle East.

CYPRESS *(Cupressus sempervirens – Cupressaceae)*

Cupressus is a genus of about 20 species of columnar evergreen coniferous trees which can grow to about 25 – 45 m (80 – 150 ft) in height. Tiny scale-like leaves are pressed against the branches and twigs; male and female flowers are present on the same tree; and the female flowers produce round cones containing small winged seeds. *C. sempervirens* – the Mediterranean or Italian cedar – is native to Mediterranean Europe, although trees are now cultivated in much of temperate Europe and North America. Planted very close together, they act as a screen in the south of France against the *mistral*, and they appear in many southern French, Greek and Italian gardens.

Cypress was known to the Ancient Egyptians; many different papyri record its medicinal uses, and sarcophagi were made from the wood. The Ancient Greeks dedicated the tree to Pluto, god of the underworld, thus the frequency of the trees in cemeteries. Hippocrates recommended cypress for severe cases of haemorrhoids with bleeding. In fact almost every mention of cypress I have unearthed has recorded its efficacy as a haemostat. Dioscorides and Galen, for instance, recommended macerating the leaves in wine with a little myrrh for a fortnight; this was to be drunk for bladder infections and internal bleeding. As such it was also highly recommended by doctors Leclerc and Cazin.

THE ESSENTIAL OIL

Description: *This is produced by steam-distillation of the fresh leaves and cones. It is colourless or a very pale yellow, with a woody and balsamic, agreeable amber scent.*
The principal constituents: *Terpenes (65 per cent, in particular β-pinene and terpineol), cedrol, cypress camphor, some acids and tannin.*

ITS USES

In illness

Dr Leclerc has also confirmed that cypress acts as a vaso-constrictor, and should be prescribed for all **circulatory problems** like **varicose veins** and **haemorrhoids**. For varicose veins, mix together 50 ml (2 fl oz) grapeseed oil, 3 drops wheatgerm oil and 15 drops cypress. Massage the legs every day. As a decoction for the same problems – and for **menopausal symptoms**, cypress is *wonderful* at this time – boil 15 g (½ oz) crushed cypress cones for a few minutes in 1.1 litres (2 pints) water. Infuse for 10 minutes and then drink a cup full three times a day.

Dr Jean Valnet used to use cypress in hospital for **coughs** and **bronchitis**: a few drops of the oil on the patient's pillow stopped the coughing. I've found this effective too. In France, cough pastilles were once made from crushed cypress cones.

(*See also* **arthritis, bruises, dysmenorrhoea, fatigue, fever, frostbite, menstrual cycle problems, oedema** *and* **pneumonia**.)

In beauty

Broken veins or capillaries are another circulatory problem that cypress can benefit. Mix 5 drops of cypress oil into 25 ml (1 fl oz) almond oil and 3 drops wheatgerm oil. Massage gently into the cheeks twice a day, morning and night, until the symptoms improve.

(*See also* **cellulite**.)

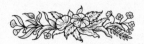

ELEMI *(Canarium luzonicum – Burseraceae)*

The oleoresin known as elemi or gum elemi comes from large trees which originated in the Philippines, but which are found in many varieties in Australia, India, South and Central America, and Africa.

Elemi became popular as a medicine in Europe around the sixteenth century, and was referred to as '*resina elemnia*'. It was used for ulcers and skin infections, being added to many skin creams and ointments such as the French *baume de Fioravanti* and *baume paralytique*. Another French cure using elemi was *l'emplâtre* (plaster) *diachylon*: this was used externally to help knit bones. J J Wecker, an early seventeenth-century doctor, found elemi very successful in the treatment of head injuries and wounds. Soldiers of the time were treated with elemi too; sword wounds were deep, but elemi speeded the healing process.

THE ESSENTIAL OIL

Description: *The white oleoresin exudes from the tree bark. It is very similar to turpentine, but of a much thicker consistency. As the oleoresin ages, it becomes waxy and yellow, losing most of its balsamic smell. The essential oil is obtained by distillation of the oleoresin, and is colourless or a very pale yellow. It smells strongly balsamic, hot and aromatic, due to its main constituent, phellandrene.*

The principal constituents: *Phellandrene; other terpenes are dipentene, limonene and pinene; and there is 60 – 70 per cent of resinous matter consisting of alcohols and triterpenic acids.*

ITS USES

In illness

Elemi mixed into a cream for external application on the broken limbs of older patients is very successful. Rubbed every day into the affected part, I have noted very good results, so avoiding **rheumatic pains** thereafter (a common occurrence after fractures).

This massage cream is most effective if applied to a **fracture** as soon as injury has occurred. Add 20 drops of elemi to 50 g (2 oz) thick cold cream slightly warmed. If possible, apply straight to the fresh injury

95

gently massaging it in, then cover with a thick pad of cotton wool and a bandage. Leave for a few hours to achieve a slow penetration.

After a few weeks – perhaps when the plaster cast has been removed – make up the following oil, and massage in twice a day, covering the affected part with a light bandage to keep it warm. Mix 50 ml (2 fl oz) soya oil, 3 drops wheatgerm and 20 drops elemi.

Other uses

Some varieties of elemi are used commercially in the manufacture of plasters, ointments, varnishes and inks.

EUCALYPTUS *(Eucalyptus* spp. *– Myrtaceae)*

All the eucalyptus trees – of which there are 600 or so species – originate from Australia. They have now been successfully transplanted to many other warm parts of the world, notably Central Asia, North Africa and California (where they have almost become a pest, threatening many native species). Sub-tropical on the whole, there are only a few species which grow well in more northerly areas. They grow very tall and very rapidly – 21 – 27 m (70 – 90 ft) in about 20 years – and one tree in Australia is said to be the tallest non-conifer in the world.

The evergreen eucalyptus trees are known commonly as gum trees because the bark can exude a sweet-smelling gum. It is the leaves, however, which contain droplets of essential oil, and those of the Tasmanian blue gum, *E. globulus*, are the most esteemed in therapy. The leaves of young trees are rounded and silvery (those seen in florists' shops), but these change as the tree matures, to very long ovals, generally of a deep blue-grey-green colour. The flowers of the blue gum are like tiny pots from which a lid pops off, with fragrant white flower stamens unfolding.

Commercial distillation of the oil began in Australia in 1854, and has been continued there and in other countries where the tree has become acclimatized.

The first works on the antiseptic and antibactericidal properties of the oil were published in Germany by doctors Cloëz (1870), Faust and Homeyer (1874). They classified it then as being sudorific, a stimulant, anti-catarrhal, and astringent. It was prescribed for all respiratory system conditions such as bronchitis, 'flu, asthma and coughs. These properties are still the best known, and many French prescriptions and commercial preparations for colds include eucalyptus in various forms.

THE ESSENTIAL OIL

Description: *The twigs and leaves of young and more mature trees are distilled for the oil. The more mature trees yield more oil, with better aromatic qualities. The oil has a very fluid consistency, and is a pale clear yellow. Its aroma is fresh, balsamic and agreeable.*
The principal constituents: *Cineol or eucalyptol, from 70 – 80 per cent; then there are various aldehydes, ketones, sesquiterpenic alcohols and terpenes. There are approximately 250 different constituents in eucalyptus so it is extremely difficult to reproduce synthetically.*

ITS USES

In illness
Eucalyptus oil is highly antiseptic, and it is a favourite remedy for **colds** and **'flu, coughs, bronchitis, catarrh** and viral infections. There are many ways in which it can be used for these ailments.

As an inhalation, add 3 drops to a bowl of hot water and inhale for 5 minutes. Do this three to four times a day. Put a few drops on a handkerchief and inhale from time to time. Add a few drops to a warm bath. Make up an oil containing 50 ml (2 fl oz) soya oil, 2 drops wheatgerm oil and 15 drops of eucalyptus, and massage torso and abdomen three times a day.

The same oil can also help nervous disorders and fatigue, and convalescents. Massage on sacrum area (lower part of the back), solar plexus and top of hands a few times a day. It acts as a stimulant of the nervous system.

Rheumatic conditions can benefit from eucalyptus as well (another familiar use of the oil in commerce is as part of embrocations): mix the oil as above, but use 8 drops eucalyptus and 4 drops thyme oil instead of 15 drops eucalyptus.

The leaves can also be used therapeutically for **colds** and **'flu**. Add 15 ml (1 tbsp) dried leaves to 600 ml (1 pint) boiling water and infuse for 10 minutes. Add a little honey if desired, and drink this tisane throughout the day, at least six to eight cups. An infusion of the leaves in hot water can act as a fumigant, either in public rooms or a sickroom.

Research by a Dr Trosus has revealed hypoglycaemic properties in eucalyptus, and he has prescribed it for high blood pressure and diabetes. By drinking infusions of the leaves, he says the sugar in urine can drop to a normal level.

Eucalyptus winter syrup

This is a wonderful stand-by for when **colds** and **'flu** are about. It is also extremely good for **asthmatics.**

> *20 g (¾ oz) dried eucalyptus leaves*
> *300 ml (½ pint) water*
> *300 g (11 oz) fructose or honey*

Prepare a very strong infusion by boiling the leaves in the water for 10 minutes. Leave to infuse for 20 minutes, then strain and add the fructose or honey. Store in a dark bottle, and take a teaspoon a few times a day when colds threaten.

(*See also* **abscesses and boils, asthma, burns, bursitis, chest infections, cuts and wounds, cystitis, fever, hayfever, neuralgia, pneumonia, sinusitis, stiffness** *and* **stings and bites**.)

Other uses

The trees are said to keep insects away. Oil from *E. citriodora*, the lemon-scented gum (the leaves of which contain citronellol), is used in perfumery, and the leaves in pot-pourris. Much of the oil produced is used in commerce for products as apparently diverse as disinfectant and boot polish. The bark of some eucalyptus – which is as deciduous as most trees' leaves – yields a beige dye; the leaves a red dye.

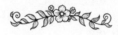

FENNEL (*Foeniculum vulgare – Umbelliferae*)

Like the other umbellifers, fennel is native to southern Europe, particularly around the Mediterranean. It has become naturalized in many other non-tropical parts of the world – Japan, Persia, India and the USA – growing mostly beside the sea. It was introduced to northern Europe by the Romans, and to the USA by early European settlers (it has become a weed in California). It is a hardy perennial, with a haze of blue-green feathery leaves, and umbels of yellow flowers followed by seeds. A relative developed in Italy is the Florence fennel or *finocchio* (*F.v. dulce*): this is an annual, and produces the plump stalk bulbs eaten raw in salads, as well as feathery leaves and seeds.

The herb fennel has been known since the very earliest days, the Chinese, Indians and Egyptians all using it both as condiment and medicine. Theophrastus and Pliny preferred it to anise, and Dioscorides and Hippocrates both said it promoted the flow of breast milk (a property still appreciated today). Pliny valued it as an eye herb too. The Romans used it for its digestive properties, making the last course of a meal something like a cake which included fennel and other seeds (much as the Indians do today, offering *paan*, a selection of seeds including fennel, at the end of a meal). The Greeks believed fennel was a slimming herb, and as it is slighly diuretic, this may well have had some basis in fact. Charlemagne ordered that fennel be one of the plants grown in his gardens, and St Hildegarde praised the plant for many medicinal properties. The first mention of fennel as an essential oil was in a book *On the Art of Distillation*, written by Jerome Brunschwig in 1500. In the nineteenth century doctors Cazin, Bodard and Bontemps classified fennel as a tonic, stomachic, galactagogenic, emmenagogic and carminative. More recently, Dr Leclerc and Dr Maury recorded cases of gout, rheumatism and kidney disfunction (especially stones) that had been successfully treated with fennel.

THE ESSENTIAL OIL

Description: *Although all parts of the plant are aromatic, it is the seeds which are crushed and distilled for the essential oil. This is usually colourless, sometimes a very pale yellow. It has a very characteristic and strong aroma reminiscent of anise, but which is softer and more camphor-like.*

The principal constituents: *Anethol, up to 60 per cent; others are anisic aldehyde, camphene, d-fenchone, dipentene, estragol, fenone, phellandrene and pinene.*

Dangers: *The combination of anethol and estragol (methyl-chavicol) – as in anise, see page 38 – would seem to be dangerous. I have never seen any bad reactions to the oil, but sensitive people should, of course, be very careful.*

ITS USES

In illness
Fennel has long been associated with **digestion**, and it is an ingredient, along with its fellow umbellifer, dill, of baby gripewater. (If a baby has **colic**, some boiled carrot and fennel water could help.)

Fennel is marvellous as a tonic for muscular energy, particularly useful for athletes and people who practise a lot of sport. It is also good for convalescence after illness. There is enormous benefit to be had from eating the herb and its vegetable relative as often as possible and from drinking fennel tisanes.

For a fennel tisane, put 7.5 ml (½ tbsp) crushed seeds in a teapot, and pour on 600 ml (1 pint) boiling water. Let it stand for 7 minutes before straining and drinking. Sweeten with honey if you like (good for athletes) and drink as a tonic in the morning or during the day.

For a tonic bath, add 10 drops of the essence to the hot water while it is running, then lie in it and relax for 10 minutes. (This is also good for urinary problems, such as **cystitis**.) Afterwards, massage legs, arms, torso, back of the neck and feet with a body oil consisting of 50 ml (2 fl oz) soya oil, 4 drops wheatgerm oil and 15 drops fennel oil.

(*See also* **appetite, loss of, constipation, dysmenorrhoea, halitosis** *and* **muscular pains**.)

In beauty

An infusion of the seeds can be cleansing and gently toning for the skin.

Fennel is also very helpful for **eye inflammations, puffiness** and **conjunctivitis**. Boil 15 ml (1 tbsp) crushed seeds in 600 ml (1 pint) water for a few minutes. Leave to infuse and cool then strain. Use in an eye bath and clean both eyes several times. If you do this several times a day, the problem should disappear fairly rapidly. Consult your doctor or ophthalmologist if symptoms persist.

In cookery

Fennel is the herb most associated with fish: the feathery leaves are used in fish sauces, soups and salads; the dried stalks are often placed under a whole fish to be grilled on the barbecue. The leaves can be used to flavour herbal oils and vinegars, and make a wonderful white sauce for asparagus along with parsley. The seeds flavour an Italian salami and are one of the Chinese five spices. They are often used in curries, baked on breads, and can flavour a pounded sea salt as does lovage. The seeds go particularly well with cucumbers, and can also be mixed with cheese and sprinkled over steamed vegetables. The stalks can be cooked as celery, and the roots were once candied.

The plant and the oil are used in some alcoholic drinks, mainly of the aniseed or *pastis* variety (which usually use star anise). A French herb liqueur, La Tintaine, is sold in a bottle with a fennel stem.

The bulb fennel possesses many of the properties of the herbal plant, and can be eaten raw in a salad or cooked. To eat raw, trim (keeping the feathery leaves for use as a herb), and cut into slices. Sprinkle with chopped parsley, first-pressing olive oil and some salt and pepper to taste. This is a good side salad, for fish especially.

BRAISED FENNEL   *Serves 4*

This can be eaten as a main dish, or as an accompaniment to game, veal or chicken.

> *4 large fennel bulbs*
> *salt and freshly ground pepper*
> *1 garlic clove, peeled and halved*
> *about 85 ml (3 fl oz) first-pressing olive oil*
> *100 g (4 oz) Gruyère cheese, grated*

Trim the bulbs well, cut them in half, and boil them in salted water for 30 minutes. Drain well. Rub a dish with the cut clove of garlic, and sprinkle with some of the olive oil. Place the half bulbs in the dish and sprinkle with some more olive oil. Season with salt and pepper and sprinkle with the grated cheese. Cover with greaseproof paper and cook in the oven preheated to 180 – 200 °C (350 – 400 °F) Gas 4 – 6 until brown – about 35 minutes.

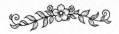

FRANKINCENSE (*Boswellia carteri – Burseraceae*)

Frankincense, often known as olibanum, is an aromatic gum resin obtained from African and Middle Eastern trees of the genus *Boswellia*, chiefly *B. carteri*. The tree is small, growing to a height of 3 – 7 m (10 – 23 ft), and is related to the tree which produces myrrh.

Frankincense has been used since ancient times in religious ritual and, indeed, is still used today, as a major ingredient of church incense. It was very highly valued by many early cultures – thus one of the three gifts from the Magi to the infant Jesus – and it is believed that the Phoenicians zealously monopolized its trade for a quite considerable time.

Dioscorides and others mention the therapeutic use of the gum in the treatment of skin disorders, in ophthalmology, haemorrhages and pneumonia. Soldiers were treated with frankincense: a sixteenth-century surgeon, Ambroise Paré, noted that it stopped the blood flowing out of wounds, and helped scar tissue to form quickly. He also said it was good for breast-feeding abscesses. This century, a French doctor, Professor Cabasse, recorded frankincense's effectiveness in treating skin cancer.

THE ESSENTIAL OIL

Description: *Deep incisions are made into the trunk of the tree, from which white resinous matter exudes in large 'tears', ovoid in shape. These dry and fall to the ground where they are collected. The tears are whitish yellow, milky and waxy. I tasted one in Muscat: it melted slightly on contact with my tongue, and was like a mix of turpentine and butter. Commercially, it is usually supplied in yellowish blocks covered with white dust; it is also available powdered.*

The oil is steam-distilled from the gum, which contains approximately 3 – 8 per cent essential oil. This is colourless or pale yellow; it has a balsamic fragrance, subtly lemony, and sometimes with a note of camphor.

The principal constituents: *Ketonic alcohol (olibanol), resinous matters (30 – 60 per cent) and terpenes (camphene, dipentene, α- and β-pinene, phellandrene).*

ITS USES

In illness

Like other resins, frankincense is said to be bechic, a sedative, pectoral and a good antiseptic. It is effective in inhalations for **catarrhal discharge** and **respiratory congestion**. Put 2 drops of the oil into a bowl of hot water and inhale for 7 minutes, head covered with a towel. Mix together 10 ml (2 tsp) soya oil, 2 drops wheatgerm and 6 drops frankincense oil. Use this to massage the sinus area, the ganglions behind the ears when sore, temples and chest. Do this a few times per day.

(*See also* **coughing, dermatitis, gout** *and* **nails.**)

Other uses

Frankincense can help meditation at home. Place a few drops on a piece of cotton wool near a warm radiator or light bulb, or in a dish of hot water. Do your exercises, yoga or otherwise, nearby, closing your eyes and breathing deeply.

Frankincense has been used in many pot-pourris and burning perfumes throughout the centuries.

GAIAC *Guaiacum officinale – Zygophyllaceae*)

Gaiac oil comes from a small evergreen tree, known as *Lignum vitae* or 'tree of life', which can grow to a height of about 6 m (20 ft). It produces large numbers of crooked branches, and has a very pronounced dome-like shape. The flowers are blue, produced in axillary clusters of five to ten, and fruits are fleshy and orange. It has a very hard, dense bark, which does not rot – the part used in aromatherapy – and is reminiscent of the box tree. It grows in South America especially the Argentine (in the province of Gran Chaco, and along the Rio Berjamo) and Paraguay. In many old books it is known as *palo santo* (healthy wood) or *palo balsamo*. It also grows in the Caribbean: it is the national tree of the Bahamas, and its flower is the national flower of Jamaica.

The *conquistadors* introduced venereal disease to the South American Indians, and it was the latters' use of the bark to cure the new maladies, especially syphilis, that promoted its introduction to Europe. The natives used shaved bark in decoction for both drink and applying as a poultice on affected parts. Later research by Ambroise Paré in France, in 1585, notes the sudorific, stimulant and healing effect of the bark in viral disease, especially syphilis. Gum guaiacum, as the product of the tree is known, was used in the Caribbean and elsewhere until very recently in the treatment of arthritis and syphilis.

THE ESSENTIAL OIL

Description: *When cut, the bark is whitish, but after exposure to the air turns a greenish-yellow. The bark has a high content of resin which normally exudes naturally. This is viscous, brownish, and has an exotic and aromatic smell – reminiscent of jasmine, vanilla and tea. The resin crystallizes into a solid block and has to be warmed to a temperature of 40–50 °C (104–122 °F) before melting.*

The principal constituents: *Guaiacol (around 20–30 per cent), gaiaretic acid, gaiol, resinols and terpenic hydrocarbon.*

Dangers: *It is not recommended for self help, and should only be used by practitioners. There are a number of reasons for this. As the oil has a hard consistency, it must first be dissolved. The provenance of the oil, too – the certainty that it is unadulterated – is vital, as treatment could be disastrous. The age and sensitivity of the patient have to be taken into consideration, and the dosage is very important. Research done by Dr Perrot in 1971 found that doses which were too large could provoke colitis, enteritis, heavy bleeding in women, and severe dehydration as a consequence of heavy sweating.*

Gaiac oil is often mixed with geranium oil, for instance, to imitate

Bulgarian rose. And gaiac itself is often replaced by synthetic gaiacol imitating the suave smell of linalool.

ITS USES

In illness

Gaiac is one of the strongest sudorifics in aromatherapy. It is a diuretic, anti-rheumatic, a stimulant and antiseptic. It is useful for **gout, skin** and **urinary problems**, and for **virus infections.**

GALBANUM *(Ferula galbaniflua – Umbelliferae)*

Galbanum is a resinous gum obtained from some species of *Ferula*, a family of perennial giant fennels. The plant has the typical umbrella flower and seed head of its more familiar relatives, a thick stalk, and can grow to about 2 m (6½ ft) in height. It is native to southern Europe, North Africa and western Asia and is said to have originated in Iran. *Ferula foetida* is a very close relative, the plant which produces the resin asafoetida, used both as a medicine and as a condiment in Eastern, particularly Indian, cooking.

Galbanum was used in religious ceremonies by the Ancient Egyptians, and in embalming – traces of it have been isolated from the bandages of mummies. The Hebrews used it as well in annointing oils. Dioscorides and Pliny mentioned galbanum, noting its sedative, antispasmodic, emmenagogic and diuretic values. Lemery in the seventeenth century classified it as emmenagogic in his treatise on simple drugs.

THE ESSENTIAL OIL

Description: *To obtain the resinous gum, incisions are made in the stalk near the roots, from which the gum runs like brown tears. This is sometimes viscous, sometimes dry, depending on the species. Approximately 14 – 25 per cent of essential oil is obtained by steam distillation from the gum. The oil is thick and yellow with an agreeable aromatic smell which is a bit earthy.*

The principal constituents: *50 – 60 per cent is carvone, sesquiterpenes (cadinene and myrcene) and sesquiterpenic alcohol (cadinol) and terpenes (limonene and pinene).*

ITS USES

In illness

The plant grows especially well in Iran and India, and even today the resin is applied as a plaster to skin ulcers, snake and insect bites, abscesses and **skin inflammation**. I find galbanum useful for **skin disorders** such as abscesses or inflammations, and it is particularly effective for encouraging the **formation of scar tissue**. Mix together 5 ml (1 tsp) each of wheatgerm and almond oils, and 5 drops galbanum. Apply four to six times a day, until better, covering with a piece of gauze each time.

(*See also* **ageing skin, dermatitis** *and* **nails.**)

Other uses

Galbanum is used as a fixative in perfumery.

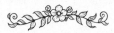

GERANIUM (*Pelargonium* spp. – *Geraniaceae*)

Pelargoniums, commonly called geraniums, should not be confused with the European genus *Geranium*, which includes crane's bill or Herb Robert. Pelargoniums – the name comes from the Greek *palargos*, stork, because of the beak-like fruits – originate from South Africa, and were first formally recorded in Europe in 1690; they are now a popular, familiar and widespread garden plant in frost-free areas. Although there are more than 200 species, only a few are cultivated for the production of essential oil, and these include *P. graveolens* (rose-scented geranium), *P. roseum, P. odoratissimum, P. capitatum,* and *P. radula.* The main areas of flower cultivation and production are Réunion, Madagascar, the Congo, Egypt and most other North African countries; Spain, France, Italy and Corsica produce on a smaller scale, and other species of pelargonium are cultivated in China, India and Russia. The best quality oil is from Réunion, once called Île de Bourbon (another name for the essence is 'gernanium Bourbon-la-Réunion'), and that from Egypt is good as well. Climate and soil are vital factors in the quality of the plant and of its essential oil.

There is scant mention of geranium in old manuscripts, although there are references in Dioscorides to 'geranion', but is it the same plant? It could be something quite different. There was nothing at all about the oil until the work by Recluz, the chemist responsible for the first distillation of the leaves in 1819; later Demarson, a chemist and botanist, made a study in Paris as to the best varieties to cultivate for the production of essential oil (that of rose geranium began in France in 1847). These researches introduced the oil to therapy.

THE ESSENTIAL OIL

Description: *The oil is steam-distilled from the aromatic green parts of the pelargonium, especially the leaves. The plant must be freshly cut just before the flowers open. About 300–500 kg (675-1,125 lb) of plants are needed to obtain 1 kg (2¼ lb) essential oil so it is quite expensive (though not as much so as rose). The worldwide annual production of the oil is estimated to be in the region of 300 tonnes, an enormous quantity, mostly used in perfumes (of which the oil is the most important ingredient). The oil is limpid, and fairly colourless, although there is a faint tinge of green. It has a wonderful aroma, and that of rose geranium is rather like rose oil: this also contains geraniol and citronellol, which is why geranium is often used to falsify the more expensive rose oil.*

The principal constituents: *Alcohols (terpenic geraniol, about 75–80 per cent, borneol, citronellol, linalool, terpineol), esters (acetic, butyric, valerianic), ketones, phenols (eugenol) and terpenes (phellandrene, pinene).*

Dangers: *The best-quality geranium oil is quite expensive, so it in turn is often falsified with artificial esters, cedarwood, turpentine or lemongrass. These falsifications can easily be detected by an expert, but are sold as true geranium to the public. These falsified oils will obviously not give good results in therapy, so buy very carefully.*

ITS USES

In illness

Geranium oil is one of the most important oils in aromatherapy – almost a first-aid kit in itself. It is vulnerary, a tonic, an antiseptic and a haemostatic, and is good for tiredness, general fatigue and convalescence. It can be used for children too, but as always, the remedies must be at half strength or less.

It is particularly useful for many **skin disorders**, and can help heal cuts and bruises, burns, frostbite, fungus infections, **athletes foot** and **eczema**. Apply neat on cuts and bruises as you would any antiseptic, and cover with a gauze. Repeat a few times per day when changing the dressing.

For **haemorrhoids**, add 1 drop geranium oil to a small jar of cold cream or 5 ml (1 tsp) wheatgerm oil. Apply with a gauze, leaving this in place if possible, and repeat several times a day or whenever painful.

Athlete's foot remedy
Before applying the oil below, have a foot bath of warm water and sea salt, with 5 drops of geranium oil mixed in.

15 ml (1 tbsp) soya oil
3 drops wheatgerm oil
10 drops geranium oil

Mix well and put in a dark bottle. Apply on the feet morning and night, massaging it in well.

Geranium tonics
Diffuse the tonic aroma of geranium through the room where you have to study or work late. Apply a few drops of essential oil on a piece of cotton wool or folded tissue, and leave beside the heat of the lamp on your desk. Take a deep breath from time to time.

If feeling very exhausted, and needing a pick-me-up before starting to work – or play – mix 10 ml (2 tsp) soya oil and 5 drops of geranium. Massage this into the temples, back of the neck, sinus area, back of the hands and clockwise into the solar plexus. Rest on the floor for 5 minutes, then you will feel refreshed, with renewed energy. This is particularly effective for when you return from work and haven't time for a proper relaxing bath before dashing off out again.

(*See also* **abscesses and boils, anthrax, bruises, bursitis, colds, cramp, dental abscess, headaches, pediculosis, shingles, stings and bites** *and* **throat, sore.**)

In cookery
Rose geranium leaves can give a rosewater fragrance, but many other varieties of scented leaves are available – orange, lemon, apple and nutmeg. Elizabeth David uses leaves in blackberry jelly as a flavouring, and in lemon water ice. Use leaves fresh or dried in cakes and puddings.

Other uses
When travelling, geranium oil can be a wonderful insect repellant – rather more attractive than most proprietary products. Make a simple body oil in the proportion of 20 ml (4 tsp) soya oil to 16 drops geranium, and massage your body with it. If bitten, apply geranium oil neat to the

bite, and repeat several times a day to stop the itching. (You can use this on the face but never too near the eyes.)

A few drops of neat oil can be left on a piece of cotton wool or tissue beside your bed at night to keep insects away.

GINGER (*Zingiber officinalis – Zingiberaceae*)

Ginger, one of the most familiar of spices, is a tropical herbaceous perennial which grows to a height of about 60 – 90 cm (2 – 3 ft). It likes water, humidity and heat, and its long spiky leaves are similar in appearance to reeds. The flower is yellow with a purple lip, rather orchid-like, but it is the underground rhizomes or tubers which provide the spice. These are known as 'hands' as they often consist of several finger-like protuberances.

The plant is thought to have originated in India, and was one of the first spices to reach Europe from Asia. The Spanish *conquistadors* introduced it to the West Indies, where it quickly naturalized, and Jamaica in particular became one of the major world producers of the spice. Ginger is now grown in many countries with suitable climates, among them India (50 per cent of the world production), Malaysia, Africa, Japan (where 40 species have been recorded), China, Queensland and Florida.

Ginger has been used for centuries in India, China and Japan for its medicinal properties and features largely in those traditional cuisines. The Ancient Egyptians grew ginger and used it in their cooking to keep epidemics at bay. The Greeks and Romans also used it both medicinally and in cooking. Dioscorides recommended it as a stomachic, to help a sluggish system, and as a stimulant of the digestion, giving it similar virtues to those of pepper. The Romans, interestingly, used ginger in ophthalmics: for advanced cataracts, a ginger preparation was made up and applied on the eyes several times a day. St Hildegarde, a twelfth-century healer, recommended it as a stimulant and tonic, and reiterated its effectiveness for eye diseases. She also said it had aphrodisiac properties, especially for stimulating the vigour of older men married to young women! Ginger was used in the Middle Ages to counter the Black Death; it provoked sweating (much as does the spice when used in a good curry).

To the natives of the Pacific island of Dohu, ginger is sacred, and they use it in abundance in cooking, magic ritual and medicine. The witchdoctor chews the roots, and spits it on to his patients' wounds and burns. The islanders believe it has remarkable healing effects. A story is also told on the island about the actions of fishermen when there's a storm at sea: they too chew the ginger roots, but spit them out into the winds to make them abate. It works apparently!

THE ESSENTIAL OIL

Description: *The oil is distilled from the rhizomes. It is more or less fluid, and yellow, sometimes pale, sometimes dark. It is very aromatic, and camphory with a lemon note, and very peppery, rather like pimentoes.*
The principal constituents: *Sesquiterpenes (camphene, d-phellandrene, zingiberene), sesquiterpenic alcohols (isoborneol-linalool), and terpenes, with citrol and resins.*
Dangers: *The essential oil should never be applied or rubbed neat on the skin, or added neat to a bath, as the skin could react badly, with a nasty rash, followed by blisters. It must always be diluted in a pure cold-pressed vegetable oil base.*

ITS USES

In illness
Ginger is well known as a warming **stimulant** and as an aid for digestion and **digestive problems**. It is also good for **colds, coughs** and **sore throats**. A little of the oil mixed with a vegetable oil makes an effective warming rub for swellings caused by water retention or for **rheumatism**.

(*See also* **dyspepsia**.)

Ginger aphrodisiac
It is perhaps most revered for its reputed aphrodisiac properties (known to the Romans who would ginger up their wine for this purpose!).

10 ml (2 tsp) soya oil
3 drops ginger oil
3 drops wheatgerm oil
2 drops savory oil
2 drops clove oil
1 drop rosemary oil

Mix together and massage gently into the spine for a few minutes, concentrating on the lower part.

Follow this with a tisane, made with hot water, some grated ginger, a pinch each of dried savory and rosemary, and a stick of cinnamon. Infuse for 5 minutes and add honey if desired.

In cookery

Ginger stimulates the gastric juices, which in turn facilitates good digestion. Ginger's antiseptic action was once used to protect against meat bacteria, but now its flavour is best known as a vital ingredient of many curries and Chinese stir-fry dishes. In the western world it is used primarily in sweet preparations – gingerbreads, cakes and biscuits feature in the cuisines of many European countries – but it is also used in preserves, confectionery, ginger beer and ginger ale.

Fresh ginger is now freely available (the rhizomes can stay viable for quite some time), as is dried ginger (which should be bruised before use to release the fragrance). Ginger preserved in syrup is prepared largely in China, and it can also be crystallized in sugar, pickled, and stored in a strong spirit or sherry. Ginger is conveniently bought ground, but the essential oil which gives it flavour is easily lost.

Use ginger in a number of dishes in the winter to give warmth and help those suffering from coughs and colds: add a little to milk puddings, and a slice of fresh to spiced hot drinks, ranging from hot chocolate to a wassail bowl at Christmas.

Other uses

Ginger can be used for its aroma in spicy pot-pourris, but its most unusual use must be in an unscrupulous French veterinary practice. To impress clients or judges, horse dealers rub grated ginger under the horse's tail. As the heat becomes unbearable, so the horse raises its tail, thus giving the illusion of vigorous health and fitness!

HORSERADISH

(*Cochlearia armoracia* [also known as *Armoracia rusticana*] – *Cruciferae*)

Horseradish is a hardy, long-lasting perennial plant belonging to the cabbage family, grown for its edible roots. It is thought to be native to eastern Europe, and is commonly cultivated in northern countries, but it has spread and now grows wild in many parts of Europe and North America. It is found in some parts of Brittany, especially in damp coastal areas, and grows successfully on the roughest ground; Richard Mabey in *Food for Free* says that 'British Rail could probably pay off their deficit if they cropped the plants growing along their cuttings.'

The plant can reach a height of nearly 1 m (3 ¼ ft), and has a rigid stem with large, rough, dark-green leaves rather like dock; in summer a spike of small, white, cross-shaped flowers is produced. It has a thick, long, tapering tap root: if the plant is grown as a perennial, these root systems expand and can become invasive; many gardeners grow them as an annual, digging them up and storing through the winter in sand.

The plant has been known since the time of the Ancients. Young horseradish leaves were one of the five bitter herbs Jews were enjoined to eat at the Passover. Theophrastus mentioned the roots as being a diuretic, and named many varieties. Dioscorides praised it for intestinal disorders, as a digestion stimulant, and advised it to be eaten with fatty meat dishes by stout people! Galen found it a good diuretic and emmenagogue, recommending it for women suffering from menstrual problems such as amenorrhoea and fluid retention. In 1567, one Jean Wien of Basle wrote a book on therapeutic plants – *Medicarum* – and classified the plant as antiscorbutic (preventing scurvy).

All the above properties have been recognized in this century, and doctors Cazin, Leclerc and Mme Maury classified it as a stimulant of the gastric functions, endorsing it also for all lymphatic and chronic rheumatic conditions.

THE ESSENTIAL OIL

Description: *The oil is steam-distilled from the oil-rich roots. It is a pale yellow, and not too fluid. The smell is reminiscent of hot mustard seed oil. The pungency of horseradish is found in the outer part of the roots, is quickly dispelled when the root is grated, and is not formed at all if the root is cooked.*

The principal constituents: *The main ingredient is sinigrin, a glycoside which, combined with water, yields the so-called mustard oils or isothiocyanates. Other constituents are the isothiocyanates, allyl and butyl.*

Dangers: *The essential oil is difficult to obtain, but when I have found a source I have only used it externally. Taken internally it can be quite toxic, caustic even, and can cause inflammations.*

ITS USES

In illness

Once the grated root was used as a rub on the torso in cases of pulmonary problems and complications (like the old-fashioned mustard plaster).

Marguerite Maury would advise patients suffering from **slow digestion** to eat the root grated on crudités and on fatty meat. For other digestive problems she would recommend this wine. Boil 1 litre (1¾ pints) good quality white wine with 400 g (14 oz) fructose for a few minutes, then add 30 – 50 g (1 – 2 oz) peeled horseradish cut into small pieces. Put the mixture into a bottle and store in the dark for 2 – 3 weeks, shaking the bottle occasionally. In winter, to avoid coughs and colds, drink 30 ml (2 tbsp) a few times a day. For **pre-menstrual retention of fluid**, take 15 ml (1 tbsp) wine mixed with mineral water before meals. In cases of **bad digestion** or **flatulence**, drink 5 ml (1 tsp) diluted in a glass of hot water.

For **rheumatic conditions** and aches and pains, boil 15 – 30 g (½ – 1 oz) peeled chopped horseradish in 1 litre (1¾ pints) mineral water for 7 – 10 minutes. Leave this, covered, to macerate in a dark and cool place for 24 hours, then drink two to three cups per day between meals, with a little honey if desired.

For **gum diseases** such as inflammations and receding gums, eat the fleshy root slowly. Rub thin pieces around the gums to firm them. Do this as often as you can. Together with peeled dogwood shoots, this was particularly popular as a gum massager in North America.

In beauty
For **hair problems**, the oil is one of the most important oils for the scalp, being a wonderful stimulant. If used when hair begins to be lost, it is an excellent remedy. Make an oil consisting of 10 ml (2 tsp) soya oil, 40 ml (1½ fl oz) grapeseed oil, 2 drops of wheatgerm oil and 30 drops of horseradish oil. Apply to the scalp and massage in with the fingertips. Leave for a few hours, then wash off with a mild shampoo.

(*See also* **alopecia**.)

In cookery
The root is scrubbed then peeled – usually in the open air, as it is more pungent than the strongest onion. It is then grated and mixed with some other ingredient, usually to make a condiment sauce. Yoghurt, cream and vinegar are all bases for these sauces, most of which probably originate from Germany and Scandinavia, but which have reached their
peak in the sauce served in Britain with roast beef. Horseradish sauces were once served with eggs, chicken and sausages and are particularly

good with smoked fish. The young leaves can be used in a salad. The roots can be macerated in vinegar, and can be sliced and dried.

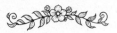

HYSSOP *(Hysoppus officinalis – Labiatae)*

The name comes from the Greek, *hysoppus*, itself derived from the Hebrew *ezob*, meaning good scented herb. A hardy green bushy plant with narrow dark leaves similar to those of lavender and rosemary, it grows to around 30 – 60 cm (1 – 2 ft) in height. It originated in southern Europe and was introduced to Britain by the Romans (and then to America by early settlers). It grows wild in France in rocky soil and on old ruins; in Britain it is often found in garden borders or hedges, mixed with rosemary, catmint and lavender. Its beautiful flower tops are usually royal blue, but can be white or pink. The flowers are highly aromatic and attractive to bees and butterflies.

Hyssop, both flowers and leaves, has been highly valued since ancient times for its therapeutic properties, and was one of the bitter herbs mentioned in the Old Testament (used in the Passover ritual). Hippocrates, Galen and Dioscorides favoured its bechic and pectoral properties. In pagan religious ceremonies, hyssop was sprayed on worshippers to purify them. The Romans used it medicinally and culinarily, the latter both for protection against plague and for its aphrodisiac effect in conjunction with ginger, thyme and pepper. Thomas Tusser in *500 Points of Good Husbandry* (1573) recommended hyssop as a strewing herb, and by the time of the great herbals of the Middle Ages, the herb was so well known that their writers felt no need to go into too much detail about it.

THE ESSENTIAL OIL

Description: *The plant is cultivated for its essential oil in different parts of France, in the regions of Doubs (Jura) and Haute Saône in particular. This oil has a very aromatic, pleasant odour, and is dark-yellowish.*

The principal constituents: *Alcohol, geraniol borneol, thuyone phellandrene and, in large quantities, a terpenic ketone, pinocamphone.*

Dangers: *It is the pinocamphone that can cause the use of the oil to have toxic effects, and hyssop essential oil should not be sold to the public, only prescribed by doctors or reputable aromatherapy practitioners. Much research – by Cadéac and Meunier (1889), by Dr Leclerc and Professor Caujolle (this century) among others – has proved that the oil can cause*

113

epileptic fits if the dosage is not properly respected. It should never be used on sensitive people, as its action on the nervous system can be fatal. Some deaths have been registered in France due to the wrong dosage, and as a result the Ministry of Health has limited its sale to prescription only. I use the oil with enormous care, mainly in combination with other plant essential oils as an inhalation. You can, however, safely use the plant itself.

ITS USES

In illness

Hyssop is pectoral, an expectorant, decongestant, stimulant, sudorific and is carminative. It is recommended for **coughs, colds, 'flu, bronchitis, asthma** and **chronic catarrh**. To alleviate the effects of these, pour 1 pint (600 ml) boiling water over 15 g (1 tbsp) of young green tops and flowers of fresh hyssop, infuse for 10 minutes, and take three cups per day between meals.

Hyssop can also be used externally, and one of the recurring recommendations is as a poultice of young bruised leaves on a **bruise, cut or wound**. Boil 50 g (2 oz) of the young leaves in 600 ml (1 pint) water, let it stand for 15 minutes, then apply with cotton wool on the affected part.

Hyssop syrup

This is also good as a tonic after illness, for 'flu, coughs, bronchitis and for a gargle when you have a **sore throat**. Gather the fresh flowers and leaf tops at the end of July, beginning of August.

100 g (4 oz) flowers and leaf tops
1 litre (1¾ pints) boiling water
1.5 kg (a good 3¼ lb) sugar or 1 kg (2¼ lb) fructose

Mix together until the sugar has dissolved, then leave to marinate for a few weeks in a dark bottle, well corked, and exposed to the sunlight. Take 2 tsp of the syrup per day, morning and mid-afternoon.

(See also **depression**.)

In cookery

Despite the warnings about oil, hyssop can be used as a culinary herb, and indeed has been so since the Middle Ages – there is mention of it in old French recipes in poultry and game stuffing, in stews and potages (soups). Its slightly bitter, minty flavour counteracts the fats of some meats and fish, and a few leaves can be scattered in salads. My grandmother used to serve us a real feast in August when we were little: slices of lightly toasted wholemeal bread were brushed with a garlic clove, covered with buttermilk (you could use fresh yoghurt instead), then sprinkled with a little salt and some finely chopped fresh hyssop leaves.

LEEK AND HYSSOP SOUP   *Serves 4*

An opera singer client swears by this soup, finding its throat properties invaluable before a performance, or before her strenuous singing practice.

> *1 medium onion, peeled and chopped*
> *2 medium leeks, cleaned and chopped*
> *1 garlic clove, peeled and crushed*
> *600 ml (1 pint) water or goats' milk*
> *salt*
> *15 ml (1 tbsp) olive oil*
> *a bunch of fresh hyssop, washed and chopped*

Boil the vegetables in salted water or milk until just soft. Add the oil and chopped hyssop leaves, stir well and serve warm. (You could add a little milk to the water-based soup if you like.)

Other uses
Hyssop is one of the ingredients of some eau de colognes, and it is also used in the making of absinthe and vermouth. It can be infused in the rinsing water for linen.

JASMINE *(Jasminum officinale – Oleaceae)*

Jasmine is a genus of some 300 species of tender and hardy, deciduous and evergreen shrubs and climbers, most of whose flowers have a beautiful fragrance. The leaves of jasmine are mostly pinnate, and the generally white flowers are tubular and borne in clusters or panicles. The genus originated in India, China and Persia, and the name derives from the Persian 'Yasmin'.

Jasmine is one of the most important plants for perfumery (it forms the middle notes), and it is cultivated in many countries: the annual world production of the plant is from 12 to 15 tonnes, Egypt, the largest producer, exporting about 6–8 tonnes, followed by Morocco and India; smaller quantities come from France, Italy and China. The most common variety used in the west is *J. grandiflorum*, and about 40 varieties, many of them grafts, are cultivated.

The plant arrived in southern Europe in about the middle of the sixteenth century and became well acclimatized. Most will survive happily a bit further north, as long as they are sheltered from cold winds and frost, but some require greenhouse cultivation. The flowers do not come to full capacity until about two years after grafting, then they are cropped from July to October. Those appearing from August to the end of September are the most fragrant, when they are at their peak in odoriferous molecule content.

There has been a lot of controversy about jasmine's place in therapy. In the early nineteenth century, the US dispensatory recorded a child poisoned by the fruits of jasmine; the symptoms were coma, dilated pupils, difficult respiration, pale colour, weak pulse, convulsions and paralysed limbs. But later on, in the 1830s, a syrup made with flowers was prescribed as a medicine for coughs and hoarseness.

THE ESSENTIAL OIL

Description: *Until recently the plant was used in three different forms: as an essential oil, as an absolute, or as a concrete (see pages 11 and 12), and all required different methods of extraction. The essential oil was the most expensive, as the flowers yield comparatively little oil, and was extracted by steam distillation. Today it is virtually impossible to obtain the essential oil.*

The principal constituents: *The main one is ketone jasmone, which is responsible for the wonderful smell; others are α-terpineol, benzyl acetate, benzyl alcohol, indol, linalool and linalyl acetate. The ketone jasmone has echoes of orange blossom, daffodils and osmanthus (a Chinese evergreen tree with apricot-smelling flowers), but is really quite distinctive, and so exquisite that it is worth buying the best quality, and ignoring the expense!*

The indol in Spanish and North African flowers is much stronger than that of French flowers. This reaches its greatest strength at night so is picked at that time.

Dangers: *Since the late 1980s essential oil of jasmine has not been available, since distillers have switched from the expensive method of steam distillation to extraction by solvents. The absolute produced by this method is unsuitable for use in therapy. It is likely that any jasmine labelled as essential oil is really the absolute and is only suitable for use as a fragrance.*

ITS USES

In illness

In Indonesia, the flowers of *J. sambac* are boiled; the strong tea is used to bathe **infected eyes** and to use as a compress. In Cochin China, a decoction of the leaves and twigs of *J. nervosum* was taken as a blood purifier. Another species, *J. floribundum,* is used to treat people suffering from tapeworm; the leaves and twigs are sometimes added to the mixture to increase its effect.

I believe that jasmine plays little part in therapy, but undoubtedly its fragrance is so exquisite that merely to smell it can lift the spirits: plant some near windows or doors to perfume the air (but preferably not by a bedroom as the fragrance is stimulant and could keep you awake). I also know that many people feel better after they have drunk a jasmine tea – green China tea perfumed with dried jasmine flowers. Many of my clients say it is helpful for migraine and has a calming effect. Conversely, I find it a stimulant, so it seems that people respond differently to the constituents fixed in the flowers.

In beauty

In Indonesia, India and China, a tradition of the women was to roll jasmine blossoms up in their newly washed and oiled hair. Left all night or day, the perfume of the flowers, basically by the process of enfleurage, would be retained by the hair for quite some time.

Other uses

Jasmine's place in the perfumery industry is obvious, but the blooms can also be used in pot-pourris and in rinsing water for linen – Louis XIV apparently liked jasmine-scented sheets.

JUNIPER (*Juniperus communis – Cupressaceae*)

There are about 60 species of juniper, but the one which yields berries for culinary and medicinal use is *J. communis*. This is an evergreen prickly shrub or tree, depending on location and habitat; it sprawls or is prostrate in exposed situations, and as a tree it can reach 2 – 4 m (6 – 12 ft) high. It is widespread over all the northern hemisphere, growing freely in chalk and limestone, in Swedish, Korean and Canadian forests, and Hungarian and Scottish mountains. In Britain, since the decline of rabbits due to myxomatosis, other hardier shrubs have tended to take over from the juniper, and it is now rarer than it once was. The trees are unisexual, the flower 'cones' of the female trees developing into green berries which turn blue-black during the second or third year.

Often there are green and black berries on the tree at the same time which might be one explanation of the name – from the Latin *juniores*, referring to the constant new berries. There is disagreement among experts, though, some claiming the name developed from the Celtic *gen*, meaning small bush, and *prus*, meaning bitter hot. This latter is more likely to be the basis of the European names – *genièvre* in France, *genever* in Dutch – from which developed the word *gin*, the spirit flavoured by juniper berries.

Juniper berries were known to the Ancients. They were found in prehistoric Swiss lake dwellings, and mentioned in Egyptian papyri. They were burned in ancient Greece to combat epidemics – as was the wood rather more recently, in French hospitals during the smallpox epidemic of 1870. The Romans also used it as a strong antiseptic; and in cooking, they flavoured with juniper berries instead of the rare and expensive pepper. Pliny and Galen favoured juniper berries, especially for liver complaints, and recommended it instead of pepper for heavy eaters. Cato the Elder considered the berries to be diuretic – one of their principal proven properties – and formulated a diuretic wine recipe: a large quantity of berries crushed and heated in some old red wine, bottled then stored for ten days. A glass first thing in the morning was said to work wonders!

In the Middle Ages, juniper was considered a panacea for headaches and kidney and bladder problems. St Hildegarde prescribed it for pulmonary infections if crushed in a hot bath, and for high temperatures, advice echoed later by the School of Salerno. In Britain, juniper berries were considered more magical than medicinal: sprays of berries hung on doors kept witches away on May Eve; smoke from a juniper wood fire kept demons away, and an infusion of the berries was thought to restore lost youth.

The German Renaissance botanist, Fuchs, considered juniper a universal remedy, recommending it for virtually any complaint, later echoed by the French writers René Bretonnayau and Guillaume Burnel. Dr Lemery gave an interesting recipe for a plague preventative in his medical dictionary: he advised the *confiseurs* of France to make juniper dragees – crushed berries instead of almonds in a sugar coating – for people to take several times a day to avoid infection. These Dragees St Roch became very popular.

Throughout the seventeenth and eighteenth centuries, doctors and herbalists advocated the properties of juniper, and later Dr Leclerc composed a formula which contained a large amount of berries. This '*apothème diuretique*' also contained horsetail and elderberries. Another juniper remedy called *huile d'harlem* contained some linseed oil and turpentine, and was sold for liver complaints.

THE ESSENTIAL OIL

Description: *The oil is distilled from the fresh black, ripe berries. The further south the berries grow, the more essential oils they contain, and the better the flavour. Those from Italy are said to be the best.*

The oil is transparent, fluid and colourless, sometimes with a tinge of greenish-yellow. The aroma is similar to that of pine, but more peppery, hot and balsamic, with a burning, somewhat bitter taste.

The principal constituents: *It is rich in α-pinene, borneol, cadinene, camphene, isoborneol, a bitter principle called juniperine, terpenic alcohol and terpineol.*

Dangers: *The oil is often adulterated with turpentine, so beware when buying.*

ITS USES

In illness

The principal properties of the oil are antirheumatic, antiseptic, depurative, diuretic, emmenagogic, stomachic, carminative, sudorific and tonic. Used externally, it is a parasiticide.

For **rheumatism** or **aching joints**, mix together 10 ml (2 tsp) soya oil, 2 drops wheatgerm and 10 drops juniper. Massage on the stiff joint, the back of the neck, solar plexus and spine twice a day until better. Massage in until the oil is completely absorbed.

To alleviate the **retention of fluid** before a period, put 5 drops juniper oil in a warm bath. Follow this with a massage using the oil above (but increasing the soya to 20 ml [4 [tsp]), from the feet to the top of the legs, tummy and hips. The bath also helps **cystitis**.

Juniper is good for some skin conditions. For **acne**, mix 5 ml (1 tsp) each of soya and grapeseed oils with 5 drops juniper, and 1 of wheatgerm. Apply a few times a day when the acne is bad.

For large acne boils with pus, dip a cotton wool bud in pure juniper essence and apply morning and night. This acts as a very strong antiseptic, and will help with the inflammation. It can be repeated two to four times a day when symptoms are at their worst.

For weeping **eczema**, mix 10 ml (2 tsp) almond oil, 5 drops wheatgerm, 6 drops juniper and apply immediately, repeating every four hours until symptoms are better. Cover with a dressing – a piece of gauze will allow the skin to breathe.

(*See also* **abscesses and boils, arthritis, backache, chest infections, cystitis, headaches, leucorrhoea, lumbago, pediculosis, pneumonia** *and* **sciatica.**)

In beauty
A couple of drops of juniper in a bowl of warm water makes a good facial sauna for **greasy skins**.

In cookery
Juniper berries are always associated with game: they can be cooked with game, or their flavour can make milder meats taste somewhat like game. The French for instance are very fond of Provençal game birds which eat the berries: this makes their flesh very succulent and full of flavour. As a result, poultry is stuffed with juniper berries to emulate the 'naturally flavoured' birds. Use the berries in marinades for wild boar, pork or venison. They also go well with veal and, crushed with garlic and rock salt, make a wonderful flavouring for fresh cabbage. They are traditional in *sauerkraut*, and many pâtés.

The berries were a food source of the American Indians of the Pacific North West. They ground them to make into cakes, ate the inner bark of the tree in times of famine, and made tea from the stems and leaves.

The wood and berries can be burned on barbecues, and salmon smoked over juniper is said to have a deliciously winey flavour.

The berries are added to many drinks, to wines and liqueurs like Chartreuse. They make a herb tea in Lapland, a conserve and herb beer in Scandinavia, and were once roasted and ground as a coffee substitute. The most famous drink flavoured by juniper is gin. This originated in Holland 400 years ago when a Dutch apothecary experimented first with wine, then with spirits, calling his product *genièvre*, 'gin' in English, *geneva* or *genever* to the continentals. It was originally produced for purely medical reasons as a diuretic. In England, the cheap gin became a scourge, being called 'mother's ruin', perhaps referring to the belief that juniper berries acted as an abortificant. (Many herbalists still advise that juniper remedies should not be taken during pregnancy.) All gins have juniper flavouring to a greater or lesser degree, the exact proportions being secret, as are those of the other 'botanicals' – such as angelica, aniseed, caraway, cardamom, cassia bark, coriander and orange peel.

Other uses
Juniper wood is a good wood to carve, with pink heartwood and white sapwood. It makes a fragrant firewood, and is also used to make fragrant pencils. The berries can be used for brown or khaki dyes.

LAUREL *(Laurus nobilis – Lauraceae)*

No tree has been as much praised for its elegance, fragrance and therapeutic properties as the laurel, sweet bay or bay laurel, to list but a few of its names in English. *Laurus* is a genus of unisexual, hardy, evergreen shrubs or trees which originates from Asia Minor, but has been well established in all the Mediterranean countries and further north for many centuries; the tree was introduced to Italy before the time of Christ, for instance. It arrived in Britain around the sixteenth century, and can flourish, although it is smaller in size than in warmer habitats (where it can grow as high as 19 m [65 ft]). In Greece, wild bay trees are very common, as they are in south and west France.

The bay laurel has blackish green bark, and evergreen, shiny, lanceolate leaves which exude a wonderful aroma when crushed. The insignificant, creamy-yellow flowers form in clusters in April on both male and female trees, but it is only the female which produces the small blackish-blue berries. Other aromatic trees of the laurel family are the camphor laurel (*Cinnamomum camphora*) of south-east Asia, the Californian laurel or Oregon myrtle (*Umbellularia californica*), and the sassafras (*Sassafras albidum*) of the eastern United States. *Laurus nobilis*, the true laurel, must never be confused with the tree called the common laurel, which is an evergreen ornamental cherry (*Prunus laurocerasus*) and can be poisonous (the leaves contain a small proportion of prussic acid).

The Greek name of laurel – Daphne – salutes the nymph who, on being pursued by Apollo, asked the other gods to help. They turned her into the laurel tree which has, ever since, remained under the protection of all the gods in Olympus. The French, however, often call the tree the 'laurier d'Appollon', and many sources speak of the tree as dedicated to Apollo, the god of music and poetry. The tree also became a symbol of military glory for the Greeks, and generals would encircle their heads with a crown of laurel and carry a twig in one hand. From this derives the British 'Poet Laureate', and the French *baccalauréat*. This latter originated in the the Renaissance, when gifted scholars would be crowned with laurel as in days of yore. Other phrases in English are 'to win or gain one's laurels', and 'to look to one's laurels'.

The greeks also believed the laurel had powers of divination and prophecy, and that it could protect against thunder and lightning, evil and contagious disease. Asclepius, the god of medicine, was always depicted crowned with the magic leaves.

The Romans, too, believed laurel had great powers. Pliny's *Natural History* records an amusing anecdote of how a white hen bearing a twig of laurel in its beak landed in the lap of Augusta, Caesar's fiancée. This was considered very propitious, and the twig was planted and quickly became a very beautiful tree. Later, Caesar, triumphant in battle, wore a garland of leaves from the same tree – although many thought the crown was for another purpose, to hide his bald patch!

In medicine, the tree has been attributed with many therapeutic values from the very earliest times. Dioscorides considered the leaves to be vomitive, the fruit to be pectoral, and the roots to help dissolve kidney stones. Galen thought the tree to be a good remedy for liver complaints, stimulating and warming the vital functions. In the Middle Ages, St Hildegarde, the abbess of Bingen, described laurel as a universal remedy for a number of ailments, including fever, asthma, migraine, gout, palpitations, angina pectoris, and liver and spleen complaints. She also echoed some of the earlier beliefs: she claimed that it could keep evil 'at bay', and that people should wear it or go under its branches to protect themselves from thunder and lightning. A medieval French saying, quoted by Corneille in *Horace*, was *'foudre ne chiet sur le lorier'* ('lightning does not fall on the laurel').

THE ESSENTIAL OIL

Description: *The leaves are distilled to produce a greenish-yellow essential oil. It has an agreeable odour reminiscent of cajuput although the latter is softer and more acrid.*

The principal constituents: *Cineol up to 50 per cent, and α-pinene, eugenol, geraniol, linalool, phellandrene, sesquiterpene and sesquiterpenic alcohol.*

Dangers: *Because of the eugenol content, laurel oil can corrode metal. Do respect recommended quantities.*

ITS USES

In illness

Last century, Dr Cazin classifed laurel as a carminative, expectorant, diuretic and sudorific, and prescribed it for **flatulence**, slow and difficult **digestion, asthmatic conditions** and **bronchorrhoea** (a chronic form of bronchitis, with a great amount of phlegm). More recently Dr Leclerc recommended its use for **chronic bronchitis, 'flu** and **'flu fevers, dyspepsia, flatulence** and virus infections; his remedy was an infusion of the leaves or berries.

I prescribe laurel tisanes for the ailments mentioned by Dr Leclerc. Use 5 g (¼ oz) leaves, 10 g (½ oz) organic orange peel and 300 ml (½ pint) boiling water: infuse for ten minutes, strain and then drink with honey if required. It is a wonderful sudorific – promoting sweating – and can really help in the case of 'flu.

To help counter **rheumatic aches and pains**, add 10 drops of laurel oil – or some fresh leaves – to a hot bath and relax for a while. After the bath, rub the affected areas with an oil made from 20 ml (4 tsp) grapeseed oil and 12 drops laurel; wear a thick, warm dressing gown and lie on your bed for at least half an hour.

A soya and laurel oil is very useful for a stiff neck: add 5 drops laurel to 10 ml (2 tsp) soya oil and use to massage all over the neck until absorbed then wear a thick scarf for at least 20 minutes, resting your head on a pillow. You could use leaves as well: boil for 10 minutes, then dip a small towel or nappy in the liquid and place around the neck. Either of these remedies can also be used for sprains.

The essential oil can also be used for **pediculosis, scabies** and **loss of hair** after an infection.

In cookery

Bay laurel leaves may be used fresh, when they are rather bitter, or dried, when the aroma is still present but the bitterness has softened. (Really old bay leaves will taste of nothing at all.) Bay leaves are used in cooking all over the world, but particuarly in Europe to flavour stocks, *court-bouillons*, marinades, sauces, *bouquet garnis*, and in and on pâté mixtures. The *tej-pat* of Indian cookery is not bay, as is so often thought, but dried cassia leaf (that of laurel's not-too-distant relative, *Cinnamomum cassia*).

Bay can also be used in sweets, boiled in the milk for a pudding or custard, for instance.

Meat marinade

Marination helps tenderize meat of any sort, and using plenty of aromatics helps to prevent putrefaction.

500 ml (18 fl oz) dry white wine
1 sprig each thyme and savory
4 – 5 shallots
3 – 4 bay leaves
3 – 4 garlic cloves, slightly crushed
2 cloves

Mix the wine, the herbs and spices together in a large bowl, and immerse the meat in it. Leave for 24 hours, and then drain, season, and cook in the normal way.

Other uses

Laurel leaves were used as a strewing herb in the time of the Elizabethans. Bay leaves are placed in boxes of figs to keep away weevils; and a leaf or two in jars of flour or pulses will similarly discourage insects at home.

Laurel essential oil has been and still is used in a great many medicaments, for bath lotions, and in antiseptic soaps, as well as in food flavouring, and perfumery. In veterinary practice, it is included in cleansing ointments for farm animals.

LAVANDIN (*Lavandula fragrans/delphinensis – Labiatae*)

The essential oil called lavandin is obtained by the steam distillation of a hybrid lavender, a cross between lavender and aspic. Hybridization occurs naturally as bees convey the pollen from one lavender to another. The plants grow at the same sort of altitudes as lavender and aspic, reaching about 60 – 80 cm (2 – 2 ½ ft) in height. The flowers are dark blue, very highly scented and larger than true lavender.

This is the plant which is most valued by commerce as it has many advantages for the producer: the plant is more resistant to hard weather and disease; as it is taller than lavender, it is easier to cultivate; and it produces more flowers. True lavender distils 500 – 600g (18 – 21 lb) essential oil from 100 kg (220 lb) of organic flowers whereas the lavandin bush will produce 3 kg (6 ½ lb) of oil from 100g (220 lb) of flowers.

Lavandin is primarily cultivated in France, Spain, Italy, Switzerland and Hungary. In 1991, the production of lavandin in South East France was approximately 750 – 900 tonnes while that of lavender was 50 – 200 tonnes. France accounts for three-quarters of the world production of lavandin oil. The USA imports approximately 100 tonnes per year, the EC 5 – 600 tonnes, followed by Japan at 40 tonnes.

THE ESSENTIAL OIL

Description: *The essential oil is yellow to dark yellow and smells acridly aromatic and a little camphory. It is very similar to lavender oil, but is less subtle.*
The principal constituents: *Borneol (40 – 50 per cent), camphor (10 per cent), cineol (10 per cent), geraniol, linalool and linalyl acetate (15 – 35 per cent). It differs from lavender in its content of camphor, its greater proportion of borneol and its lesser proportion of linalool.*

Dangers: *Lavandin is less therapeutic than lavender but is often sold* as *lavender.*

ITS USES

I don't use lavandin in therapy, but it is wonderful as a home fragrance. Use it to perfume the linen cupboard, or clothes (add a few drops of oil to the rinsing water). It has the same calming effects as lavender, so a few drops could be put in a bowl or on a piece of cotton wool next to a radiator or the bulb of a lamp.

Lavandin, like aspic, is used extensively in soaps, household goods, and cheaper perfumes.

(*See also* **frostbite**.)

LAVENDER (*Lavandula augustifolia/officinalis – Labiatae*)

Lavender is an evergreen and fragrant shrub native to southern Europe, especially around the Mediterranean. The majority of the commercial crop is grown in France, Spain, Bulgaria and the Soviet Union. Some is also grown in Tasmania, and there is a minor, but flourishing, industry in Norfolk, England.

Lavender can grow at considerable heights – one organic Provençal grower calls his product 'Lavande 1100' from the height in metres (3,600 ft) at which his plants are cultivated. Individual plants grow up to 1 m (3 ft) in height, and can become very woody and spreading. The narrow leaves are grey and downy; the flowers are blue-grey, borne on long slender stems. The oil glands are in tiny star-shaped hairs with which the leaves, flowers and stems are covered; rub a flower or leaf between your fingers to release some oil (it has a short-lived aroma).

There are several varieties in the genus, chief among them *L. angustifolia*, *L. stoechas* and *L. spica*. Lavender oil comes from *L. angustifolia*, also known as *L. officinalis* (medicinal lavender) and *L. vera* (true or Dutch lavender, although some say this latter is a separate and compact form of *L. spica*). *L. spica* itself (spike or Old English lavender) produces aspic oil. Lavandin oil is produced by distillation of a hybrid, a cross of true lavender and aspic lavender. (See also Aspic and Lavandin.)

Lavender has been used since ancient times as much for its delicate perfume as for its medicinal properties. The oils of aspic and stoechas were mentioned by Dioscorides, Galen and Pliny. The Romans added lavender to their bath water (the name comes from the Latin, *lavare*, to wash). It was an established plant by the twelfth century as St Hildegarde awarded it a whole chapter in her medical treatise. It was also a plant grown in medicinal monastery gardens in Europe in the thirteenth and fourteenth centuries.

Lavender was grown at Hitchin in Hertfordshire in 1568, being commercially cultivated after 1823. In the eighteenth century, the perfumery company, Yardley, were making lavender soaps and perfumes, with fields at Mitcham in Surrey. Like so many other plants which produce essential oils, the trade is recorded in street names in towns and cities – Lavender Hill in south London among them. Norfolk is now as famed for its lavender fields as is Provence, particularly the mountains near Grasse, in France.

All lavender varieties were once distilled together without distinction, many calling the resultant oil sticadore or oil of spike. In 1760, however, the plants' botanic characteristics started to be classified separately.

The ancients classified lavender as a stimulant, tonic, stomachic and carminative. Matthiole, the sixteenth-century botanist, regarded lavender flowers as a most effective panacea, mentioning lavender cures for epilepsy, apoplexy and mental problems; one of his recipes to prevent fluid retention involved boiling flowers in wine and drinking two glasses of this a day. The French used to make a herbal tea with lavender, cinnamon and fennel; this would cure jaundice as well as act as a cardiac tonic. Lavender is valued for containing many of the same properties as sage, rosemary and the other members of the labiate family: as well as those indicated by the ancients above, lavender is also credited with being an antispasmodic, diuretic, antiseptic, vulnerary and circulatory plant. All in all, it is one of the most commonly used, valued and prescribed oils.

THE ESSENTIAL OIL

Description: *The flowers are steam-distilled in the fields where they have grown, and approximately 100 kg (220 lb) are needed to obtain 500 – 600g (18 – 21 lb) essential oil.*

The oil varies in colour from dark yellow to dark greeny-yellow, and smells very highly scented. The content and quality of the oil depends greatly on climate, soil and altitude. The French lavender is considered better than the English, for instance, because it is richer in linalyl acetate: this gives a fruitier and sweeter note, considered pleasanter than the camphoric English lavender with its higher proportions of lineol.

An oil can also be produced from the stalks, but the scent is less subtle than that from the flowers.

The principal constituents: *Alcohols such as borneol, geraniol and linalool, esters such as geranyle and linalyl, and terpenes like pinene and limonene. Lavender also contains a high proportion of phenol, so is a strong antiseptic and antibiotic.*

Dangers: *Lavender is one of the least toxic oils, but care must still be taken. Lavandin (see page 124) is often sold as lavender, because it is cheaper to produce. No remedy will work if lavandin is inadvertently used instead of lavender. The price should be your guide: lavandin is one-third the price of lavender. There is so much adulteration, and one must be very sure of the oil's provenance. It is however easy to make your own lavender oil (see page 27).*

ITS USES

In illness

Lavender is *the* oil most associated with **burns** and healing of the skin. Anyone who is at all interested in aromatherapy will have heard the story of Dr R M Gattefossé, one of the founding fathers of the therapy, and lavender. When he severely burned his hand in the laboratory, he plunged it accidentally into the nearest bowl, full of essential oil of lavender. The pain ceased and the burn healed very quickly thereafter. At home, apply pure oil on a burn and cover with gauze of muslin (to let the skin breathe). Or, if there is no oil available, get some lavender flowers or leaves from the garden, apply to the burn, and wrap as above. It is also good for other skin problems, see below.

Lavender is very effective in treating **cystitis**, vaginitis and **leucorrhoea**. Make a herbal tea with 5 ml (1 tsp) dried lavender flowers and 600 ml (1 pint) boiling water, infuse for 5 minutes, sweeten with honey and drink six times a day until the symptoms have disappeared. The tea can also be added to cold water in the bidet for the same problems, for urinary infections, and for those who have problems after intercourse (or add 3 drops of the oil to warm water in the bidet).

The herbal tea above is also good as a morning tonic for convalescents, as a **digestive** after meals, and for **rheumatic conditions**, and at the first appearance of a **cold** or 'flu. For the latter, gargle tea with a couple of drops of the oil added and drink, at least five times a day.

Because it is so gentle, lavender can be used during **pregnancy** (although its smell gave two of my clients nausea). To prevent circulatory problems such as **varicose veins**, massage the legs with an oil consisting of 3 drops cypress, 2 drops each of lavender and lemon, and 25 ml (1 fl oz) of soya oil.

Lavender is reputed to cure **headaches** (pickers used to put a sprig

127

under their hats). Shakespeare recorded its possible aphrodisiac use: Perdita in *The Winter's Tale* offers 'hot lavender, mints, savory, marjoram ... these are flowers of middle summer, and I think they are given to men of middle age.'

(*See also* **abscesses and boils, anaemia, arthritis, backache, bronchitis, bruises, colic, coughing, cuts and wounds, fatigue, gout, menopause, oedema, pediculosis, shingles, stings and bites** *and* **stress**.)

In beauty
Just as lavender can help heal burns quickly, so it can help problems such as **bruises, frostbite, acne, dermatitis** and **swelling**. Add 3 drops to 10 ml (2 tsp) soya oil, and apply. Use the oil in a facial sauna for acne. Add some drops of the oil to a warm bath to help **cellulite**.

A lavender tea as above is good for **oily skins**, and the plant helps normalise the secretions of the sebaceous glands. Lavender water (available from chemists, or make you own) is a good toner for the skin for the same reason. It is also useful for oily hair (especially dark hair) as a rinse.

Other uses
The leaves of young lavender were eaten by the Elizabethans in salads, and they have been substituted for mint in savoury jelly.

The plants were used as hedging in Elizabethan knot gardens, and as strewing herbs: Thomas Tusser's list included 'Lavender, lavender spike, lavender cotton [santolina]'. Ladies would sew sachets of lavender into their skirts, and use the flowers in pot-pourris (lavender is second only in popularity to rose). In the fourteenth century, Charles VI of France would sit on lavender-stuffed pillows. Lavender bags for scenting clothes and linen are still as popular today as in Elizabethan times, if lavender smelling salts and vinegars have somewhat waned. Bunches of lavender were used to scrub floors, and the oil to polish furniture. Even today, lavender is the most common fragrance in perfumes, soaps, furniture and floor polishes.

Lavender can deter dog and cat fleas and moths.

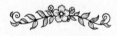

LEMON (*Citrus limon – Rutaceae*)

The lemon tree is a relatively small member of the *Citrus* family, reaching up to 5 m (16 ft) in height. Like most of its relatives, it originated in South-East Asia, in India, China and Japan, but is now grown extensively in hot countries around the Mediterranean, in Spain, southern Italy, Sicily, and the south of France. Lemons are also grown in California. They are the least hardy of the citrus trees. Although small, an individual tree can produce up to 1,500 fruit per year. The white flowers have the most exquisite perfume.

The fruit is thought by some not to have reached Europe until the Middle Ages, but it was known to the Greeks and Romans, if rare. Virgil wrote of it as the Median apple, because lemons came from Media near Persia. The ancients used the peel to perfume clothes and act as a pesticide. A well-known Roman agronomist, Palladius, started cultivating lemons on a large scale in the fourth century. Lemons were planted in the Sahara by Arab invaders in the eighth and ninth centuries; the Moors introduced them to Andalusia in southern Spain during their eight centuries of occupation.

The therapeutic values of lemon began slowly to be recognized. Nicolas Lemery in his book on simple drugs in 1698 mentioned them. They were classified as digestive (helping flatulence), as a blood cleanser, and as helping sweeten the breath after a heavy meal. They reached the height of their therapeutic fame when they were issued to counteract the effects of scurvy on the British Navy (resulting in the erroneous nickname of 'limey').

With oranges, lemons are the most important citrus fruit. Linnaeus thought the lemon was a variety of citron (the earliest *citrus* fruit to reach Europe) and classified it as *Citrus medica* var. *limonum*; but it has now achieved its own classification as *C. limon*. Essence of lemon is second only to orange in its world production and use. There are a great number of tree varieties cultivated for their essential oils, and each oil is different, depending on provenance, culture, climate and method of extraction. The annual world production of the oil is 2,000–2,500 tonnes (1987 figures). The principal producers are the USA, Argentina, Italy, Sicily, the Ivory Coast, and Brazil. Australia is beginning now to cultivate lemons. Western Europe is the most important market for the oil, importing some 750 tonnes per year.

THE ESSENTIAL OIL

Description: *Like bergamot, the oil is obtained from the oily rind of the fruit. This is pressed from the skin by sponges; the oil gathers in the sponge and is then squeezed out. Although slow, this old-fashioned method produces an oil of a better quality than that obtained by more modern methods. The oil is pale yellow, sometimes even green, with a nice fresh smell.*

The principal constituents: *Limonene (up to 90 per cent) and citral*

129

(3 – 5 per cent); others are coumarines (bergamotine and limettine), and flavones (diosmine and limotricine).

Dangers: *Like most citrus oils, the essential oil does not keep well, and if left open or in the light, can quickly become cloudy and pale with a disagreeable smell. When buying, check the date mark very carefully, and do not buy if it is cloudy. Certainly never use an old oil on your skin as it could cause terrible allergic reaction – and it won't have any therapeutic value anyway. Lemon oil is restricted by IFRA and causes dermatitis if there is exposure to sunlight after use.*

ITS USES

In illness

A remedy for **eye infections** that has long been used in my own family for as far back as I can remember involves putting several drops of pure lemon juice in the eyes five or six times a day. I still use it myself when I have an eye infection. I must warn you, however, that it is extremely painful, with a burning sensation that persists; the eyes do calm down after a while, and they feel much better. A drop in each eye is sufficient a few times a day.

Lemon essential oil is called '*polyvalent*' (cure-all) by French phytotherapists, who classify it as being a tonic, stimulant, stomachic, carminative, diuretic, antiseptic, bactericidal and antiviral. It was still being used as an antiseptic and disinfectant in hospitals up to the First World War.

Lemon is very useful for all vein problems, **varicose** or **broken capillaries**. Either eat a lemon per day, or drink the juice of one mixed with mineral water and 5 ml (1 tsp) honey twice a day, hot or cold.

Lemons also help the symptoms of **PMT** and **insomnia**. Every day for the seven days leading up to a period, drink a hot, freshly squeezed lemon drink last thing at night and first thing in the morning. For period pain massage an oil made from 20 ml (4 tsp) almond oil and 8 drops lemon oil on the stomach clockwise.

Lemon is a well-known and popular remedy for **colds, bronchitis** and **laryngitis**: like its citrus relatives, it contains vitamin C. Drink a few hot lemon drinks throughout the day, and for a **sore throat**, gargle with pure lemon juice in a little hot water.

(*See also* **catarrh, chilblains, fatigue, melanosis** *and* **oedema**.)

In beauty

Lemon juice is used a lot in various beauty preparations – pure lemon juice makes a simple pore-refining toner: use on a **greasy skin** or on blackheads. It makes a good rinse for fair hair and it can help **psoriasis** and **dandruff**. For dark or hard-skinned elbows stand each elbow in half a lemon.

I have found lemon most effective for its rejuvenating properties. Mix some pure lemon juice with some distilled or mineral water, and massage gently on to wrinkles until dry, especially around the mouth and eye areas. This is also good for stomach **skin during pregnancy**, for the breasts and for the nipples, improving circulation.

Lemon beauty mask
Mix together beaten white of an egg and the juice of a half lemon. Apply on the face and neck, leave for 10 minutes, then remove with mineral water. Finish off with a few drops of the oil given opposite for PMT.

Lemon hand cleanser
Pure lemon juice is a wonderful hand cleanser. After preparing vegetables or when hands are stained or smelly, rub them well with a half lemon. Rinse in cold water, then rub in some almond oil. I can guarantee that your hands will be clean, and remain young-looking, with white healthy nails; better than any expensive hand cream. (The juice also acts as a bactericide, very important in the kitchen when preparing food.)

(*See also* **ageing skin, cellulite** *and* **circulatory problems**.)

In cookery
Lemon is one of the most important citrus fruits, but an anomaly exists in that it is the only major food not eaten complete, by itself – it is *parts* of it, the peel and the juice, which are used. Lemon juice is the most common souring agent in Western cooking, and slices appear in a variety of drinks from tea to gin and tonic, and as ubiquitous garnishes. Lemon juice is used to acidulate water to prevent cut or bruised fruit or vegetables turning brown. It is used in salad dressings instead of vinegar and in meat and poultry marinades where it has a tenderizing effect. Lemons are used in many pickles, primarily by the Indians who preserve young fruit in mustard oil and spices, and the Moroccans who salt-preserve small, thin-skinned lemons and tart bergamot lemons in their famous *Citrons Confits*.

Other uses
Lemon essential oil is used in enormous amounts in commercial drinks and beverages – in sodas, lemonades and squashes. It is also used in the food, perfumery and pharmaceutical industries. Certain of these

industries prefer deterpened essential oil (that is, with the terpene removed) as it is more concentrated: high in aldehydes, it has more aroma and keeps better.

Dried lemon peel can be used in pot-pourris, and lemons can be studded with cloves (like oranges) for a sweet-smelling pomander.

LEMONGRASS *(Cymbopogon citratus* and *flexuosus – Gramineae)*

Lemongrass is a fragrant tropical grass closely related to palmarosa and citronella (and once known, like them, under the generic name of Andropogon). It is native to tropical Asia, and is cultivated in India, Sri Lanka, Indonesia, Africa, Madagascar, the Seychelles, South and tropical North America. The oil is produced by two types of lemongrass. *C. citratus*, the plant which is the culinary flavouring, is not dissimilar to citronella (see page 82) in general appearance, but can be distinguished by the distinct lemony odour of the leaves and by its less robust growth, from 30-50 cm (12-20 in). It is also variously known as melissa grass, fever grass, citronella grass and geranium grass. *C. flexuosus* is a taller grass bearing large, loose, greyish panicles, and is known also as Malabar or Cochin grass. Lemongrass is propagated by root division, planted during the rainy season, and is ready for cutting about six to eight months afterwards.

THE ESSENTIAL OIL

Description: *The two distinct types of lemongrass are important in therapy.* C. citratus *is known in France as* 'Lemongrass Indes oriental'; *C.* flexuosus *is known as* verveine des Indes. *The oil from both is yellow-brown with a light tinge of red, and has a very pronounced lemon odour and flavour.*

The principal constituents: *Both* C. citratus *and* C. flexuosus *contain a high proportion of citral (from 70-85 per cent).* C. flexuosus *also contains citronellol, dipentene, farnesol, geraniol, limonene, linalool, methylheptenol, myrcene, n-decylic aldehyde and nerol.* C. citratus *differs* *slightly, containing caprylics, citronellol, dipentene, farnesol, furfurol, gera-niol, isopulegol, isovalerianic aldehyde, l-linalool, methylheptenone, myrcene, n-decyclic aldehyde, nerol, terpineol and valeric esters.*

Dangers: *Because lemongrass oil is fairly inexpensive, it is often used, with geranium and citronella, to imitate rose (which contains geraniol and citronellol as well) and verbena.*

ITS USES

In illness
Lemongrass has long been used therapeutically, especially in Ayurvedic medicine in India. There it is given as an antidote to infectious virus or high fever, especially in the treatment of cholera. It is considered to be stomachic, carminative and digestive, and is given in cases of enteritis, **colitis, flatulence** and slow **digestion** due to stress.

Because of its high proportion of citral, the oil is remarkably antiseptic, and it is useful for some **skin problems** and for **athlete's foot** (see below). It is also wonderful used to deodorize a room in which people have been or are ill, and to protect against air-borne infection. Put 250 ml (8 fl oz) warm water and 5 ml (1 tsp) lemongrass oil in a vaporizer bottle, shake well and spray the room several times a day. The oil can be used neat in kitchen, bathroom and bedroom cupboards, to keep parasites away (they don't like the smell).

Athlete's foot remedy
A good footbath for athlete's foot or excessive perspiration can be made by adding a few drops of the oil to a bowl of warm water. After bathing the feet use the following oil.

200 ml (7 fl oz) almond oil
5 drops wheatgerm oil
10 drops lemongrass oil

Mix together and rub between the toes. Use morning and night.

(See also **dental abscess** *and* **migraine**.)

In cookery
Lemongrass features largely in south-east Asian cookery, especially in that of Thailand, and has become more popular in the West in the

133

last few years. It is available fresh as bulbous base and stem, with overlapping leaves. The bulbs and stems should be crushed before use, and then removed from the dish. It is not eaten. Lemongrass is also available dried, when it should be soaked for 2 hours before use. Powdered lemongrass is found in ethnic shops as *sereh*.

Lemongrass adds a unique lemony pungency to many fish soups, rice and *dhal* dishes and curries: if it is unavailable, substitute lemon peel, the outer part of which also contains citral.

Other uses
Lemongrass is mildly insect repellant (though much less so than its relative citronella), and is used in commercial preparations. The oil is also extracted for use in the soap and perfume industries.

LOVAGE *(Levisticum officinale – Umbelliferae)*

Lovage is a hardy herbaceous perennial, native to southern Europe, which can grow to about 2 m (6 ft) in height. It looks similar to other umbellifers (fennel, coriander, parsley, etc), with large umbels of yellowish-green flowers followed by seeds. It has a sturdy, thick and hollow stem, and its large leaves are like those of celery and, indeed, taste like them. For this reason lovage, or *livèche*, is also called bastard celery in France. In English, lovage is also known (hopefully) as love parsley. An old generic name for the plant was *Ligusticum officinalis*, perhaps deriving from Liguria in Italy where the plant grows abundantly. I have also seen it growing wild in the mountains in the South of France. There is a related species, *Ligusticum scoticum*, which is known as Scottish or sea lovage: this grows wild around the northern coasts of Britain and the northern Atlantic coasts of America.

Lovage was used by the Greeks and Romans as much for its thera-peutic as for its culinary values. Galen, Dioscorides, Pliny and Apicius all mentioned it, and the Roman legions brought it to northern Europe and Britain. It is said to have grown in profusion in the Emperor Charlemagne's gardens. St Hildegarde recommended it in the twelfth century for coughs, abdominal pains and heart problems. The School of Salerno praised its use in all liver complaints, echoed centuries later by Dr Leclerc who prescribed it for jaundice and all other liver disfunctions, as an infusion or tincture.

THE ESSENTIAL OIL

Description: *Although all parts of the plant – root, stem, leaves and seeds – have medicinal properties, it is the roots which are distilled for the essential oil. Depending on whether the roots are fresh or dried, the oil obtained can be yellow or dark brown; it is a little resinous and thick, and has a strong aroma, reminiscent of angelica with a touch of bitterness and a hint of celery.*
The principal constituents: *Cineol, limonene, selinene and terpineol, with traces of guaiacol and isovalerianic and palmic acids.*

ITS USES

In illness
As a tisane, lovage is a natural blood cleanser and should be used for all hepatic disfunctions and for **skin eruptions, gout,** and **rheumatism**. It is also digestive. To cleanse and detoxify the body after over-indulgent festivities, drink a tisane of lovage leaves: infuse 15 ml (1 tbsp) leaves in 600 ml (1 pint) boiling water for 7 minutes, then drink several cups throughout the day. The flavour is very agreeable, more like a broth than a tea.

For liver problems, you can make up a poultice with linseed adding 8 drops of lovage oil. Place this hot on the area of the liver, keep warm, and repeat twice a day. Fast for the day as well, drinking only 1-2 cups of the above tisane, mixed with mint, at each of the three mealtimes.

Because it cleanses the blood, lovage is also good for the skin. It is said to have deodorizing properties as well.

In cookery
Lovage can be bought as dried leaves, as whole seeds, or in root form; it is easy to grow in the garden to have all three, plus the delicious fresh leaves. These can be used for their yeasty celery flavour in soups,

stocks and casseroles when meat is short – in fact they're most useful in vegetarian dishes and salads. The stems can be blanched and eaten as a vegetable with a cheese sauce (an old French recipe); they can also be candied like angelica. The roots can be peeled and boiled as a vegetable, but they are very strong in flavour; they were once ground and used as a bread flour. The seeds can be sprinkled on bread or biscuits before baking, and they can be ground in a mortar with rock or sea salt to make an extremely aromatic seasoning.

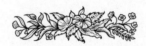

MANDARIN (including Tangerine)
(Citrus reticulata, syn *C. nobilis* – *Rutaceae)*

Another member of the orange family, the mandarin orange tree is smaller and more spreading than the orange tree, with smaller leaves and fruits which are slightly flattened or compressed at both ends. They are distinguished from other varieties of orange by their loose skins, and segments which are easy to separate. They are the most delicately flavoured of citrus fruits, but are also the most hardy. Mandarins have been cultivated in China for centuries, and the origins of the name are debated: they are thought either to have been given to mandarins as gifts, or the size, colour and shape of the fruit is thought to have recalled the buttons on hats of those Imperial Chinese officials. There is also debate about the relationship between mandarin oranges and tangerines. Some believe they are the same; many say the latter is a variety of mandarin, which acquired its name through being shipped from Tangiers; while in Ceylon, for instance, they have distinct names, mandarin being *Jama-naran*, tangerine being *Nas-naran*.

Although mandarins and other loose-skinned oranges had been long popular in Japan and China, they didn't reach Europe until the latter part of the nineteenth century. They are now grown in the Mediterranean regions of Europe and North Africa, and in South and North America. Many hybrids have been developed, including the Temple orange (a mandarin/sweet orange cross), the tangelo (a mandarin/grapefruit cross) and clementines (thought to be a tangerine/sweet orange cross).

Essence of mandarin came originally from Italy, and that of tangerine from the USA. Brazil, though, now dominates the market in both essential oils, exporting over 200 tonnes per year (1987 figures). The State of São Paulo is the most important region of cultivation. The olfactory notes of both Brazilian oils are less subtle and not valued as highly as those from Italy. The major consumers in Europe are Germany, France, Spain, Britain and Holland.

THE ESSENTIAL OIL

Description: *It is the oil-rich rind of the fruits which is sponge-pressed like lemon, for the essential oil. The oil is golden with a lovely blue-violet luminosity (even more noticeable if alcohol is added to it). The perfume of the oil is reminiscent of both lemon and orange simultaneously, but is sweeter and more agreeable.*

The principal constituents: *The constituent particularly responsible for its fluorescent colour (and for the perfume to a great extent) is methylanthranilate. The oil also contains limonene and some quantities of geraniol and terpenic aldehydes (citrol and citronellol).*

Dangers: *Mandarin oil is often adulterated with orange and lemon essential oils, so beware. It deteriorates quickly, like all citrus oils.*

ITS USES

In illness

Therapeutically, both mandarins and tangerines have the same properties as oranges – tonic, stomachic, slightly hypnotic and they act as a sedative for the nervous system. They are very good for **stress** and irritability. Drink the juice instead of orange juice.

Nervous people who have **difficulty in sleeping**, should eat a few mandarins after dinner in the evening. The bromine content, a substance sedative to the nervous system, is higher in mandarins than in any other citrus fruit. The fruit is also rich in vitamin C.

(*See also* **backache** *and* **oedema**.)

Other uses

The essential oils are used in the food and perfumery industries. The peel of both mandarins and tangerines can be dried and used in cooking – once a favoured flavouring of some Chinese dishes. Make sure the fruit are organic, with unsprayed and unwaxed skins. A couple of liqueurs are made from the peels of mandarins and tangerines. The Belgian *Mandarine Napoléon* is said to be made from the recipe with which Napoleon wooed his favourite actress, Mlle Mars.

MARJORAM *(Origanum majorana – Labiatae)*

Marjoram is thought to have originated in Asia, but is now grown all over Europe. It grows in abundance in Tunisia – where it is known as *khezama*, the Arab name for lavender – carpeting the fields between almond and olive trees. There are three major varieties: sweet or knotted marjoram (*O. majorana*), pot marjoram (*O. onites*), and wild marjoram (*O. vulgare*) or oregano; marjoram and oregano have been confused throughout history. Sweet or knotted is a small sub-shrub of about 50 cm (1¾ ft) in height; it has reddish stems with hairy, oval, greyish leaves. Knot-like clusters of pink, white or mauve flowers open from June to September. The origin of the name marjoram is obscure, but is thought to have derived from the medieval Latin 'majorana' and Old French 'mariol', the latter alluding to the knots of flowers which look like little marionettes.

The plant was considered sacred to Shiva and Vishnu in India, and to Osiris in Egypt. To the Greeks it was '*amarakos*', a symbol of love and honour, and young married couples would be crowned with flowers. Aphrodite used it to cure her son Aeneas' wounds (it had been scentless, apparently, until she touched it). Ointments were made with it to retain the natural colour and lustre of hair and eyebrows.

Dioscorides made a pommade called '*amaricimum*' with marjoram for nervous disorders; Pliny prescribed it for stomach disorders and flatulence. In the Middle Ages, St Hildegarde warned people not to touch the plant as she considered it a remedy only for leprosy, and that it could initiate other skin disorders. The School of Salerno classified marjoram as an antispasmodic and a good expectorant, and prescribed it for easing and facilitating labour.

In Renaissance times, pots of the herb were grown, and jams and perfumed sachets were made for chest infections; marjoram mixed with honey was taken for coughs. A poultice of marjoram applied externally helped jaundice and other liver afflictions. In the seventeenth century, a famous Danish physician called Fabricius received 200 gold *écus* for curing the soldier Wallenstein of a cold and rheumatic pains. Later, the apothecaries of the eighteenth century classified marjoram as sternutatory (causing sneezes)!

In 1720, J B Chomel, head of the Academy of Medicine in France, recommended that it be inhaled in dried and powdered form to fortify the brain and reduce fatigue; the herb added to a wine would help the nerves and circulation. F J Cazin, in his history of natural drugs in 1876, prescribed marjoram for nervous disorders such as apoplexy, paralysis, dizziness, epilepsy and loss of memory.

THE ESSENTIAL OIL

Description: *The oil is distilled from the flowering heads. When fresh it is a greenish-yellow which turns brown with age. The smell is very aromatic, reminiscent of camphor, thyme and cardamom with a little peppery note.*

The principal constituents: *Over 80 per cent phenols (carvacrol and thymol), with borneol, camphor, cineol, cymene, pinene, sabinene and terpineol.*

Dangers: *For some conditions, the oil works better on older people, as it can occasionally provoke the opposite effect on the young. Always measure out doses very carefully, and I advise that it never be used on young or sensitive people or children without proper prescription.*

ITS USES

In illness

Marjoram is a stomachic, expectorant, and sedative, good for treating **insomnia, migraines, dysmenorrhoea** and **diarrhoea**. It is also a good antiseptic, but not as strong as its sister oregano.

It is particularly good when you are tired or suffering from sleeplessness or nervous tension. Dr Leclerc confirmed its sedative or stupefacient properties, as did Dr R M Gattefossé and his team, and it has been classifed as such. There are several ways in which marjoram can be used. For lack of sleep and nervous fatigue, add 5 drops marjoram oil and 2 of orange to a warm bath. Follow with a massage oil made from 10 ml (2 tsp) soya oil, 6 drops marjoram and 4 drops orange. Another effective massage oil for the same symptoms consists of 10 ml (2 tsp) soya oil, 2 drops wheatgerm, 4 drops nutmeg, 3 drops rosemary and 8 drops marjoram. For insomnia, drink a tisane made from a pinch each of dried marjoram and dried lime flowers, half an hour before going to bed. One drop each of marjoram and orange oils on a tissue beside your bed can also calm you and help you sleep.

Marjoram is very effective in **mouth disorders** because of its antiseptic properties. For **thrush** or **gum infections**, or the **sore throat** at the start of a cold, make a mouthwash from 300 ml (½ pint) warm boiled water and 1 drop marjoram oil. If you haven't any oil, make a strong decoction of leaves and flowers and use as a mouth rinse.

I use it too for **earache** caused by a cold. Warm a bottle of almond oil under the hot tap, then mix 1 drop of marjoram oil with 5 ml (1 tsp) warmed almond. Dip a small piece of cotton wool in this and insert inside the affected ear. Leave overnight and repeat in the morning if the pain has not gone.

(*See also* **anorexia nervosa, asthma, bruises, cuts and wounds, depression, flatulence** *and* **stress.**)

In cookery
Fresh marjoram's smell reminds me a little of basil; in flavour it is rather like thyme, but sweeter and more scented. Pot marjoram is not nearly as sweet, being rather bitter. (Oregano is more pungent than both.) Marjoram features in many Tunisian, Italian, Portuguese and Provençale dishes, and is one of the most important culinary herbs. It can be dried successfully.

The Ancient Egyptians used it to enhance the flavour of meat and help assimilate the minerals from it, and it is very useful still in marinades, bouquet garnis and stocks. Towards the end of the cooking time, add it to stews, meat dishes, stuffings for meat or vegetables, omelettes, to cooked vegetable dishes (it will help the digestion of vegetables like cabbage or beans), and salad. Its therapeutic properties can also be enjoyed by making herbal oil and vinegar for dressings and cooking.

Other uses
Used once as a strewing herb, the dried leaves and flowers can be used in pot-pourris, or in scented and sedative herb pillows.

MELISSA *(Melissa officinalis – Labiatae)*

Commonly known as balm or lemon balm (as well as bee balm and sweet balm), melissa is a hardy herbaceous perennial native to southern Europe. It was introduced to northern Europe by the Romans. It has wrinkled and toothed, pale-green, nettle-like leaves, with tiny white flowers in June and July. The whole plant is fragrant, with a strong lemony smell. It makes a good garden plant, but it also grows wild in Europe, carpeting fields and woods, particularly around Angers in France.

The name *melissa* derives from the Greek word for bee because the plant is irresistible to bees and has been grown for this purpose for centuries.

Melissa has been known and appreciated since the time of the ancients. Theophrastus and Dioscorides wrote of *melissophyllon* (bee leaf) as being emmenagogic, a sedative and vulnerary. Avicenna recommended it because it was cheering, a property still very much part of the plant's effect: other Moslem and Arab writers considered it very important for treating melancholy and heart conditions. Melissa's fame continued in France, as it was *the* ingredient of Carmelite water, the *'Eau de melisse des Carmes'* distilled in Paris since 1611 by monks. An early version of eau de cologne, the water was used medicinally as a digestive and antispasmodic, and it still finds a place in many French households.

THE ESSENTIAL OIL

Description: *The plants are harvested in France in May or June just before the first flowers appear for the aroma is less interesting when the plant is in bloom. The oil is steam distilled from the leaves and tops, and is pale yellow with an agreeable and subtle, warm, lemony aroma. Melissa oil is not common and it is very expensive because 7 tonnes are needed to produce 1 kg (2¼ lb) oil. It is very special.*

The principal constituents: *Citral, citronellol (responsible for the lemony smell), geraniol, limonene, linalool and pinene.*

Dangers: *The expense of manufacturing melissa oil leads to falsifi-cation, usually with citrus oils or lemongrass (itself sometimes called melissa grass). As a result, you should buy melissa very carefully, as the remedy is more or less useless if the oil is not pure. Melissa is often confused with citronella.*

The oil is classified in France as a 'stupéfiant' (narcotic), thus great care must be taken with its use. Research in the nineteenth century by Cadéac and Meunier revealed that the oil taken internally without food could provoke most unpleasant reactions – severe headache, sudden low blood pressure, and difficulty in breathing.

The oil must be administered extremely carefully, especially so with children, and I do not advise its use by non-practitioners.

ITS USES

In illness

Melissa is antispasmodic, emmenagogic, a stimulant for the nervous system, and a tonic for the cardiac system. It is extremely good for **headaches, depression**, nervous anxiety, **palpitations** and **insomnia.**

Although I don't advise you to use essential oil, you can take advantage of the plant itself, either making a tea from the leaves, eating it in salads or infusing it in alcohol. For a general tonic and a simple remedy for **migraine, depression, PMT** and **menopausal symptoms**, macerate 50 g (2 oz) melissa leaves for 48 hours in 1 litre (2 ¼ pints) good white wine: strain and drink 30 ml (1 tbsp) whenever symptoms appear.

Melissa tonic

This old family recipe is slightly more complicated than the above mixture, but it is more effective.

> 1 litre (2 ¼ pints) vodka
> 50 g (2 oz) melissa leaves
> 15 g (½ oz) lemon peel
> 15 g (½ oz) ground nutmeg
> 10 g (⅓ oz) raw angelica
> 10 g (⅓ oz) cloves
> 5 g (⅙ oz) powdered cinnamon or sticks

Macerate the herbs and spices in the vodka for a fortnight, keeping the bottle tightly corked and in the dark. Filter, pressing all the ingredients well, and then cork firmly again. Drink a coffee spoonful – no more – whenever symptoms appear.

Melissa tea

This is slightly sedative (because of the citronellol) and is good for insomnia due to high blood pressure around the time of menstruation or menopause. It is also very good for nervous tension and depression. Put a good 15 ml (a heaped tbsp) of leaves in the teapot, add 600 ml (1 pint) boiling water and infuse for 10 minutes. Drink two to four times a day with a little honey if desired. It is a very pleasurable drink and I have found it very helpful, especially as a tonic in the morning.

(*See also* **anaemia, anorexia nervosa, colic, coughing, cramp, dysmenorrhoea, stings and bites** *and* **stress.**)

In cookery

Lemon balm leaves have traditionally been used in wine cups and iced summer drinks – for those merry-making properties presumably! The young shoots and leaves give their lemony flavour to stuffings, savoury or fruit salads, sauces and omelettes; they are used in Spain in soups, and with fowl, game and fish dishes. A few fresh leaves can replace lemon or lemongrass in most recipes. It is a *sweet* herb, so can be used in desserts like syllabub. In Spain it perfumes milk – *leche perfumada con melissa* – so could be used in milk puddings. The leaves can be crystallized and added to jams and jellies.

Other uses

Melissa leaves have long been an ingredient of pot-pourris because of their cheering effect. They were also used as a strewing herb, in rinsing water for linen, and in herb pillows and bags. In France, the plant is also called 'bee's pimento', and many believe the bees revive after taking the nectar from the flowers! Certainly, the association between bees and balm has been appreciated for years: Pliny noted that hives were rubbed with balm leaves to attract and keep swarms. Balm oil was also added to a syrup to attract queens, and many orchards were traditionally planted with balm to encourage bee pollination. And, very usefully, if your lemon balm attracts bees and you get stung, balm will also soothe the pain – simply crush the leaves and rub them on the area.

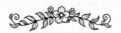

MINT (*Mentha piperita – Labiatae*)

The numerous varieties and hybrids of mint, about 20 in all, are native to the Mediterranean area and Western Asia, but now grow in termperate climates all round the world. Mints include water, corn, horse, eau de cologne and spearmint varieties, but *M. piperita*, peppermint – thought to be a hybrid between water mint and spearmint – is the one used in therapy.

As with all members of the *Labiatae*, mints are characterized by their square stems; they have paired leaves, and small flowers in summer, ranging from purple to white. The leaves and hairy stems contain the oil glands. Mints can be propagated by seed, but can also swiftly take over a herb bed by creeping underground root systems. Mints are perennial, dying down in the winter.

Mints were well known to the ancients: from hieroglyhics dedicated to the god Horus in the temple of Edfu, we learn that mint was used in a ritual perfume. There are several references to mint in the Bible, and in Greek and Roman mythology and poetry. The name itself comes from the myth of the nymph Minthe, as told by Ovid, who was surprised by Persephone in the arms of her husband Pluto; she was metamorphosed into a herb to be trampled underfoot (probably *M. pulegium*, or pennyroyal, which has a creeping habit). Hippocrates, in his medical treatise on plants, mentioned mint for its diuretic and stimulant properties. Galen thought of it as an aphrodisiac; others suggested the opposite, that it diminished sexual appetite. The Romans looked upon mint as a carminative, helping flatulence and the digestion of heavy foods.

Peppermint was not discovered in Britain until 1696, in Hertfordshire, and thereafter it was cultivated, particularly at Mitcham in Surrey. Mitcham mint is as famous as its lavender, and it was soon included in the English pharmacopoeia and many other national codices.

In modern therapy, many practitioners, doctors and scientists have confirmed the therapeutic values of mint as being stomachic, carminative and antispasmodic, a tonic and stimulant; as being good for nervous disorders, nervous vomiting, flatulence and colitis (Dr Leclerc). Dr Cazin prescribed it successfully for intestinal problems, and for liver and kidney deficiencies. It is especially recommended for old people for its digestive values, and for convalescence, fatigue and anaemia.

The USA is the largest producer of mint essential oil, followed by eastern countries and Japan. The oils most favoured for their aroma are those produced from the Mitcham mint and a variety grown in the south of France, known as 'Franco-Mitcham' mint. Japanese essential oil is less agreeable to connoisseurs as it has a strong camphory note, being utilized mainly for the extraction of menthol.

THE ESSENTIAL OIL

Description: *Peppermint is defined as black (with purple stems) or white. The leaves and flowers are picked just before maturity when the essential oil content is at its greatest, and steam distilled. The oil is colourless or of a very pale yellow. The smell has an agreeable freshness, strong, penetrating, giving that feeling of being able to breathe deeply. Fresh, the oil is very fluid, but it thickens and darkens as it ages.*

The principal constituents: *The main constituent is menthol, approximately 40-70 per cent, but this depends on the plant, the soil, the country of origin. Menthol is a very unusual substance, white and crystalline, which causes a sensation of cold in the mouth. Other constituents are, depending on the plant, 20-30 per cent carvone, cineol, limonene, menthone, pinene and thymol, traces of aldehydes, and acetic and valerianic acids.*

Others mints are distilled for their oils. M. *pulegium or pennyroyal, which is the creeping variety found all over Europe, has a ketone, pulegone, as its principal constituent.* M. *spicata, or spearmint, is distilled mostly in the USA: its oil is rich in carvone. Another US mint,* M. *citrata or eau de cologne mint, an offspring of peppermint, contains linalool and linalyl acetate.*

Dangers: *Take care when using mint essential oil. Observe the following guidelines:*

- *Never use mint oil undiluted, as it could provoke a bad reaction.*
- *Never use mint oil as a bath essence on its own.*
- *Never rub the oil on its own over the entire body. Because of the menthol, you will feel like a block of ice, and that could be dangerous.*
- *Don't use mint oil at night as it could keep you awake.*
- *Avoid using mint remedies in conjunction with homoeopathic remedies. Mint acts as an antidote.*

ITS USES

In illness and beauty

The essential oil is good for the nervous system, acting as a regulator and sedative; menthol is well known as a cardiac tonic in pharmaceutical preparations.

It is a good blood cleanser, because it is antiseptic and antibacterial. Drink mint tea often if you have **acne** or spots. A tea is good, too, if you feel **nauseous**: add 30 ml (2 tbsp) chopped fresh or dried mint leaves to 600 ml (1 pint) boiling water, leave to infuse for 5 minutes, and add honey if desired.

For **bruises** and swellings, mix up an oil made from 20 ml (4 tsp) soya oil and 15 drops of mint oil and apply immediately. Repeat a few times over the next few hours.

If you have **swollen gums, mouth thrush** or **mouth ulcers**, mix together 10 ml (2 tsp) cognac or whisky, 5 drops mint oil and 300 ml (½ pint) hot boiled water. Gargle with this several times throughout the day until finished, leaving the liquid in the mouth as long as possible each time.

If you have a **toothache**, mint is a sovereign remedy. Put a few drops of the neat oil on a piece of cotton wool and place on the tooth. It acts as an analgesic and anaesthetic – those wonderful menthol properties – and you will feel relief from the pain. The antiseptic properties of the oil will help disinfect the cavity as well. But don't forget to go to the dentist.

If your shoes are too small, or you suffer from swollen ankles, mix 10 drops of mint oil and 10 ml (2 tsp) grapeseed oil, and rub into the soles of your feet before putting on your socks or stockings, tight shoes or boots. This is especially effective if you are going dancing, or have to stand for a long time. Don't forget to wash your hands well with soap afterwards.

(*See also* **abdominal pains, anorexia nervosa, colic, coughing, cramp, dysmenorrhoea, stings and bites** *and* **stress**.)

In cookery
Peppermint is rarely cooked, but mint has been used as a raw flavouring since antiquity – the Romans introduced spearmint and mint sauce for lamb to Britain. Mint is famously digestive: 'The smell of mint stirs up the mind and appetite, to a greedy desire for food', according to Pliny. Sprigs of mint are traditional too with new potatoes, peas and many vegetable dishes; leaves also flavour jellies, icecreams, stuffings and fruit dishes. Mint is used a great deal in Middle Eastern and Indian cooking, combined with yoghurt and coconut in relishes and chutneys, and in the famous cracked wheat salad, *tabbouleh*. Mint mixed with Chinese green tea leaves makes the famous mint tea of Morocco. Many refreshing summer drinks are enlivened by fresh mint, most notably mint juleps; mint liqueurs like Crème de Menthe are well known too. A strong decoction of fresh mint will make the most delicious home-made peppermint creams.

Other uses
Mint essential oils are used widely in pharmaceuticals – in toothpastes, mouthwashes, massage cream – and menthol is even used in conjunction with tobacco in cigarettes.

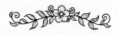

MUSTARD (*Brassica nigra* and *Brassica juncea* – *Cruciferae*)

There are three varieties of mustard which produce seeds used as a condiment. The first two are very closely related: *Brassica nigra* or black mustard (probably native to the Middle East) and *Brassica juncea* or brown mustard (probably native to China and India). The seeds of these are the ones distilled for use in therapy. The third variety is *Sinapis alba*, also known as *Brassica alba* or white mustard (native to the Mediterranean), which is the seed grown for the seedling mustard of mustard and cress (usually now that of rape). All are members of the cabbage family and are characterized by cross-shaped flowers (thus the name *Cruciferae*); these are followed by smooth erect pods containing the seeds. *B. nigra* is the largest variety, reaching to 2.4 m (8 ft) in height. All three are grown throughout the world.

Mustard seeds were found in Ancient Egyptian tombs along with other offerings such as coriander, parsley and lotus seeds; the plants and seeds were mentioned on stele and papyri dating from as early as the first dynasty. Sanskrit mentions date back to 3000BC, which suggests that mustard must be one of the oldest recorded spices. (Some sources claim that mustard was cultivated in the Stone and Iron Ages.) The Greeks and Romans, too, knew mustard: according to classical tradition, it was introduced to man by Aesculepius, the god of medicine, and Ceres, the goddess of agriculture and seeds. The Romans steeped the seeds in must – new wine – calling the result *mustrum* or *mustum ardens* (burning must), from which the name in English is thought to derive. They brought the seeds to Britain, and early emigrants introduced the plant to North America.

Both England and France were and are famed for mustard production. Monks in St Germain des Prés were famous for growing the plants over 1000 years ago, and mustard making and eating has been recorded in Burgundy as early as 1336: the city of Dijon was granted exclusive rights to mustard manufacture in 1634. England had known mustard since Roman times, and the centre for production at the time of Shakespeare was Tewkesbury. At the beginning of the eighteenth century, Durham became important, and a hundred years later, with the entry into the mustard business of one Jeremiah Colman, the British mustard industry became centred on Norwich and East Anglia.

THE ESSENTIAL OIL

Description: *The seeds of mustard contain 30-35 per cent of oil. Seeds have to be crushed and macerated in warm water to release the oil through fermentation, before the process of distillation can take place. This maceration is necessary because the so-called mustard oils, or isothiocyanates, are inactive in the live plant: only when the tissue is broken and wetted, do enzymes release the oils.*

The essential oil is very fluid, with little colour, perhaps a yellow tinge. It has a very hot, strong smell which makes the eyes water (like horseradish). In

147

daylight, the oil becomes a reddish-brown, and it leaves a fatty deposit coating the inside of its container.
The principal constituents: *Allyl isothiocyanate (allylsenevol).*
Dangers: *The essential oil is not easy to obtain. It is very strong and many have reported that it can burn the skin if not used in the right proportion. The use of the oil should be avoided by those suffering from nervous or allergic conditions, as it can provoke even worse skin reactions.*

ITS USES

In illness
Used externally, the essential oil can be used for **neuralgia** and all the aches and pains of **rheumatism, sciatica** and **lumbago**. If you are confident you won't have a reaction, massage a little oil gently on the affected areas a few times a day, and relief will be felt very quickly. (The theory is that by irritating the skin, mustard oil draws blood to the surface, thereby actually relieving inflammation in deeper tissue.) You could do the same with the fresh mustard seeds crushed into a paste and applied on a poultice (see page 24). The poultice can also be used on the torso to help **chest infections** such as **coughs** and **colds**, and pulmonary problems. The lazy way is to use mustard powder.

Try to avoid letting any mustard oils near the eyes, as this can be very painful. If it happens, wash the eye out with cold water, and follow with a chamomile or rose compress.

Mustard foot baths have been traditional for centuries in both Britain and France, and a paste of mustard seeds and other ingredients is reputedly sold as winter foot warmers in the States to skiers and hikers.

(*See also* **bronchitis, pneumonia** *and* **respiratory system problems.**)

In cookery
It is the seeds which are used culinarily although the leaves are edible: the greens of the Deep South of America have been developed from an African variety of mustard. Most seeds are ground and powdered for the various types of mustard, those which are darker having retained the seed coats. Mustard may be a traditional condiment with meat because it disguises possible spoilage; the seeds are preservative, though, thus their inclusion in pickles. Mustard seeds and mustard oil are used a great deal in Indian cooking.

To make up dry English mustard, mix with cold water (hot would inactivate the enzymes), then leave for 10 minutes or so for the enzymes to release the pungency of the oils. If adding mustard to food while it is cooking, add it late and cook very gently.

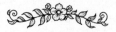

MYRRH *(Commiphora myrrha – Burseraceae)*

There are many species of *Commiphora*, spiky, knotted and stunted shrubs and bushes native to the Middle East, North Africa and North India. They grow in abundance, wild and cultivated, along the Red Sea, in Iran, Libya, Abyssinia and along the coast of Somalia. The small trifoliate leaves, which are scanty, are covered with fluff, and the oil is distilled from an oleoresin exuding from the stems and shoots of the bushes. The true myrrh or *myrrhe hérabol* is cultivated in Arab countries, and is also called *karam* or Turkey myrrh. The myrrh from Abyssinia and Somalia is called *bisabol* or *bdellium* (*C. abyssinica*). This is similar to the Indian myrrh, called Indian *bdellium*, which produces an oil of inferior quality to true myrrh.

Myrrh was well known to the ancients. It was an ingredient of incense used for religious ceremonies and fumigations by the Ancient Egyptians. Called '*punt*' or '*phun*', it was an ingredient of a famous Egyptian perfume '*kyphi*', was prescribed to counter hayfever, and was an important ingredient in embalming as well. Moses was enjoined to take myrrh with him from Egypt so that the Children of Israel could continue their worship, and myrrh was one of the three gifts to the infant Jesus from the Magi. In *The New Testament*, Nicodemus ordered 100 lb of myrrh and aloe to annoint the body of Jesus (as was the custom among Jews at that time). The Hebrews would mix myrrh in their wine and drink it to raise their state of consciousness before participating in religious ritual. The same mixture was given to criminals a few hours before execution to ease their mental suffering.

There are many mentions of myrrh's therapeutic properties in the *Old* and *New Testaments*, in the *Koran*, and in Greek and Roman texts. Herodotus, Theophrastus and Plutarch sang its praises, and Dioscorides and Pliny classified it as healing, recording many therapeutic salves.

The essence was being distilled in 1540, and Valerius Cordius and Conrad Gesner described how to prepare ointments from the resin. They classified it for external usage, as a vulnerary (wound healing). Later remedies – called in France '*l'elixir de Carus*', '*baume de Fioraventi*', '*baume du commandeur*' or '*baume du samaritain*' – were all based on myrrh. These healed cuts, burns and wounds, and were used as an expectorant for catarrhal discharge and bronchitis, and in fumigation. In 1608, Dr

149

Philippe Guybert's *Médécin Charitable* recorded that 'myrrh warms at the same time dries, cleans, strengthens, gets rid of the old cough, brings the late period to women. It is a wonderful remedy.' In his *Traite des Drogues Simples* (1699), Nicolas Lemery confirmed that myrrh was a good emmenagogue and recommended it for hastening labour and facilitating birth. He also included myrrh in a recipe for treating hernias. Cartheuser in *Matière Medicale* in 1765 confirmed the above, but also recorded myrrh's properties in treating skin ulcers and other skin diseases: mixed with sage it could fortify the gums and was a good antiseptic for rotten teeth. In Ayurvedic medicine in India, myrrh is still used for this purpose, in parallel with conventional medicine. In the 1928 *Officine de Dorvault*, a list of drugs officially dispensed over a certain period, myrrh was recorded as being used in hospitals for bed sores (a formula for 'Myrrholine' still exists).

THE ESSENTIAL OIL

Description: *There are still many unanswered questions about the origin and identity of the various species of* Commiphora, *especially botanically. The bushes exude the resin naturally from fissures in the bark, but they can also be tapped. The resin is a pale yellow, but becomes reddish as it hardens into a thick irregular mass, often with white lines. It has a strong balsamic smell in which camphor can be detected. It is acrid and bitter at the same time. Some producers add some ammonia to the resin when distilling to increase the yield: this naturally deprives the oil of all therapeutic value, and so great care must be taken to obtain the purest form. Myrrh can be bought as an oil, as a simple tincture (like benzoin), and powdered.*

The principal constituents: *Acids (acetic, formic, myrrholic, palmitic, triterpenic, etc), alcohols, aldehydes (cinnamic, cuminic, etc), sugars (arabinose, galactose, etc), phenols (eugenol, m-cresol), resins and terpenes (cadinene, dipentene, limonene, pinene, etc).*

ITS USES

In illness

As long as myrrh is pure, it is a great healer for all **skin problems, scars, skin infections** and **ulcerations**. For treating skin problems such as **acne** and **dermatitis**, and to reduce inflammations, mix 10 ml (2 tsp) soya oil with 2-4 drops myrrh and apply externally.

Used with another essential oil for flavour, like mint or cardamom, it makes a good mouthwash and is antiseptic and balsamic for all **throat and gum problems**. Add 1 drop of myrrh and 1 drop of mint or cardamom to a glass of water. Use to rinse the mouth and gargle, but do not swallow. It also makes a good antiseptic inhalation during **sinusitis**, say.

(*See also* **halitosis**.)

In beauty
A simple tincture of myrrh, like benzoin (see page 50), can be used as a **toner**, to close pores.

(*See also* **nails**.)

Other uses
Myrrh is one of the principal ingredients of incense, and it can be used at home as a 'burning perfume'. Like benzoin, it is also a good fixative, and is an ingredient of many pot-pourris and pomanders.

MYRTLE (*Myrtus communis – Myrtaceae*)

This aromatic evergreen shrub originates from Africa, and grows all around the Mediterranean. It was introduced to Britain in 1597, but generally only flourishes in the south, or under glass (it can also be grown as a pot plant). It has small, shiny, dark green leaves which contain vesicles full of essential oil. The flowers are fragrant and white, five-petalled with a spectacular spray of thin stamens. These are followed by purple-black berries. In its natural habitat, myrtle can grow to virtual tree height, up to about 4 m (14 ft).

The Ancient Egyptians knew of the therapeutic properties of myrtle, macerating the leaves in wine to counter fever and infection. Theophrastus later confirmed its place in therapy, adding that the best and most odiferous tree came from Egypt. Dioscorides also prescribed a wine in which the leaves had been macerated: this fortified the stomach and was effective for pulmonary and bladder infections, and for those who were spitting blood.

In 1876, Dr Delioux de Savignac advocated the use of myrtle for bronchial infections, for problems of the genito-urinary system, and for haemorrhoids. Despite this enthusiasm, it was only last century that the therapeutic properties of myrtle were properly investigated; in his thesis about myrtle, one M. Linarix reconfirmed all the properties listed in the old texts, and judged myrtle the best tolerated of all the balsamic plants.

Venus was ashamed of her nudity on the island of Cythere, so hid behind a myrtle bush. In gratitude, she took the plant under her protection, and it became her favourite.

In Biblical times, Jewish women wore garlands of myrtle on their heads on their wedding day as a symbol of conjugal love, and to bring them luck. It is still often carried with orange blossom as a traditional bridal flower. Women in the south of France used to drink an infusion of the leaves every day to keep their youth and beauty.

To protect one's house from the evil eye in the south of France, a myrtle tree was planted nearby. However, this was apparently only effective if the tree were planted by a woman.

THE ESSENTIAL OIL

Description: *Only the fresh leaves are used for distillation. The oil obtained is liquid, and a clear yellow to greenish-yellow. It smells camphory and peppery green, rather like bay.*

The principal constituents: *Camphene, cineol, geraniol, linalool, a compound called myrtenol and pinene. The oil also contains a lot of tannin.*

ITS USES

In illness
Because of its astringent action, due to the high tannin content, myrtle is very effective against **haemorrhoids**. Add 6 drops myrtle to 30 g (1 oz) cold cream, and mix well. Apply a few times per day, when the pain and swelling are at their worst.

(*See also* **haemorrhoids, shingles** *and* **stings and bites**.)

In beauty
Because the leaves are astringent, they were used in the sixteenth century to clean the skin. A special perfumed water called '*eau d'anges*' was prepared in France and used for its tonic and astringent action.

Myrtle is very effective in bad cases of **acne**, especially when there are painful boils with white heads. Mix 10 ml (2 tsp) grapeseed oil, 1 drop wheatgerm and 7 drops myrtle, and apply a few times per day until better. Cleanse the skin before and after applying the oil with a lotion made from 50 ml (2 fl oz) rosewater and 5 drops myrtle. This has a particularly astringent action on the greasy skin which is so often associated with bad acne.

In cookery
Meat and the small birds which are a delicacy in Mediterranean countries can be wrapped in or stuffed with myrtle leaves: these impart their flavour after the meat or bird is cooked. Myrtle branches and twigs can be burned on a fire or barbecue beneath meat. The berries are edible, and were once dried like pepper: they can be used much like juniper, although they are milder.

Other uses
Myrtle has an anti-insect effect much the same as eucalyptus, and it would be worth planting a few shrubs for this purpose if you suffer from mosquitos, for example. Not only will you be bite-free, but you will also purify the room with the fresh, clean, camphory fragrance, which will be beneficial to the respiratory system.

Myrtle flowers can be dried for use in pot-pourris; the oil-rich leaves were once used as an aromatic polish for wooden furniture; and the bark and roots (presumably because of the tannin content) were used in tanning.

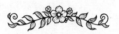

NEROLI (*Citrus aurantium bigaradia – Rutaceae*)

Neroli is an essential oil extracted from the fragrant flowers of the bitter, sour or Seville orange tree, also known as *Citrus bigaradia* or bigarade orange. In their favoured Mediterranean or sub-tropical climate, bitter oranges can grow to a height of 9 m (30 ft). (*See also* Bergamot, Orange and Petitgrain.)

Although oranges had been known since the first century, it wasn't until the late seventeenth century that neroli oil was discovered; it is thought to have been named after Anna Maria de la Tremoille, Princess of Neroli (near Rome). The oil and the therapeutic properties of the flowers were particularly valued at this time by the people of Venice, who used it against the plague and other fevers, drank it as a tisane, and rubbed a distilled water into their bodies twice a day. At one time, neroli was used as a perfume by prostitutes in Madrid (customers could recognize them by the smell), but now orange perfumes have undergone a sea change, signifying purity, and blossoms are worn in bridal headdresses.

153

The principal commercial producers of the trees and oil are Italy, France, Tunisia, Egypt and Sicily. The best oils come from Tunisia, Sicily and France, but the volume from the latter has decreased in the past few years. Worldwide the annual production does not exceed 2 tonnes; 1 tonne of flowers is needed to produce 1 kg (2 lb) of oil – thus neroli is highly expensive.

THE ESSENTIAL OIL

Description: *This is obtained by the steam distillation of the flowers of the Seville or bigarade orange. The fresh essence is yellowish but turns reddish-brown if exposed to light and air making it unsuitable for use in therapy. The smell is wonderful, very sweet and orangey, with a bitter undertone.*

A by-product of distillation is orange-flower or orange-blossom water – a solution of neroli in water – which is used in pharmaceutical preparations and in cookery.

The principal constituents: *Acetic esters, dipentene, terpineol, farnesol, geraniol, indol, jasmone, l-camphene, α- and β-pinene, nerol, and nerolidol, plus traces of benzoic acid and a few hydrocarbons.*

Dangers: *Because of its very high price, petitgrain is often added to neroli, which of course decreases the therapeutic value of neroli.*

ITS USES

In illness

The properties of neroli are sedative, antispasmodic, tranquillizing, anti-toxic, and slightly hypnotic. It has always been one of my favourite essential oils, because of its wonderful perfume, and its therapeutic properties, particularly those which treat the nervous system. Anxiety and nervous **depression** can be banished virtually instantaneously by the use of a little neroli – just 3 drops mixed into 10 ml (2 tsp) soya or almond oil. Rub this clockwise on to the solar plexus, nape of the neck and temples, breathe deeply and relax for 10 minutes. There is a great feeling of peace, and the nervous tension disappears. This calming and relaxing effect can be particularly valuable in **pregnancy**: a bowl of warm water with a few drops of neroli in it can be placed beside the bed during **labour** too. And a new baby could safely be bathed in water containing ¼ drop of the oil: mix 1 drop of oil in a capful of baby shampoo, then add just a quarter of this to the bathwater.

For **insomniacs**, the slightly hypnotic effect of the oil can induce sleep, acting as a natural tranquillizer; put a few drops of the oil into a warm bath taken just before going to bed. Or make a tisane from the dried orange blossom – known as bigaradier – and drink before sleep (this is digestive as well). Or simply have an orange tree in a pot nearby (see Petitgrain).

Neroli is also good for **bad circulation**, when the oil, as above, is massaged in every day. The blossoms, taken as a tisane, are a good natural blood cleanser. And baths containing a few drops of the oil are also effective for the symptoms of **PMT**.

(*See also* **backache, fatigue, oedema, palpitations** *and* **stress**.)

In beauty
Orange flowers were a constituent of Hungary Water, and, together with bergamot oil, neroli oil was used in the first eau de cologne in the early eighteenth century.

Neroli can be useful in **acne** conditions: mix equal quantities of neroli and another oil (juniper, lavender or clove), and add 3 drops of this to a kettleful of hand-hot water in a bowl. Cover the head with a towel and lean over the bowl so that the aromatic vapours can reach the skin.

Orange-flower water is a good toner. Marie Antoinette is said to have used it to improve her rather sallow skin.

In cookery
Bitter oranges are the ones that should be used in cookery, despite the fact that the sour flesh is virtually inedible. Sevilles are the oranges for marmalade making, and their juice and peel is that used in Sauce Bigarade, a classic French haute cuisine accompaniment to duck. Because the peel of bitter oranges is particularly aromatic, it is candied, used in syrups and dried; the latter is included in *bouquet garnis* in France for beef and veal stews, and some fish dishes. (It is always best to use the peel of bitter oranges; that of sweet oranges is often dyed and sprayed for marketing purposes.) Peel and oil from bitter oranges are used in the making of orange liqueurs such as Curaçao, Grand Marnier and Cointreau.

Neroli orange-flower water can sometimes be obtained from Greek or Greek-Cypriot shops; other orange-flower waters can be found in chemists (check they are suitable for use in cooking). Orange-blossom water is used in many North African and Middle Eastern recipes (as is rose water), and blossom jams are also known. Use the water – or make your own decoction from the flowers – to perfume cakes, creams, custards and pancake batter. It will also make them more digestible.

NIAOULI (*Melaleuca viridiflora* – *Myrtaceae*)

M. viridiflora is a variety of the tree which produced cajuput, and it grows principally in New Caledonia and Australia. Like *M. leucadendron*, it is evergreen, has a spongy bark which flakes off, linear, lanceolate leaves of an ash colour, and white flowers on a long spike. The leaves are extremely aromatic and the essential oil is distilled from the fresh leaves and twigs. The oil is often called Gomenol, because distillation once took place near the port of Gomen in New Caledonia.

Like cajuput, it does not seem to have appeared in Europe until the seventeenth century, although it was very highly valued by the locals, who used it for reducing fever and healing wounds and considered it good for diarrhoea and rheumatism.

THE ESSENTIAL OIL

Description: *This is very liquid, and is pale yellow which can become dark yellow (depending on the copper content of the soil, and which can be traced in the oil). It has a strong hot smell, very balsamic with a note of camphor. It is similar to cajuput in aroma and therapeutic properties.*

The principal constituents: *Eucalyptol (50–60 per cent) plus a few esters (butyric and isovalerianic), limonene, pinene and terpineol.*

ITS USES

In illness

Niaouli is considered a strong antiseptic, and is prescribed by phytotherapists and aromatherapists for the urinary system (cystitis and leucorrhoea), and for pulmonary trouble (bronchitis, catarrh, runny or stuffy nose). Many people can tolerate it without suffering any side effects.

I always use the oil in combination with others – especially eucalyptus, pine and myrtle – for pulmonary problems, respiratory problems, **colds** and **'flu**. An inhalation is best for the latter: fill a large bowl with hot water, add 2 drops niaouli, and 1 drop each of eucalyptus and myrtle, and inhale under a towel. Follow this with an oil rubbed on to the chest, sinus area, temple and nape of neck: mix 10 ml (2 tsp) soya oil, 5 drops niaouli, 2 drops eucalyptus and 1 drop myrtle.

For **cystitis, leucorrhoea** and irritations, niaouli is invaluable. When using the bidet, add 2 drops of niaouli and a few flakes of a natural, scent-free soap (or 15 ml [1 tbsp] sea salt). Then make an oil to rub on the stomach and lower back three to four times a day: mix 5 ml (1 tsp) soya oil and 5 drops niaouli. These two remedies can also be very helpful for women who have **inflammation and cystitis after intercourse**.

To protect against air-borne infections, make a room spray by mixing 300 ml (½ pint) warm water with 5 ml (1 tsp) niaouli in a spray bottle. This is particularly effective sprayed in public places like waiting rooms.

(*See also* **catarrh, chest infections, dental abscess, dermatitis, fever, hayfever, headaches, neuralgia, pneumonia, sinusitis, stiffness, stings and bites** *and* **throat, sore**.)

Veterinary use

In France, many vets use the essential oil on dogs: diluted with cooled boiled water it is effective on infected wounds and all skin irritations. It is also rubbed neat into rheumatic canine limbs.

I use niaouli on my two Persian cats, because they tend to have respiratory problems due to their flat noses. I brush them well, then after rubbing my hands with a little neat niaouli, I brush my hands over their fur, back, sides and front. This not only protects them from cat fleas, but helps them breathe, and builds up their immune systems.

NUTMEG and MACE (*Myristica fragrans – Myristicaceae*)

The trees which produce both nutmeg and mace are large evergreens native to the Moluccas but which are now grown elsewhere in the tropics, notably Grenada in the West Indies. The trees can reach a height of 18 – 24 m (60 – 80 ft), and are either male or female. One male per ten to twelve female trees is the norm in plantations, resulting in them being known as harem trees! The trees do not flower or fruit until about eight or nine years old (thus cannot be sexed until then) and yield about 100 fruits; by the time they are 30 years old, they can yield an average crop of 3 – 4,000 fruit a year. Trees can bear for a good 70 years.

Yellowish flowers are followed by large yellow apricot- or plum-like fruits. When they split open, these reveal the black seed (the nutmeg) wrapped in its red lacy aril (the mace). Both spices are dried separately, and the major producers are the Moluccas and Grenada, the latter exporting some 2,000 tonnes to the US each year. Nutmeg has always been more available and popular than mace, which is much more expensive; this is not surprising as mace equals one-fifth of the weight of the whole seed, and only 75 g (3 oz) mace are gained from 100 nutmegs.

It is thought that the ancients knew nutmeg and mace, but by the twelfth century, the spices had definitely reached the Mediterranean, brought by Arab traders. Not long after, the School of Salerno recorded the poisonous effect of using too much nutmeg; they praised its cardiac effects, but recorded haemorrhage and fatalities if used in large doses. '*Unica nux prodest, nocet altera, tertia necat*' (One nut is good, another is less good, the third kills).

For years, both spices were the monopoly of first the Portuguese and then the Dutch, until Pierre Poivre smuggled some young trees from the Spice Islands. When the Moluccas were part of the British Empire, trees were transplanted to the West Indies, where they thrived.

In the eighteenth century, nutmeg and mace were included in French codices and in the nineteenth century, Pulligny wrote a book of 876 pages entirely devoted to the nutmeg tree and its spices.

In folk medicine, carrying a nutmeg in the pocket is reputedly a cure for lumbago and rheumatism.

The main producers of the oils are the USA, Canada and Singapore (of nutmeg respectively 20 – 30 tonnes, 5 – 10 tonnes, and 1 – 2 tonnes per year, 1987 figures). The USA is the largest consumer of nutmeg oil (30 tonnes), followed by Britain with 10 tonnes. A little is used in the perfumery industry, which leaves one with the worrying question (see below) as to how the remainder is used – by the food industry?

THE ESSENTIAL OILS

Description: *Nutmeg oil is steam-distilled from nuts crushed to a butter; oil from the islands is re-distilled in France to improve the quality. Mace is steam-distilled from the arils. Both oils are similar, very pale yellow and very fluid. Nutmeg smells spicy, pleasant and hot, mace very strongly spicy. Both oils change as they become old, turning dark brown and smelling disagreeable, acidic and turpentine-like – do not buy or use if like this.*

The principal constituents: *Both oils contains myristicine, with small quantities of borneol, camphene, cymol, dipentene, geraniol, linalool, pinene, sapol and terpineol, and acetic, butyric, caprilic, formic and myristic acids.*

Dangers: *Myristicine is narcotic, hallucinogenic and very toxic, especially* *during pregnancy (traces are also found in black pepper, carrot, parsley, and celery seeds). So, I do not recommend that anyone other than practitioners use either mace or nutmeg oils in therapy. Neither oil must be left where children could find it, and the oils must never be used in cooking. Side effects of too much of either of the* spices alone *include severe headaches, cramps and nausea (the spices have been used as a drug for their hallucinogenic properties); ingestion of the concentrated essential oil could be fatal.*

I do not use either oil much as nutmeg, in particular, is too hot for the skin, and can cause rashes and allergies. (In Indonesia, workers guard against the irritant properties of the nuts themselves by dusting their faces with sago-palm powder.) I would much rather use the undoubted therapeutic properties of both spices in cooking, than use either essential oil in any way.

ITS USES

In illness
In the eighteenth century, in France, mace was classified as a tonic and stimulant, as a cardiac tonic, as an aid for general fatigue, and as a brain stimulant. It continues to be revered for its digestive properties, for people who cannot assimilate food, for **wind**, and for **pre-menstrual pain**. Nutmeg too is a tonic, good for the heart, for convalescents, and for general fatigue. Nutmeg has a reputation as an abortificant (it was once used to ease labour in Malaysia), so should be avoided in pregnancy.

(*See also* **backache**.)

In cookery
Both spices can be used – but in moderation – to enliven food and do you good at the same time. To allay any fears, you would have to ingest at least two whole nutmegs before any hallucinatory effects were noticed.

Mace is available in blades (the dried aril itself) or as a powder (it is impossible to grind at home). It loses its aroma very quickly, so buy a little at a time. It is used in cakes and sweet dishes, and in some sausages and curry dishes. I like to use it as an aid to slow digestion, and as a good stimulant of the nervous system, in milky rice puddings, and in the egg mix for omelettes along with some coriander leaves.

Nutmeg, too, comes ground or whole, being best ground freshly from the whole nut on special nutmeg graters, for spicing of egg dishes, sauces (a white or cheese sauce for cauliflower, for instance), and cakes. It goes particularly well with onions and spinach, and mashed potatoes benefit from a good sprinkling. Nutmeg is included also in sausages, ravioli, and many spiced Eastern dishes. A sprinkling of nutmeg on a hot drink – hot chocolate, say – can have pick-me-up properties (not what you want at night, unless you need to work late).

In Indonesia, a candy is made from the tiny amount of pulp surrounding the mace and nutmeg; in the Caribbean, this outer pulp is fermented to make a brandy-like drink.

ORANGE (*Citrus aurantium sinensis* – *Rutaceae*)

Citrus is a genus which includes many evergreen or semi-evergreen trees and shrubs, originating in eastern Asia, and which is most famous for its fruit. The forebear of all today's varieties was probably *C. aurantium*, the bitter, sour or Seville orange. The other principal oranges are the sweet orange (*C. sinensis*) and the mandarin orange (*C. reticulata*); the rest of the family includes lemons, limes, grapefruit and all their sub-species and crosses. The rue family, *Rutaceae*, is huge, and only a few members of it, including *Citrus*, are trees.

Orange trees can grow to a height of 4.5 – 10 m (13 – 33 ft), depending on the species and climate. The leaves are large and a glossy dark green, and the flowers are white. The fruit can take a year to be formed, thus there is often blossom and fruit on the tree at the same time. In the tropics, oranges are green when ripe, and the characteristic orange colour of fruit grown in sub-tropical areas is, in fact, the tree's response to a slightly cooler temperature in winter. In temperate regions, oranges have to be greenhouse cultivated although, as with the famous orangeries attached to regal palaces and châteaux in the sixteenth and seventeenth centuries, they can be grown in pots outside in the summer and taken inside in the winter. Oranges and other citrus species can also be grown as house or pot plants.

Oranges were first brought to the Mediterranean by the Arabs, probably in the first century. They did not become a permanency, though, until after the eighth century, when the Moors turned a large part of southern Spain, including Seville, into one huge orange orchard. The Romans, however, did know oranges: they recorded directions for protecting the trees from cold, and an orange-flower water or decoction was drunk to avoid hangovers and indigestion.

Oranges are thought to have reached Britain in 1290 when Eleanor of Castile bought seven from a Spanish ship. Later they became so common that girls sold them in the streets of London, one of them Nell Gwynn who was valued for rather more than her fruit-selling skills by Charles II.

It was Christopher Columbus who took oranges to the New World, collecting seeds and saplings from the Canaries and planting them in Hispaniola in 1493. Oranges are recorded as growing in Florida – a major orange-growing area now – as early as 1539. The trees now grow all over the world – in North Africa, Turkey, south of France, Italy, Spain, Israel, Egypt, South Africa, the USA (especially Florida and California), the West Indies, Brazil and Mexico.

The therapeutic values of oranges and their various oils were first mentioned by the Arabs. In France, these values do not seem to have been appreciated until about the sixteenth century, as the fruit was rare and therefore expensive. Called '*pommes d'orange*' at first, they were viewed as luxuries and given as sumptuous gifts for Christmas and the New Year. By the eighteenth century, however, oranges were recorded as remedies for epileptic fits, melancholia, heart problems, asthma, colic, seasickness, labour pains and nervous illnesses of all sorts. Nearer our own time, Dr Leclerc, Dr Maury and others considered oranges to be stomachic, antispasmodic, and digestive (good for gastritis, flatulence, dyspepsia, indigestion, and the supreme remedy for constipation); oranges also reinforced the immune system, acted as a natural blood cleanser and as a sedative of the nervous system.

THE ESSENTIAL OIL

Description: *This is extracted from the skin of the fruit by expression. The essence is pale orange and smells very orangey. It is not completely clear as it contains some wax from the outer skin.*

The principal constituents: *As much as 90 per cent limonene, with aldehydes, citral, citronellol, geraniol, linalool, methyl anthranilate, nonyl alcohol and terpinol.*

Dangers: *All citrus oils are very difficult to preserve, so store in dark bottles, cork very carefully and keep in the dark. Always buy in small quantities. Orange oil can turn dark brown quite quickly, and smell so unpleasant that it has to be thrown away.*

Many commercial oranges are sprayed with ethylene to improve the colour, and some are coated with an edible wax to retain moisture; for therapeutic use, oranges must, of course, be as natural and untampered with as possible.

ITS USES

In illness and beauty

The raw fruits contain a multitude of healthy properties. They are rich in a particular bioflavoid complex (sometimes known as vitamin P), which fortifies the capillaries and vascular system and in B vitamins and vitamin C. The latter is the most famous health constituent, but only 25 per cent of it is actually in the flesh and juice, and there is more in the peel and pith. The natural sugars of the orange are good for athletes and diabetics. Oranges also contain calcium, magnesium, phosphorus, potassium, sodium, sulphur, a little copper, iron, and zinc, and traces of bromine and manganese.

As the raw fruit is so valuable, so too is the essential oil of the fruit. I would recommend that you search for essential oil of sweet or *douce* orange, or bigarade. It has been found to have many properties: it is a tonic for the muscular and nervous systems, it is good for **eczema** and **dermatitis**, and particularly good for the skin, helping to **rejuvenate the skin** and combat wrinkles.

To banish **after-sun wrinkles**, mix together 10 ml (2 tsp) hazelnut oil, 4 ml (a scant tsp) almond oil, 2 drops good wheatgerm oil and 8 drops sweet orange essential oil. Massage gently into the skin, concentrating on the wrinkles. Use it once a day, two applications, preferably in the evening (it will help you sleep too). Every now and again, you can also use freshly squeezed orange juice. Apply this to the skin, leave to dry for a few minutes, then rinse off and apply the oil as above. If you do this often enough, your skin will regain vitality quickly.

A good way of detoxifying the system after over-indulgence (Christmas, for example), is to go on an orange-only diet – juice and raw – for 1 – 2 days. Avoid bottles, tins and cartons of juice as these lack a large proportion of the natural vitamins and minerals.

Orange oil makes a good mouthwash to heal and cure **halitosis, thrush** and gingivitis. Put 2 drops in a tumbler of boiled warm water and use to gargle a few times each day.

(*See also,* **fatigue, menopause, oedema, palpitations, pre-menstrual tension** *and* **stress**.)

In cookery

Needless to say, for both health and beauty, oranges should be eaten

162

raw or drunk as juice as often as possible (although some claim that those suffering from migraine or arthritis should avoid them). Sweet oranges are best for this, but bitter oranges (see Neroli) can be used in cooking. You can, of course, use segments of sweet oranges as garnishes for savoury dishes, or in vegetable or sweet fruit salads (when the juice, like that of lemon, can prevent acidulation of cut fruit such as apples). Oranges can be used to flavour food in many ways. The peel of sweet oranges can be candied, but that from the bitter or Sevilles is better. The vitamin C of the peel can be used as zest in many recipes – above all in the luxury Crêpes Suzette. Put some orange juice in the batter for wholemeal pancakes: this gives a wonderful flavour and makes the pancakes very much more digestible.

Other uses
Orange essential oil is used in many industries – in pharmacy to flavour pills etc; in perfumery for its lovely fragrance; in confectionery to flavour sweets; and by many major food and drink manufacturers.

OREGANO (*Origanum vulgare – Labiatae*)

This plant is a member of the marjoram family, and is known also as common or wild marjoram. The name comes from the Greek, *oros*, mountain, and *ganos*, joy, after its favourite habitat. It grows wild all over Europe, particularly in Italy and Greece (where it is known as *rigani*). The plant is similar to marjoram, but with crimson flowers, a creeping habit and stems that can rise to about 30 – 45 cm (1 – 1 ½ ft) high. The flowers bloom in July and August.

Margoram and oregano have been thoroughly confused throughout history, both botanically and culinarily, therefore it is difficult to identify which herb is being discussed in old herbals and medical treatises. Theophrastus, Aristotle, Hippocrates, Dioscorides and Pliny revered oregano as a strong antiseptic for the respiratory system, and for wounds, ulcers and burns. They believed it also helped the digestion in cookery; and Apicius, the famous Roman gourmet, gave recipes using oregano, including a seasoning of salt and oregano which is still in vogue now (particularly on pizzas).

In his treatise on common plants (1837), Dr Cazin recommended oregano oil for aches and pains due to cold and 'flu, used as a friction on the body and in a hot bath; he also described it as stimulant, stomachic, expectorant, sudorific and emmenagogic. Dr Leclerc confirmed its effectiveness in the treating of ailments of the respiratory system, and also described it as a good stimulant and stomachic for those with digestive problems due to nerves or eating too fast.

THE ESSENTIAL OIL

Description: *The flower tops are distilled to make the essential oil which is dark yellow to pale brown and smells aggressively phenolic, spicy and hot.*

The principal constituents: *The plant and oil are very similar to marjoram and to thyme (country people often call oregano 'shepherd's thyme' for this very reason), and has similar properties to other plants of the* Labiatae *family.*

Oregano is the most important antiseptic oil in aromatherapy. Its proportion of phenol – the constituent responsible for the strongest antibacterial action – is the highest of all aromatic plants. The chemical constituents of the plants, however, vary from one species to another, and depend on the provenance. The soil in which it is grown is particularly important. Oregano oils are normally high, from 80 – 90 per cent, in phenols (thymol and carvacrol); there is a little borneol, pinene and terpineol, and traces of esters.

Dangers: *Buy oregano oil very carefully, and from a reputable source, as it is often falsified, frequently being completely synthetic, without a trace of the essential oil itself. If there is any doubt at all, rely on the benefits of the fresh herb instead.*

ITS USES

In illness

Oregano oil works successfully on **eczema, psoriasis** and mycosis (parasitic fungus), for **rheumatic conditions**, and the pains of **shingles** and **neuralgia**.

It is also good for late periods. Make a massage oil with 5 ml (1 tsp) almond oil and 4 drops oregano oil, and massage clockwise gently on the stomach and lower part of the back for a few minutes. Repeat three times a day, morning, midday, and late afternoon.

For a rheumatic remedy, make up a poultice (see pages 23 – 4), using 1 cup linseed, 300 ml (10 fl oz) boiling water and 10 drops oregano oil. Clean the work surface first with a few drops of oregano oil before preparing the poultice. Apply the poultice and leave in place until cool.

Afterwards apply an oil made from 10 ml (2 tsp) almond oil, 2 drops wheatgerm oil and 8 drops oregano oil, and massage gently into the affected part. This oil would also be effective for **sciatica**, tennis elbow and **lumbago**.

(*See also* **abscesses and boils, bronchitis, colic, coughing, diarrhoea, flatulence, migraine, pneumonia** and **stings and bites**.)

In cookery

Oregano can be used as marjoram, but is much more pungent. The variety grown in Italy, and sold dried in markets, is particularly strong in flavour, and the herb is very important in Italian cooking. It is the flavouring of pizzas from Naples, but is also used with tomato, cheese, bean, vegetable, fish and meat dishes.

Marguerite Maury recommended cooking mushrooms with marjoram and oregano as all fungi contain a substance called chitin which can be very indigestible. Similarly, use both herbs when cooking cabbage, pulses and turnips, which can be equally indigestible and cause wind. A wild marjoram tea, called 'red tea', is drunk in Switzerland after a heavy meal, and to help the digestion of *fondue* (this can also prevent chills in cold weather).

Other uses

To utilize the spectacular antiseptic powers of oregano at home, add a few drops of essential oil to washing-up liquid and other soapy household products. Put a few drops on a tissue or cloth and clean surfaces in the bathroom.

PALMAROSA (*Cymbopogon martini* – *Gramineae*)

Palmarosa belongs to a family of tropical grasses rich in aromatic, volatile oils, formerly known mostly under the generic name of *Andropogon*, but now included in the genus *Cymbopogon*. Close relations are lemongrass and citronella. Palmrosa grass occurs in two varieties, *Motia* or *Palmarosa*, and *Sofia* or *Rusa*: according to *Tropical Planting and Gardening* by H F

165

Macmillan (1935), the oil of the former commanded the highest price in London at that time, about 5 – 6 shillings per pound.

Originally from Central and North India, and now cultivated in Africa and Madagascar as well, the grass is slender, bearing panicles of a blue-white colour which mature to a dark red.

THE ESSENTIAL OIL

Description: *Also known as Indian geranium or Turkish geranium oil, it is distilled from the leaves and flowers of the grass. It has been distilled since the eighteenth century, especially in Turkey, to simulate or adulterate Turkish rose oil (which is very expensive).*

The principal constituents: *Geraniol (between 75 and 95 per cent), with other alcohols like citronellol and farnesol, and esters like dipentene (but in small proportions).*

Dangers: *Palmarosa oil is not too expensive, but it is nevertheless often mixed with turpentine and cedarwood, so care needs to be taken when purchasing.*

ITS USES

In illness

The plant has long been used in India, taken internally as a remedy against infection and fever – easily understandable because of the very high proportion of geraniol, a natural antiseptic and bactericide. The oil is also stomachic.

Palmarosa can relieve the discomforts of 'flu and a high temperature. A mixture of 5 ml (1 tsp) soya oil and 5 drops palmarosa massaged into the shoulders, temple, sinus area, and behind the ears, can induce an almost instant feeling of well-being. This oil can also be gently applied to **cuts and wounds** to help the healing process.

In beauty

Palmarosa is a wonderful remedy for skin conditions like **acne** because of its natural antiseptic constituents. Mix together 5 ml (1 tsp) almond or sunflower oil, a few drops of wheatgerm oil and 3 drops of palmarosa, and massage in twice a day. This can also work wonders for old acne scars, for **wrinkles** (especially those occurring after long exposure to sun) and **broken veins**. Apply palmarosa oil neat to **boils**, using a cottonwool bud. Do this morning and night.

In cookery

The plant is used in curry and meat dishes in India and West Africa, where its properties kill bacteria and help the digestion of fatty food.

PARSLEY *(Petroselinum sativum/crispum – Umbelliferae)*

Parsley is a hardy biennial herb which is native to the eastern Mediterranean. It is thought to have originated in Sardinia, but records show that seeds were imported to Britain from Sardinia in 1548; the plant had already been introduced to northern Europe by the Romans. There are several varieties of the herb. The curly leaved or moss-curled is the one most familiar in Britain as a garnish. The plain- or flat-leaved, continental parsley has heavily divided leaves, but they are not so curly; this is the plant which can be confused with another, *Aethusa cynapium* or fool's parsley, which is poisonous. Less familiar is the Neapolitan parsley from southern Italy which has thick stalks, eaten in Italy like celery (and, in fact, its French name is *'persil aux feuilles de céléri'*). All parsleys have carrot-shaped roots which can be eaten, but the Hamburg parsley (*P. fusiformis*) has been developed for its roots rather than its leaves. The common parsleys have dark green leaves, pale yellow-green flowers in umbels, followed by fruit seeds.

The name *petroselinum* comes from the Greek for rock celery, referring to the natural habitat of the plant. Interestingly, *selinum* is thought to be the same as *selinon*, the Greek name for celery; the Romans called parsley *'apium'*, also the botanical name for celery; and French fool's parsley is called *ache des chiens*, *ache* also once a name for wild celery. Celery also belongs to the *Umbelliferae* family, and possibly there have been confusions over the years.

The Ancient Egyptians used parsley, as did the Greeks, who crowned victorious soldiers with wreaths of it. Hercules did this after killing the Nemean lion, and thereafter victors in the Nemean and Isthmian games would do the same. They believed that parsley had grown from the blood of a hero, Archemorus, and Homer tells of a victory won by charioteers whose horses had renewed vigour after eating parsley. Parsley grew on Circe's lawn in the *Odyssey*.

Pliny said that no sauce or salad should be without parsley, as did Galen, and both Pliny and Dioscorides thought of it as a diuretic and emmenagogue. Apicius sang its praises too. The Byzantines used it as a diuretic and made a strong infusion to help kidney stones. Charlemagne ordered that it be cultivated in the imperial gardens as a vegetable, and it was eaten at every meal. It also found a place in monastic gardens at this time.

More recently, in the nineteenth century research was done on the emmenagogic properties of a constituent of the oil, apiol, by Professor Galligo, and doctors de Poggeschi and Marrotte. These were later confirmed by Dr Leclerc, proving to be truly efficaceous in treating cases of menstrual problems, particularly pain.

THE ESSENTIAL OIL

Description: *The oil is extracted from the seeds, roots and leaves. The seeds contain more essential oil than the leaves and roots, but an extraction from the entire plant is the most esteemed. The oil is colourless, or a very pale yellow, and it smells more bitter than the fresh plant.*

The principal constituents: *α-terpinene, pinene, and a crystalline substance, apiol, with glucoside apiin, myristicine, an oleoresin and palmitic acid.*

Apiol was discovered by Jovet and Homelle in 1850, and in 1890, Mourgues wrote a paper about many of the other chemical and physiological constituents of parsley.

Dangers: *The physiological action of the oleoresin in parsley has not yet been fully researched, but the indications are that it acts as a distinct stimulus on the nerve centres of the brain and spine. In large quantities this can produce the opposite effect to that desired, and can be dangerous. Symptons can be sudden low blood pressure, giddiness, deafness and slowing of the pulse. Apiol and myristicine have been implicated in miscarriage (see page 28).*

ITS USES

In illness

Parsley is mostly used in aromatherapy as a carminative, tonic and diuretic. Although it was used by the ancients to salute and help men, I have found it most useful in helping *women*. Echoing the findings of researches in the nineteenth and our own centuries, I find the plant a marvellous remedy for women of all ages, not only as a tonic for the nervous system, but for all the **female menstrual cycle problems** – flatulence, water retention, pain, indigestion and all other symptoms around period time. It is the supreme remedy for all of us, and we should eat parsley every day, adding it to salads, sauces and stews although it is better raw than cooked.

Make a tisane of the leaves – a large handful boiled in a litre (1 ¾ pints) mineral water for 2 minutes, then infused for 10 minutes – and drink around the time of a period. This is good for **rheumatism**, too: drink several times daily for a few days until symptoms have disappeared. With a little honey added, this tisane can also relieve **tonsillitis**.

For **dysmenorrhoea**, make up an oil to massage into stomach and lower back: 30 ml (2 tbsp) soya oil, 5 drops parsley, 2 drops chamomile and 1 drop tarragon.

For **cystitis**, mix an oil containing 30 ml (2 tbsp) almond oil, 2 drops wheatgerm, and 15 drops parsley and massage on the tummy, sacrum area and top of the hands. Baths containing parsley oils are good too for **PMT** and cystitis, and a little fresh juice extracted from parsley leaves should be drunk by sufferers of the latter first thing in the morning.

Fresh parsley juice made from crushed leaves is famed for its ophthalmic value. For conjunctivitis, or tired, sore or irritated **eyes**, put a little juice into the affected eye(s), four times a day. It will also soothe hay fever eyes. The juice can also help reduce the pain and inflammation of wounds and stings, and speed their healing.

Eating parsley is said to incease the flow of breast milk, and to sweeten the breath after eating garlic.

In beauty
Parsley is very helpful for **broken capillaries**. Boil three sprigs of fresh parsley in 600 ml (1 pint) water for 2 minutes, then leave to steep for 5 minutes. Add a drop each of rose and calendula oils, and leave to cool. Drip on to a piece of gauze or cotton wool, apply to the face, and relax for a few minutes.

An oil containing parsley oil is helpful, too, strengthening and draining broken capillaries or bruises. Mix together 10 ml (2 tsp) soya oil, 5 ml (1 tsp) wheatgerm and 1 drop each of parsley and chamomile. Massage very gently into the affected areas.

(*See also* **psoriasis** *and* **varicose veins**.)

In cookery
Parsley is the omnipresent garnish on many restaurant dishes, and all too often it is left at the side of the plate. It would probably do more good for us than the main ingredient of the meal, as 25 g (1 oz) parsley contains more iron, for instance, than 100 g (4 oz) liver. Parsley is a rich source of vitamins A, B and C; it also contains calcium, potassium and some copper. So, use and eat parsley in salads, sauces, stuffings, marinades, in herb butters, in vegetable dishes, *court bouillons* and stocks. It is an essential ingredient of a *bouquet garni* and the chopped *fines herbes* in an omelette. It helps digestion of meats, fish, eggs and vegetables.

169

Other uses

The roots of parsley were once candied, like those of fennel, to store for winter medicinal use. The leaves and stems can be used for a greenish-yellow dye. The oil from the seeds is used as a flavouring for a variety of products, from ice cream to seasonings.

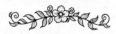

PATCHOULI (*Pogostemon cablin – Labiatae*)

Patchouli essential oil is obtained from the leaves and young shoots of an herbaceous shrub native to Malaysia, where it is called *cablan*. It is now cultivated in many places including the Seychelles, India (where it is known as *patcha* or *patchapat*), Indonesia and China. It grows to about 90 cm (3 ft) in height, and when rubbed the fresh leaves yield the characteristic earthy and woody smell of patchouli. The shrub bears flowers in terminal spikes; these are white with a tinge of mauve. The shrub is cropped two to three times a year, the leaves and shoots being dried before distillation. This is often done near the plantation as the packing of the leaves in bales for exportation can damage them. The plants weaken the soil so it has to be rotated with other crops from time to time. Replanting is apparently necessary every three to four years. Seed is rarely produced, so propagation is by cuttings.

The worldwide annual production of the oil is in the region of 500 – 550 tonnes. Sumatra produces about 450 tonnes of this; the shrub grows on the hills of Sidikolang and on the nearby island of Nias. Most of the world oil is processed through Singapore, Malaysia now exporting the essence rather than producing it. China is the second largest producer of the oil, averaging about 50 – 80 tonnes annually. This crop is more consistent than that from Indonesia, yet the oil itself is considered inferior in quality and so is very much cheaper. As the Indonesian prices and crops fluctuate, so the largest importers, the USA particularly, have had to turn to China where the production has grown in volume. India produces smaller quantities which are kept principally for local use.

The principal markets for the oil are the EEC and Switzerland (220 – 240 tonnes per year), the USA (210 – 220 tonnes, although this has increased recently), India (50 tonnes) and Japan (30 tonnes).

Patchouli has always played a large part in traditional Malay, Chinese and Japanese medicine, being attributed with stimulant, stomachic and antiseptic properties. It was *the* remedy against venomous snake and insect bites. Nowadays it is still used in its homelands as an antiseptic and insecticide. Arab doctors considered it effective against fevers, epidemics and many other illnesses.

THE ESSENTIAL OIL

Description: *After drying in the sun, the young leaves and shoots are steam distilled. The oil is liquid and transparent and is a yellow-brown or greenish-brown, depending on its provenance. Sometimes the oil can be very thick with a persistent smell, earthy and penetrating.*

Patchouli is distilled in its country of origin, often in primitive metal containers which oxidize when in contact with the oil, turning it dark brown as iron is leached into it. No research has yet been done on whether this affects the oil's curative properties. The perfume industry finds the colour of the unrefined oil undesirable, so they redistil it using a delicate process to remove the iron content. It is also not known what effects this 'refining' process has on the curative properties of the essential oil. It is hoped that in the future more of the original distillers will be able to afford the expensive stainless steel containers that do not react when in contact with the oil, so that the oil does not have to be distilled twice.

The principal constituents: *Patchoulol (from 25 – 50 per cent) and sesquiterpenes (d-gauiene, norpatchoulenol, patchoulene), with traces of benzoic and cinnamic aldehydes, cadinene, carvone, caryophyllene, coerulein, eugenol, humulene and seychellene. There is up to 35 – 40 per cent patchouli camphor in the dried leaves.*

Dangers: *Patchouli can be adulterated with cubeb and cedar oils. A synthetic patchouli has been produced, but this has not enjoyed much market success; it is now generally agreed that it is impossible to replicate patchouli exactly in an olfactory sense.*

ITS USES

In illness and beauty

The antiseptic properties of patchouli were studied in 1922 by Gatti and Cayola, by Sarbach in 1962, and by many other well-known scientists. It is recommended for many skin conditions: allergies, herpes, **impetigo**, bed sores, **burns, cracked skin, haemorrhoids,** acne, seborrhoea and **eczema**. It acts as a bactericide and can help **rejuvenate the skin**.

For bad **acne**, mix together 10 ml (2 tsp) grapeseed oil, 1 drop wheatgerm oil and 5 drops patchouli oil. Rub gently all over a clean face morning and night, and leave. Continue the usage for six months when, if it has not been successful, an alternative oil, like basil, should be used instead.

Apply patchouli oil neat on whiteheads and **abscesses**.

For seborrhoea, mix together 5 ml (1 tsp) each of soya and grapeseed oils, and 15 drops patchouli oil. Massage into the scalp for a few minutes, cover with a warm towel, and leave for at least an hour. Shampoo off with a mild shampoo. Use this twice a week.

(*See also* **bed sores, dandruff** *and* **hair problems**.)

Other uses

Patchouli has a great part to play in perfumery as it acts as a natural fixative, reinforcing the woody note of perfume and giving it even greater intensity. The dried leaves can be bought and used (sparingly) in pot-pourris; patchouli is also available as powder and shavings for this purpose. Use the powdered leaves in little sachets to perfume clothes and linen; this is traditional in India and China. Indian inks were once distinguished by their scent because they contained some patchouli; this helped fix the colour and make the ink dry quickly. To fix ink add 5 drops patchouli to a bottle of brown or violet ink. My newsagent says he always knows when I've paid my newspaper cheque as the till smells so wonderful.

PEPPER (*Piper nigrum – Piperaceae*)

The white or black peppercorns mainly used as a seasoning condiment are the fruit of a creeping perennial vine indigenous to the moist low-lying forests of monsoon Asia, from the Malabar Coast of India to the islands of the East Indies (it is also found in the West Indies). If uncultivated, the vine can grown to more than 6 m (20 ft) in height, but in cultivation for commercial reasons, it is limited to about 3 – 4 m (10 – 12 ft). It is encouraged up stakes or supports or, most economically, up shade trees such as mango or kapok. The vine has thick, dark green leaves and small white flowers which are followed by spikes or strings bearing the peppercorns. Vines can only start fruiting after 2 – 3 years, and can bear until about 15 – 20 years old. A full-grown vine can produce about 1.5 – 2.25 kg (3 – 5 lb) peppercorns annually.

Black, white and green peppercorns are the product of the same plant. The fruit are green when immature, ripening to an orange-red. For both black and green peppercorns, they are plucked green or immature; if they are dried in the sun, they become the familiar black spice; if they are canned or preserved in brine or oil they are what is known as green peppercorns. White peppercorns come from the mature berry: this is picked when red, fermented and soaked in water, and then the skin and fleshy parts are rubbed off. The inner part of the berry is then dried and it becomes the white-grey spice.

Pepper, both white and black, has long been used in cooking and medicine. It was mentioned in old Sanskrit and Chinese texts in the tenth century BC, and Theophrastus sang its culinary and medicinal praises in the fourth century BC. Pliny recorded that pepper was more expensive than gold, an attribute that was to cling to the berries for many centuries. In the Middle Ages, there was a French saying about items being 'as dear as pepper', and kings and princes would receive tribute in peppercorns (Attila the Hun was 'paid off' in cinnamon and peppercorns by a besieged Rome). There was an enormous trade in the spice – the fortunes of Venice and Genoa being made in pepper – and its value in Britain is still remembered in Pepper Street (in Southwark in London), and in the peppercorn rents paid by tenants to landlords.

Pepper was one of the spices which inspired the great voyages of exploration, and the trade was dominated in turn by the Arabs, Venetians, Portuguese, Dutch and the British.

Peppercorns seem first to have been distilled for oil in the fifteenth century, mentioned by Saladin in his *Compendium Aromatorium* in 1488. In the sixteenth century Valerius Cordius and J B Porta gave precise instructions on ways of distillation together with other spices such as cinnamon and clove.

THE ESSENTIAL OIL

Description: *The oil is steam distilled from the crushed berries (black or white), is greenish-yellow with a characteristic smell of phellandrene, a soft, spicy, hot, aromatic and piquant odour. Unlike over 80 per cent of essential oils, it is not dissolved by alcohol.*

The principal constituents: *Mainly terpenes (phellandrene, pinene and limonene in small quantity). A major constituent is the stimulant alkaloid piperine which is identical in composition to morphia. (A substance called piperonal or synthetic heliotrope derived from piperine is used in the preparation of perfumes.) It also contains starch and cellulose.*

Dangers: *The undiluted oil can be toxic and irritate the skin. Always dilute as recommended in the remedies.*

ITS USES

In illness

Pepper and its oil have long been associated with the treatment of **sciatica** and nervous conditions. It is classified as a stimulant of the digestive system – the piperine content stimulates the flow of saliva and gastric juices, thereby **aiding digestion**.

It is one of the most complete essential oils and should, I believe, be more thoroughly researched. Interesting results have been obtained when it is used, especially with **dermatitis**, aches and pains due to '**flu**, with **rheumatic conditions**, and it is truly a remarkable remedy for sciatica. For all of these, make a massage oil by adding 4 drops pepper to 20 ml (4 tsp) grapeseed oil. I have had a good response in the cicatrization of wounds: add 2 drops pepper and 2 drops wheatgerm oil to 5 ml (1 tsp) soya oil and rub gently on the wound.

I have also explored its uses in inhalations in conjunction with other plant oils. For example, I have combined it with eucalyptus to treat **catarrh**, **colds** and even **hayfever**. When I'm running out of tea tree oil, pepper is a good replacement in a gargle for a **sore throat**: use 1 drop in a tumbler of water.

(*See also* **backache, chest infections, headaches** *and* **neuralgia**.)

In cookery
Pepper is one of the seasoning spices which is constantly in use in the kitchen, in fact, has a permanent place on most tables. It should always be bought whole and freshly ground in a mill, as it quickly loses its aroma when ground (and bought ground pepper may have been adulterated). Pepper should always be added to food at the last moment for the same reason. White pepper is a little less aromatic than black (although there is debate about this), and seems mainly to be valued for its non-speckling effect in white sauces.

Peppercorns can be used in savoury stocks, marinades and *court-bouil-lons*. They can also be coarsely ground and used to coat steaks. Many people like pepper in sweet dishes – and coarsely ground black pepper is reputed to have an affinity with fresh strawberries.

Other uses
It is said that Buddhist monks in the Himalayas take peppercorns with them on a long journey; they suck them from time to time to give them strength and to alleviate the pangs of hunger.

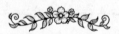

PETITGRAIN (*Citrus aurantium bigaradia* – *Rutaceae*)

Petitgrain is yet another essential oil obtained from orange trees. It is distilled from the leaves, and from the twigs and tiny green unripe fruit. Grasse in the south of France was once well-known for the large quantities of high-quality oil coming from its distilleries. The oil was particularly rich in olfactives, and was used for high-quality perfumes and cosmetics of all sorts. The Grasse industry has since diminished, and the main producer now – of an inferior and cheaper essence – is Paraguay. About 190 tonnes are exported every year, most of which goes to the food industry as flavouring for drinks, the majority of the rest into perfumery and cosmetics. Very little is destined for aromatherapy. The oil is also produced in southern Italy (that from Calabria is good), Egypt, Tunisia and other northern African countries.

(*See also* **bergamot, neroli** *and* **orange**.)

THE ESSENTIAL OIL

Description: *The pure essence smells sharp and green, with a hint of the richness of orange. For use in perfumes, the essential oil is often stripped of its terpenes and mixed with fresh orange flowers, when it acquires a very much subtler fragrance, and can then replace the very expensive neroli, as it is richer in linalyl acetate and linalool.*

The prinicpal constituents: *Genaniol and geranyl acetate, limonene, linalool, linalyl acetate, and sesquiterpene.*

Danger: *All citrus oils are very difficult to preserve, so store in dark bottles, cork very carefully, and keep in the dark. Only buy when they are fresh.*

ITS USES

In illness

The properties of petitgrain are very similar to those of neroli. It is a sedative, relaxant, tranquillizer and a cardiac tonic. Petitgrain can be used to calm anxieties, to prevent **insomnia**, and to help patients come off tranquillizers. I use it as a bath essence, as a massage oil and as a tisane.

For a tisane, simply infuse some orange leaves in boiling water for 7 minutes, then sweeten with honey (preferably orange-blossom). This is very relaxing and, diluted, can also help young children who have stomach pains or colic, or who can't sleep.

To relax after a hectic day or a long journey, lie in a warm bath containing 10 drops petitgrain, then follow that with a tisane as above.

For a massage oil to relieve **fatigue**, mix together 10 ml (2 tsp) soya oil and 10 drops best-quality petitgrain. Massage into the lower spine, nape of the neck, solar plexus, chest, stomach, hands and feet. This can be used for young children as well, but halve the proportion of petitgrain.

An even simpler solution for fatigue, tension or nervousness, is to buy a little orange tree in a pot. You get flowers and fruit, it is good to look at, and if you have it in the room near you, its perfume can act as a sedative. I once fell asleep in a grove of orange trees in blossom, and awoke amazingly refreshed.

(*See also* **backache** *and* **stress**.)

In beauty
A drop of petitgrain added to a facial sauna is good for skin problems like **acne**; it could be used in a facial oil as well. Neat, it can be applied straight on to pimples or pustules on a cottonwool bud. It is also good for **oedema** and general puffiness brought on by PMT or digestive problems.

PIMENTO (*Pimenta officinalis/dioica* – *Myrtaceae*)

The berry known variously as pimento, allspice, myrtle pepper or Jamaica pepper is the fruit of a small evergreen tropical tree which grows to a maximum height of 12 m (40 ft). It belongs to the myrtle family, therefore is related to the eucalyptus, clove, niaouli and cajuput trees, and, most closely, to *Pimenta acris*, the bay tree. It is indigenous to the West Indian islands and South America, and grows most extensively in Jamaica (thus one of its commonest names). There it grows in forests on limestone hills near the coast.

Together with red pepper and vanilla, the berry is one of the three spices which originated in the New World. It was discovered by Spanish explorers in Mexico: as one commentator noted, the Spanish were not botanists and called everything *pimienta* or pepper. It was reputedly in use in London by 1601. It has been used over the years in both medicine and cooking, primarily the latter.

THE ESSENTIAL OIL

Description: *The tree, which can go on bearing fruit until about 100 years old, first fruits when 3 years old, after a mass of flowers in June, July and August. The valuable elements of the fruit are found primarily in the outer rind of the berries, and the whole berry is ground for the oil. The berry must be picked unripe: of allowed to mature, the properties and aroma would be* *lessened. Small branches of berries are dried in the sun for some days, then the berries are removed for distillation.*

Pimento oil is a volatile, very light oil, at first yellow and gradually becoming darker (its specific colour is due to substances as yet unknown). The smell of the trees and berries is reminiscent of clove, juniper and cinnamon with a dash of black pepper. The oil is very similar.

The principal constituents: *Eugenol (from 60 – 75 per cent, even 80 per cent), phenol, and a sesquiterpene. A certain amount of resin is also present.*

Dangers: *The eugenol content means that the oil can corrode metal, so do respect dosages. Do not use the oil if your skin is at all sensitive, and avoid very dark brown oil. Also, the oil is often adulterated, so do beware. Another essential oil can be obtained from the leaves of the same tree, known as pimento leaf oil.*

ITS USES

In illness

Its prime uses in aromatherapy are for **flatulence** and **rheumatism**. For the former, use crushed berries in flatulence-causing foods.

For rheumatic conditions, add 10 drops of the essential oil to 15 ml (1 tbsp) grapeseed oil and rub gently into the affected area. For this same condition add 5 drops of pimento to a warm to hot bath.

(*See also* **alopecia** *and* **arthritis**).

In cookery

The whole berry is more pungent than ready-ground. Use the berries whole, or grind them yourself in a mill. The name 'allspice' (*toutes épices* in French) is a description of the flavour and smell, which is a combination of cinnamon, nutmeg and cloves.

In South America, allspice was once used as a flavouring for chocolate. It was used by settlers in the New World in pumpkin pies, and Jamaica and other islands of the Caribbean still use it in sweet potato dishes, soups, stews and curries. It is good in pâtés, meatloaves, long-cooking stews, vegetable dishes, marinades for meat and, in Scandinavia, in the marinade for raw herring. It can flavour North African *pilaus*, and is used in European cooking in sweet biscuits and cakes.

Other uses

Allspice, whole or ground, is found in pot-pourris, herb pillows and pomanders.

PINE *(Pinus sylvestris – Coniferae)*

Pine belongs to a genus of more than 100 species of evergreen, coniferous trees. The Scots pine or *Pinus sylvestris* is the most widespread, being native to western and northern Europe and Russia. It grows in North America as well. It is said to be the sole north European pine to have survived the Ice Ages – it can be exposed to temperatures as low as – 40°C (– 40°F). It was once very common in Scotland, but early man was responsible for the destruction of many trees; later the tall straight trunks were the favourite source of masts for sailing ships, as the trees can grow to 36 m (120 ft) in height. The needles are short and spiky, there are both male and female flowers, and cones form and mature in about two years.

Pine kernel or nut husks have been found beside Roman dwellings excavated in Britain, and it seems they were used then for food as well as medicine. Hippocrates recommended pine for pulmonary problems and throat infections. In his *Natural History*, Pliny described the therapeutic properties of pine in great detail, stressing its use in all problems of the respiratory system.

More recently, Dr Leclerc agreed about its efficacy for the respiratory system, but added that it should be used as soon as the first signs of infection appear, in cases of 'flu, bronchitis, pneumonia and asthma; he also considered it effective for all illnesses of the urinary system such as cystitis, and for leucorrhoea. Marguerite Maury considered it good for rheumatic conditions such as gout, and an effective diuretic as well as a treatment for pulmonary infections.

THE ESSENTIAL OIL

Description: *Oil can be obtained from many pines, but for therapeutic value, the best is that distilled from the needles of* P. sylvestris. *Sometimes the distillation involves the cones and young twigs and branches as well. The oil from Siberia and Finland is the most appreciated.*

The oil itself is colourless or a very pale yellow, and has a very strong aroma, a little camphory and quite balsamic.

The principal constituents: *Bornyl acetate, approximately 30 – 40 per cent, which is what differentiates it from turpentine; others are the terpenes cadinene, dipentene and phellandrene, pinene and sylvestrene.*

Dangers: *It can often be adulterated or falsified with turpentine, so beware when buying, or use an infusion of pine needles (see below).*

ITS USES

In illness

Pine is very efficient for pulmonary problems and as a sudorific. Thus it is particularly good for treating **'flu** and other virus infections.

When the first signs of a virus infection appear, mix together 50 ml (2 fl oz) soya and 5 drops of wheatgerm with 10 drops pine, 5 drops eucalyptus and 4 drops each of niaouli and myrtle. Rub vigorously on the chest and back until you have a real heat going, then wear something very warm to keep that heat in as long as possible.

You could also make a poultice of crushed linseed (see pages 23 – 4) for back and chest, adding the oils as above, but omitting the soya and wheatgerm. Apply very hot, cover with a towel to keep the heat in, and leave for 10 minutes. Then rub in the oil above on chest and back and keep warm as instructed.

I always advise an infusion of pine needles for infections as well. Infuse a pinch each of pine needles and eucalyptus in 600 ml (1 pint) boiling water for 7 minutes. Drink strained and hot, adding honey to taste.

This infusion is also very good for **cystitis** and other urinary problems, but double the quantity of pine needles. About 5 drops pine oil in the bath also helps, as does a massage on the lower part of the spine and tummy. Mix together 20 ml (4 tsp) soya oil, 2 drops wheatgerm, 12 drops Siberian pine and 5 drops cypress. Other oils which work well with pine for cystitis are eucalyptus and niaouli.

(See also **arthritis, backache, bronchitis, catarrh, chest infections, colds, colic, coughing, frostbite, lumbago, muscular pains, pneumonia, pre-menstrual tension** *and* **stiffness.***)*

Other uses

The pine nut or kernel which is eaten comes from the *P. pinea*. Pine cones can be used for yellowish dyes, or as aromatic fire kindling (the dried needles are good too). Pine needle pillows can be made to help breathing problems such as catarrh. The oil is used in many soaps, bath preparations, disinfectants and detergents.

I have heard from a Swiss friend that mattresses filled with pine needles are used for rheumatic conditions in certain parts of the Swiss Alps.

ROSE *(Rosa* spp. *– Rosaceae)*

The rose is a native of the Orient, but is now cultivated more or less all over the world, mainly in temperate climates. There are 250 different, distinct species, including wild roses, but many thousands more hybrids and varieties. There are around 30 roses which are described as 'odorata', but only three of them – and these are old roses, the 'parents' of many others – are cultivated on a large scale for their exquisite perfume. The first of these is the *R. gallica*, which is the most prolific. It originated in the Caucasus and is often called 'French rose', 'Provins rose' or 'Rose of Anatolia'. The second old rose is *R. centifolia*, which originated in Persia and is often known as 'Provence rose' or 'Rose of Ispahan': itself descended from *R. gallica*, it is parent to moss and cabbage roses. The third old rose is *R. damascena*, the damask rose, which originated in Syria, is very highly perfumed, and is the most cultivated for its perfumed oils (it is also the most valued therapeutically).

The Romans made lavish use of roses: they scattered them from ceilings during banquets; they adorned the statues of their favourite gods with roses and they wore roses to protect them from drunkenness. The gardens of Tarquin the Superb were known for their many varieties of roses, and the gardener was venerated throughout the whole city. Virgil related that Aphrodite asked for Hector's body to be embalmed with an ointment of rose essence.

The Greeks, too, venerated the rose, Homer eulogizing it in the *Iliad* and *Odyssey*, and Sappho dubbing it the queen of flowers. The Ancient Egyptians used roses in religious ceremonies, and roses have been found next to mummies in tombs.

Roses have been prized throughout history, and all over the world, for the sweetness and the soothing nature of their scent, and for the colour and shape of their blooms. They were introduced to Europe early on, and in the Middle Ages old roses were grown in monastery gardens for their medicinal properties. Until the end of the eighteenth century, the old rose varieties reigned supreme, but in 1816 the first hybrid perpetual – the 'Rose du roi' – appeared, to be followed by the numerous varieties now available.

Since prior to the French Revolution, the French have been distilling roses, mainly for their world-famous rosewater, of which the oil was a by-product.

In 1987, it was estimated that the worldwide production of rose essential oil was in the region of 15–20 tonnes. Bulgaria was the largest producer, and America the principal importer. Other countries producing rose essential oil are Turkey, France, Morocco, India and China. Bulgaria grows *R. damascena*, and steam distils to an *otto* or *attar* of roses; France distils *R. centifolia* by volatile solvents to produce a rose absolute (see page 12).

THE ESSENTIAL OIL

Description: *Not surprisingly, it is the petals which contain the most oils, although the stamens have been found to contain some as well, and these are distilled with the petals. The steam-distilled oil is a pale yellow-green, oily with a very strong, aromatic perfume. At a low temperature, shiny, long crystals of stearoptene form in a thin layer on top of the oil.*

The principal constituents: *Eugenol, farnesol and other acids, geraniol (or citronellol), linalool, nerol, nonylic aldehyde, rhodinol and stearoptene.*

Dangers: *About 5 tonnes of roses are needed to obtain 1 kg (2¼ lb) of essential oil, which is why the cost of the oil is so high, and why it is so often falsified and adulterated. Geranium,* bois de rose, *palmarosa and, more recently, gaiac, are used to adulterate rose. As geraniol is one of the principal constituents of rose oil, the essential oil is often adulterated with geraniol and citronellol. For use in therapy great care must always be taken to obtain the* purest *rose oil.*

ROSES CULTIVATED FOR ESSENTIAL OILS

Rosa Damascena

In 1888, the damask rose was cultivated at Miltitz near Leipzig. It has been cultivated in Anatolia in Turkey since 1894, and today there are many distilleries throughout the country which can be visited. Extraction of the essence with solvents started in Bulgaria in 1904, and this method has since become widespread. There is much cultivation of the damask rose in the Balkans at an altitude of 300 – 800 m (990 – 2640 ft), and many experts claim that these 'high-flying' roses give a better oil than those grown on the plains. In Russia, cultivation started in 1931, especially in the Crimea and Transcaucasus. A variety called 'Novinka' has been developed which can resist the extremely low temperatures. In Morocco, 4 – 5,000 tonnes of damask rose petals are distilled druing the short season of four to six weeks. With their modern methods of distillation, they can distil 150 tonnes per day. One part is steam distilled for the rose essential oil; the remainder is extracted by solvents.

Other roses

- When the '*rose de mai*' – a hybrid of *R. gallica* or *R. centifolia*, introduced in 1895 – is not in sufficient quantity in the south of France, 'Brenner', a very fragrant cherry-coloured rose is used.

- 'Druschky' has been introduced to Africa.
- 'Teplitz' is cultivated in India.
- *R. abyssinica* is grown in abundance in Ethiopia.
- *R. sancta* is cultivated in Eritrea.
- *R. indica* has been cultivated in China for centuries. It was discovered in the wild near Ichong in Central China, and has now spread through India and Arabia.
- *R. bourbonica*, a rose hybrid of *R. gallica* and *R. chinensis*, is characterized by the abundance of its flowers. It was introduced in 1886, and is second only to *R. damascena* in its importance in oil distillation. It is cultivated mostly in Uttar Pradesh, Kanauy, and Konpur in India.
- *R. rugosa* grows in abundance in China, Korea and Japan. In Japan it is cultivated on the coast of Hokkaido and in the north of Hunshu where the flowers are also processed. In Russia many rose varieties in the *R. gallica* and *R. rugosa* groups are being studied for their fragrance.

ITS USES

In illness

The rose has many therapeutic properties, as has the oil so long as it is grade A, Turkish or Bulgarian. Dr Leclerc valued it as a gentle laxative, and many conditions – **loss of appetite**, as in young **anorexic** girls, problems of **PMT** and **menopause** – can be treated by rose petal tisanes. The same conditions can also be treated by a body massage oil made from 50 ml (2 fl oz) almond oil and 10 drops rose oil: rub on the tummy, solar plexus, back of the neck and temples twice a day.

I have also found rose valuable for infections of the **respiratory system** – coughs, hayfever, sinus congestion, etc. Infuse 30 ml (2 tbsp) rose petals in 600 ml (1 pint) boiling water for 10 minutes, and use to gargle. This is astringent, antiseptic and healing, and if you add a drop of oil and infuse for 5 minutes, it can help to cure mouth **thrush** and ulcers (gargle twice a day until better, and then once a day for four days until symptoms have completely disappeared). The same infusion can also be used, once cooled, as an eye wash, as a vaginal douche, a compress for **skin ulcers**, and as a gargle for a **sore throat**.

Rose infusions are actually very effective for all sorts of **eye and eyelid complaints** – general inflammation, swollen eyes, eyes which are irritated or which have a discharge due to hayfever or similar. Simply applying fresh cool rose petals can help tired eyes.

Rose essential oil is good for people with a very **nervous disposition**. It seems to work on the nervous system, calming the patient, and is better received by women than men. Massage an oil into the solar plexus; apply a dilute oil after a bath; and drink rose petal infusions. Rose also helps **insomnia**.

Marguerite Maury prescribed rose for **frigidity**, ascribing aphrodisiac properties to it. Mme Maury also considered rose a great tonic for women who were suffering from **depression**.

(*See also* **circulatory problems, coughing, cuts and wounds, dental abscess, fever, mouth ulcers, oedema, palpitations, shingles** *and* **throat, sore**.)

In beauty

Rose was used in the first perfume, Hungary water, and the oil is still one of the most important in perfumery, being a constituent of some of the most expensive perfumes together with other floral fragrances. Rose essential oil was also a constituent of the earliest cold cream, a recipe recorded by the Greek physician, Galen, in the second century.

Unadulterated rose oil is a remarkable ally in the fight against **wrinkles, puffiness, broken capillaries**, even some nervous **eczemas**. Mix together 10 ml (2 tsp) almond oil and 2 drops Bulgarian or Turkish rose oil. Keep in a dark bottle. This is a wonderful oil for a maturing skin, benefitting the hands too. Tone face and neck with rose water, either bought or a home-made infusion: make up the gargle as above, then cool and use two to three times a day.

(*See also* **psoriasis**.)

Rose vinegar toner

If you omit the water, the rose-imbued vinegar can be used as a very effective gargle for sore mouths and throats. (It is also good in salad dressings!)

80 g (3 oz) pink or red fragrant rose petals
75 ml (3 fl oz) white wine vinegar
500 ml (18 fl oz) distilled water

Mix petals and vinegar together, and leave for a week, shaking it from time to time. Strain, and mix with the water.

Breast toner
Massaging the oil in the breasts after childbirth, encourages them to regain their firmness.

10 ml (2 tsp) almond oil
2 drops lemon oil
4 drops rose oil

Mix together and store in a dark bottle.

In cookery
Old-fashioned housewives would only grow scented roses like the damask or Provence in their gardens so that they could be used for making rosewater for flavouring cakes. Another common usage of petals was to put them into a cherry pie before putting on the crust. Rosewater is big business in France, but it is in Middle Eastern cuisine that the culinary use of rosewater predominates. Rose petal jam and honey come from the Balkans, and the Turkish *locoum* is flavoured with rose, as is a candy in India. In the West, rose petals are crystallized. Try making rose vinegar (page 183) to use in salads, or scatter fresh rose petals in those same salads as did the Elizabethans. Wrap butter in petals to flavour it and use petals in the syrup for crème caramel and similar dishes. Rose oil is used commercially as an additive in fruit drinks and added to jam and yoghurt recipies to give more flavour.

The Greeks steeped rose petals in wine, and a rose brandy can be made. The Chinese, Turks and Bulgarians make very sweet liqueurs from roses, and Crème de Roses is a French version.

Some roses also give rose-hips, of course, which were the source of vitamin C-rich syrup and jelly during the war years. Rose oil also contains vitamin C.

Other uses
Rose petals can be dried to use in pot-pourri or in little moth bags, and they were one of Tusser's strewing herbs. Petals or oil can be used in rinsing water for sheets, or placed among the linen. Rose oil is used to flavour some tobaccos.

To safeguard your garden roses from the ravages of greenfly, plant garlic among them. And never plant roses and carnations together; the soothing qualities of the former will clash with the activating qualities of the latter, creating an aggressive atmosphere.

LEGENDS ABOUT ROSES

Some say that the rose was created from a drop of sweat falling from the brow of Mohammed. Others say that it was due to Bacchus. He fell in love with a beautiful nymph at a banquet, and pursued her through the garden to woo her. She caught and tore her dress on a thorny bush, revealing even more of her beauty. Bacchus, in appreciation, let the bush be covered with red perfumed flowers, as beautiful as the cheeks of his timid nymph.

Cupid is said to have given the god of silence a rose to bribe him not to reveal the amours of Venus. The rose thereafter became the emblem of silence and thus the central ornamentation in the ceiling is known as the rose. This comes from the old custom of hanging a rose over the dinner table to ensure that whatever was said at the table was to be held in the strictest confidence (the meaning of the phrase, *sub rosa*, under the rose).

Rose oil, too, has a romantic origin. Dr R M Gattefossé relates the story recorded during the time of the Great Moguls, starting with the reign of Babour in 932. For her marriage, the Princess Nour-Djiban decided to surround the gardens with a canal containing rosewater. The bridal pair rowed on this delicately scented water in the sunshine, and notice an oily, greenish substance floating on the surface. This was highly aromatic – a rose oil produced by the heat of the sun bringing together the rose water's aromatic molecules. Thereafter, the production of rose oil began in earnest, in Persia, India, then Turkey and the rest of Europe.

SOLVENT DISTILLATION OF ROSES

In Grasse in the south of France a typical plantation of *R. centifolia* consists of about 1,000 rose bushes per acre, planted 90 cm (3 ft) apart in rows of the same distance. A rose plantation lasts about ten years, and each season will produce 2,000 kg (4,400 lb) of flowers from which only 400 g (14 oz) of rose essential oil can be obtained by steam distillation. Extraction by solvents, however, would produce 2.5 kg (5 ½ lb) of absolute of rose from the same quantity of flowers.

The blossoming time is in early May, when the plants are aflame with colour and the air is heady with fragrance. At the appropriate time, sometimes the middle of the night, the workers pick all the flowers into big baskets which are then taken to the distillery at the heart of the plantation. They work quickly as the flowers lose moisture, needing to be sprayed occasionally with water. Because of this necessity for speed, there are many more pickers than there are workers in the distillery.

Very strict safety regulations are observed in the distillery because of the danger of the solvents which are very volatile and inflammable. There is no electrical apparatus in the main areas: telephones are locked in special boxes; only rubber shoes are worn; and nylon is disallowed because of the static electricity. The floors, doors, walls and the large ventilating windows are all specially insulated, and would have been built under the regulations specified by the French Ministry of Health.

The distillation cylinders – like enormous pressure cookers – dominate the interior of the distillery, with yards of piping twisting and turning at all angles and in all directions. The whole place smells of roses, with just a note of synthetic: one can get high on it, the nose is so completely saturated with the perfume.

The workers bring in the heavy baskets – of 25 kg (55 lb) each – and spread the flowers on five trays layered inside each 'pressure cooker' – when the lid is closed, the solvent and water are added by opening a valve. The operation is begun, and the temperature is checked – it will reach a maximum of 45–50°C (113–122°F). The solvent and the water run continuously through the trays of flowers, impregnating them and taking with them the odoriferous molecules. These gather as a concrete, very stiff and waxy, at the bottom of the cylinder in a small bowl. Each set of trays is 'cooked' for about an hour, then the solvent-saturated flowers, now a dull grey, are discarded and replaced by fresh ones until the operation is complete and the bowls are full.

Filling the bowls normally takes about a day, and the distillery workers labour for as long as it takes, and to all hours, to utilize all the flowers and extract as much essence as possible.

Enormous costs are involved, but the quantity of rose oil produced by volatile solvents is much greater than that of the essential oil produced by steam distillation. Traces of the solvents can still remain in the oils, so they can only be used in perfumery, not in therapy, and indeed can be called an adulterated oil, not an essential oil.

ROSEMARY *(Rosmarinus officinalis – Labiatae)*

Rosmarinus (meaning 'dew of the sea') is a genus of three species of hardy and half-hardy evergreen flowering shrubs. The plant is native to the Mediterranean but now grows in many other warm countries such as Spain and Tunisia; it dies if exposed to cold winds and frost in Britain. The leaves are linear (rather similar to those of lavender), dark on top and paler beneath, and the flowers are pale blue, tubular and borne in axillary clusters; both flowers and leaves are very strongly aromatic and it seems the calyxes retain most of the volatile principles. The plant can grow to a height of about 1.8 m (6 ft).

Rosemary is probably one of the best known and most used of aromatic herbs. The Ancient Egyptians favoured it, and traces of it have been found in First Dynasty tombs. To the Greeks and Romans it was a sacred plant, and Horace, the Roman poet, composed odes to its magic properties. Both Greeks and Romans believed rosemary symbolized love and death, and this is echoed in later traditional country associations with weddings and funerals. Brides used to wear rosemary entwined in their bouquets; bridesmaids would give rosemary to the groom, and other guests would receive it too as a symbol of loyalty and love.

The association of rosemary with funerals obviously involves love and constancy, but it also refers to the herb's meaning in the language of flowers – remembrance, as referred to by the tragic Ophelia, 'There's rosemary, that's for remembrance'. Rosemary's use as a safeguard against contagion and infection might also be a reason for the funerary associations (until quite recently, sprigs would be placed in the coffin at country funerals). Rosemary was one of the strongly antiseptic herbs burned as purifying incense, carried in anti-plague posies, and strewn on floors. Another French name for the herb is, in fact, *incensier* because it was used as incense in church when incense was not available or was too costly.

Enormous claims have been made for the properties of rosemary throughout the years. A Saxon manuscript herbal recorded: 'For the sickly, take this wort rosemary, pound it with oil, smear the sickly one, wonderfully thou healest him.' Richard Banckes' 1525 *Herbal* makes even more ambitious claims: 'Take thee a box of the wood of rosemary and smell to it, and it shall preserve thy youth.' The French claim it as a universal panacea, and a traditional recipe for staying well was to always carry a sprig of the herb.

Rosemary has been used medicinally for centuries. Theophrastus and Dioscorides recommended it as a powerful remedy for stomach and liver problems; Hippocrates, the 'Father of Medicine', said rosemary should be cooked with vegetables to help overcome liver and spleen disorders, and Galen too prescribed it for liver infections, particularly jaundice. To Renaissance apothecaries, rosemary was one of the most valuable remedies at their disposal; Arnauld de Villeneuve in a thirteenth century treatise described how the essential oil was then distilled.

Morocco is one of the primary world producers of the oil: the plant grows in a semi-wild state and is extracted by numerous small distillers. The amount produced has surpassed 100 tonnes, but usually it is around 70 tonnes per year. The oils from North Africa, particularly Tunisia, are more highly rated than those from France or Spain.

THE ESSENTIAL OIL

Description: *The flowering tops of rosemary are distilled to produce the best oil, one far superior to that obtained from the stems and leaves of the plant before it flowers.*

The oil is basically colourless, but veers towards a slightly pale yellow-green. The smell of the oil is similar to that of the leaves when crushed in the fingers – camphory, and rather like incense and honey.

The principal constituents: *Up to 15 per cent borneol, camphene, camphors, cineol, lineol, pinene, resins, and a bitter principle, saponin.*

Dangers: *Rosemary oil can be adulterated, by sage, aspic and, especially, turpentine oils, so try to be sure of the provenance of any you buy.*

ITS USES

In illness

Both herb and oil are strongly antiseptic, and are stimulant, cholagogue and diuretic. They are also useful in rheumatic and respiratory conditions. I find rosemary useful for mental and physical tiredness and **depression**, for liver and **respiratory problems** and for **rheumatism** (good in a poultice, see pages 23 – 4).

To combat weariness, Dr Leclerc prescribed an infusion of the tonic leaves. You could drink this, to redynamize the whole system, or you could put a little of the essential oil in the bath – 10 drops or so – which will be stimulant and tonic. Another way of combating tiredness or depression (rosemary has always been thought of as a cheering herb), is to store some of the fresh herb or a few drops of the oil on a tissue, with your clothes and bedlinen: in bed and during the day, you will be comforted by the aroma.

Rosemary tea is good for liver problems, major and minor. After a heavy or fatty meal, for instance, drink two cups of rosemary tea instead of coffee. Also massage the stomach and liver regions: use a mixture of 2 drops each of chamomile and rosemary oils in 20 – 25 ml (4 – 5 tsp) soya oil. This oil can also be used to relive **rheumatic aches and pains**, and is tonic and stimulant for children and old people who have been ill.

To counteract the breathing problems of **asthma**, you can include fresh rosemary in little pillows to have near you when you sleep. When symptoms are at their worst, a little essential oil, rubbed gently into the chest, solar plexus, forehead and sinus areas can help.

(*See also* **abscesses and boils, anosmia, backache, bronchitis, bursitis, constipation, coughing, cuts and wounds, fever, headaches, lumbago, menopause, muscular pains, oedema, palpitations, shingles, stiffness** *and* **throat, sore**.)

Rosemary wine

One of the herbals advised: 'If thou have a cough, drink the water of the leaves boyled in white wine and ye shall be whole'.

When taken in small quantities, this can act as a tranquillizing cordial for palpitations, a weak heart, headaches and tiredness.

1 litre (1¾ pints) Chablis or Muscadet
200 g (7 oz) fresh rosemary, chopped.

Warm the wine and herb together gently, *do not boil*, and then transfer to a glass container. Leave for a few days, then strain, bottle and seal.

In beauty

Rosemary is used a great deal in eau de colognes and eau de toilettes – indeed it was a major constituent of the first perfume, known as Hungary Water because it made a Queen of Hungary so well that she, although aged 72, managed to ensnare the King of Poland!

Rosemary was in ingredient of the first skin lotion sold commercially in Britain in the seventeenth century, and it is very stimulating for the skin. In *Garden of Herbs*, the reader is enjoined to 'Boyle the leaves in white wine and washe thy face therewith and thy browes and thou shalt have a fair face'.

Drops of the oil can also be used in the bath to help itchy skins (about 10 per bath), and a few drops in the bidet can act as a natural antiseptic for mild irritations.

Rosemary is perhaps best known, though, for its effectiveness as a **hair treatment**. It is tonic and conditioning for dark hair especially, and helps retain the colour. A little oil can be added to shampoos or rinses (or the fresh herb can be infused for a final rinse). Rosemary shampoo lotions can help hair problems such as dandruff and alopecia.

Rosemary hair oil

This is good for such **hair problems** as greasy hair and an itchy scalp.

80 ml (3¼ fl oz) soya oil
2.5 ml (½ tsp) wheatgerm oil
10 ml (2 tsp) rosemary oil
5 ml (1 tsp) cedarwood oil

Mix the ingredients together and shake the bottle. Let rest for a few days before applying. Put a little on the scalp a few hours before shampooing. Massage gently for a few minutes, cover hair with a warm towel to help absorption, then wash off.

In cookery

As a culinary herb, rosemary goes well with poultry, rabbit and lamb, and because of its antibacterial properties protects against possible putrefaction, and helps digestion of the fat. (The Romans used the herb in cooking to protect against cholera.) Add whole sprigs to meat marinades, stews and braises, but remove before serving; the leaves are tough and disliked by many, and only the tenderest shoots and flowers can be eaten raw. Rosemary can also give its powerful flavour and therapeutic properties to herb oils and vinegars, to salutary ales and wines (a sprig added to a less than perfect red wine will improve the bottle's bouqet); to jars of sugar (rather like vanilla pods); and milk infusions for milk puddings. Place rosemary under meat or fish to be roasted or baked; and burn a few sprigs on the coals while barbecuing meat.

Other uses

Rosemary can contribute to pot-pourris and as it promotes well being it would be valuable in a herb pillow. Rosemary's perfume is a safeguard against moths and other vermin. Banckes' *Herbal* advises: 'Also take the flowres and put them in a chest amonge your clothes or amonge bokes and moughtes [moths] shall not hurte them.' Rosemary could be used in the rinsing water of clothes or bedlinen, or linen could be dried over rosemary bushes to permeate them with the fragrance. Rosemary was used to scrub floors, both to perfume and purify: when James I visited the Bodleian in Oxford in the seventeenth century, the floors had been rubbed with the fresh herb. Writing inks were once perfumed with herbs, rosemary one of them.

Rosemary bushes can be planted among vegetables to discourage pests.

SAGE/CLARY SAGE *(Salvia officinalis/Salvia sclarea – Labiatae)*

The herbs sage and clary sage belong to a genus of some 448 species which are hardy evergreen sub-shrubs native to southern Europe. Both have grey-green and wrinkled ovate leaves (clary sage's are very much larger), and tubular flowers: those of sage are violet-blue and bloom in June and July; those of clary are blue-white and bloom in August. Sages hug the ground but can grown up to 60 cm (2 ft); clary can grow to a height of 90 cm (3 ft), and is sufficiently decorative to be grown in a flower border. There are other varieties, which include variegated and pineapple-scented.

S. officinalis, garden or common sage, is a plant familiar to most of us, and has been cultivated for centuries for its culinary and medicinal properties, the best reputedly coming from Dalmatia. *S. sclarea* is less well known, but it is extensively cultivated for its oil which is valuable both medicinally and cosmetically. Other varieties used for distillation are *S. verticulata* and *S. candelabrum*. All yield oils which are similar in composition and therapeutic properties. The world annual production of the essential oil is about 100 tonnes.

Sage's medicinal properties were known to the Romans and it was they who introduced the herb to Britain. The name derives from the Latin *salvere*, to save, and another name was *salvia salvatrix*, the plant which saves and heals. An aphorism recorded from the School of Salerno runs: '*Cur morietur homo, cui salvia crescit in horto?*' (how can a man die who has sage growing in his garden?). The Greeks too valued sage: it was one of the 400 simples of Hippocrates, and Dioscorides praised it for its effectiveness in treating liver diseases. The Ancient Greeks also considered it good for helping diminution of senses and loss of memory; today a tea made with sage leaves is still drunk in Greece. The Ancient Egyptians gave it to women who were unable to bear children, and used it as a remedy against the plague.

In the Middle Ages, the great herbals all praised sage, and clary sage was on the list of herbs ordered by a Winthrop newly settled in the New World from a London supplier in 1631. In 1639, Simon Pauli wrote a book of some 400 pages, all of them on the subject of this remarkable herb; and Saint-Simon at the court of the Sun King related that Louis was daily prescribed this panacea. An old French saying goes; 'Sage helps the nerves and by its powerful might/ Palsy is cured and put to flight'. A cure-all indeed!

The name of clary sage derives from the Latin *clarus*, meaning clear, and it became 'clary' meaning 'clear eye', because clary was once so valued in eye treatments. The seeds were collected and infused to use on tired, strained eyes, or on those suffering from blurred vision. The seeds were also used as a mucilage applied on inflammations of the skin such as swellings and abscesses.

Apart from its historical reputation, research done in 1938 by biologists Kroszcinski and Bychowska showed sage to be a plant healer because of its emmenagogical properties: they recommended it for frigidity, congestion of the ovaries, and for aches, pains and heavy sweating associated with menstruation or menopause. Its therapeutic properties in women's problems were echoed by many French therapists, including Dr Leclerc, who praised sage as an emmenagogue, tonic and stimulant, and for being antisudorific, antispasmodic, a blood cleanser, carminative and strong antiseptic.

THE ESSENTIAL OIL

Description: *The oil of S. officinalis, the true Dalmatian sage, is steam distilled from the leaves. It is a pale yellow-green, and it smells very aromatic, sometimes with a camphor note.*

The best clary sage oil is steam distilled from the green parts of the plants, especially the flowering tops. The oil is similar in colour to sage, but has a more winey, ambergris-like odour. The plant used to be extensively cultivated in France for the oil, but now Russia is the main supplier, distillation taking place in the Crimea and probably the Ukraine.

The principal constituents: *Borneol, camphor, cineole, α-pinene and salvene. The oil is chiefly characterized, however, by its thujone content, which can vary from 22 – 61 per cent in the Dalmatian product. Italian and American sage oils also have high thujone contents. The main constituents of clary sage oil are linalool and linalyl acetate; there is no thujone content.*

Dangers: *I advise self-treatment with* clary sage *essential oil only, and check very carefully that it is* pure *and from a reputable source.*

Because of its high thujone content, sage oil should not be used, particularly by sensitive or young people; taken internally it can be fatal. (Other plants and oils which contain thujone are thuja, tansy and wormwood, the plant once used in the making of absinthe, now banned.) I find it alarming that the bulk of sage oil, formally classified as a convulsant (similar to oil of wormwood) is used in the food industry for flavouring table sauce, canned and packed foods, soups, meat and especially sausages.

ITS USES

In illness

Clary sage is an all-round panacea. It can help debility of the nervous system, general **fatigue**, irritability, and **depression**, weakness of digestion, all the women's complaints, liver trouble and congestion, **asthmatic** conditions and **rheumatic fevers**, aches and pains. It can also be used in the treatment of **cuts, burns, eczema, thrush** and herpes. Merely drinking a tea made from clary sage leaves can help a variety of ailments ranging from **sore throats** and **headaches**, to **promoting menstruation** and preventing the pain of labour (take the tea daily for four weeks prior to delivery).

(*See also* **abscesses and boils, amenorrhoea, catarrh, gum disease, hair problems, palpitations** *and* **stress.**)

Massage oil for women's problems

For those suffering from anxiety, from swelling or puffiness, due to **PMT** or the **menopause**, simply mix together 10 ml (2 tsp) grapeseed oil and 3 drops of clary sage oil. Massage this on the stomach and solar plexus twice a day.

Leg remedy

This is ideal for all those people who have to stand for several hours each day, and who suffer from heavy, swollen and congested legs. Mix together 10 ml (2 tsp) soya oil and 4 drops of clary sage oil. In the evening, take a warm (not hot) bath, and starting from the ankles, massage upwards with the oil to the knees until the oil is absorbed. Then lie back on your bed or on the floor, with your legs raised on a thick cushion, for 10 minutes.

In beauty

Clary sage oil is used a great deal by the perfumery industry as a fixative; it is generally added to floral compositions, and gives body as well.

Sage in general is famed for its hair and mouth properties. Sage leaves have been used for centuries by the Arabs as a tooth cleanser; rub leaves over the teeth to polish and scent them, or crush leaves with salt for a for remedy yellowing teeth. A sage decoction is also good as a mouthwash or gargle for **sore throats**, or infected **gums** or **mouth ulcers**.

Pre-shampoo conditioner

Sage leaves are tonic, and good for hair, conditioning and darkening it; thinning and greying hair can benefit particularly. The following is an excellent pre-shampoo conditioner. The quantities given make a month's supply.

30 ml (2 tbsp) grapeseed oil
3 drops wheatgerm oil
8 drops clary sage essential oil

Mix together and store in a dark bottle. Rub a little into the scalp and roots of the hair very briskly for a few minutes. Wrap hair in a towel and leave for an hour or more. Shampoo out completely (you may need two or three applications of shampoo to remove it). For split ends apply to the ends of the hair only.

A useful decoction can be made from simmering a large handful of sage leaves in 600 ml (1 pint) water for 4 – 5 minutes; remove from the heat then cover and leave to infuse for half an hour before straining and cooling. This will keep for two to three days in the fridge and can be rubbed into the scalp for greying hair. Do this daily, saturating the hair and roots, and leaving it to dry. It also makes a conditioning hair rinse to be used after shampooing.

In cookery

Any of sage's benefits can be obtained by eating the fresh leaves of the plant. Add them to salads as the Elizabethans did (sparingly perhaps, as many people find the flavour too strong), to simple vegetable soups, and to traditional stuffings for rich meats such as pork and goose (the famous sage and onion), to help their digestion. Garnish egg, tomato and cheese dishes with sage, indeed some English cheeses are flavoured and coloured by sage leaves (Sage Derby, for example). Sage goes well with pork, and finds its way into many of the best pork sausages but it must be the fresh leaf (see page 192). The Italians use sage a lot more than the French, wrapping leaves and ham in slices of veal for *saltimbocca*, and cooking it with liver (the herb helps fix the iron in the liver, and helps its digestion as well). In many countries, small wild birds are cooked in a wrapping of sage leaves, and in Germany the herb lends its flavour to dishes of eel. In the Middle East, sage is used a lot in salads, and between chunks of lamb in kebabs.

Sage leaves can be crystallized, and one of the major exports of Yugoslavia is a superb sage honey. Add leaves of a sage – pineapple-scented, say – to savoury jellies, or use in mulled wines or ales. Clary sage was used once in combination with elderflowers to give wine the flavour of muscatel (thus the German name meaning muscatel sage, *Muskatellersalbei*). It is also used in the making of vermouth.

CLARY SAGE FRITTERS   *Serves 4*

> *24 large clary sage leaves, washed and dried*
> *300 ml (½ pint) fresh milk*
> *4 eggs*
> *75 g (3 oz) plain flour*
> *1 lemon*
> *salt, freshly grated nutmeg and black pepper*
> *corn oil for deep frying*

Make a good stiff batter with the milk, eggs and flour, adding a little grated lemon rind, nutmeg, salt and pepper. Cut away the stalks from the leaves, then drop the leaves into the batter, making sure they are well coated on both sides. Deep-fry in hot oil, turning once, until a light brown, then drain well. Serve sprinkled with some fresh lemon juice as a starter or first course – easy and delicious.

Other uses

Sage can be included in pot-pourris. The flowers are very attractive to bees – thus the Yugoslav honey – and if you plant sage among vegetables, you will discourage many insect pests.

SANDALWOOD *(Santalum album – Santalaceae)*

Towards the end of 1989 I was able to visit a sandalwood plantation and distillery in India. I was attending a holistic conference in Bangalore, which is not too far from the district of Karnataka and its main town of Mysore, the heart of the sandalwood-growing areas. After obtaining government permission – for all plantations and distilleries are government controlled – I and my good friend Helen Passant were taken by an Indian friend to Mysore. Even before hitting the outskirts of the town, we could smell the sandalwood fragrance in the warm air; in fact everything – hair, skin, clothes, the silk manufactured in Mysore – is permeated by it.

This fragrance grew more intense and sweet as we approached the plantation and factory. The manager, Mr Chandraskharaian, described to us the plant's history and the processes it goes through.

The true sandalwood – *S. album* – is an evergreen, semi-parasitic tree native to southern Asia, growing particularly well in the south Indian highlands at heights of 600 – 24,000 m (2 – 80,000 ft). Other varieties in the genus grow in the Pacific Islands and Australasia. The tree is medium sized, about 12 – 15 m (40 – 50 ft) high when mature, which is at the age of 40 – 50 years. This is when the heartwood – the centre of the slender trunk – has achieved its greatest circumference and greatest oil content. It is this heartwood and the roots which are fragrant and contain the oil, the bark and sapwood are odourless.

The tree grows from sandalwood fruits which look like small black cherries. Germination from the seeds of the fruit takes about 20 days and then the roots of the seedling attach themselves to nearby trees, bushes and grasses. For seven years the young tree depends on other plants for nourishment (causing the hosts to die), before it can survive by itself. It then requires well-drained, loamy soil, and a minimum of 75 cm (25 in) rainfall per year. The Indian government controls 75 per cent of the total output of sandalwood in the world. Rules and regulations are very strict and every sandalwood tree has to be registered: they are not allowed to be felled indiscriminately, a necessary measure when the subject involved requires up to 50 years to achieve full productivity. These safeguards have been frequently abused, however, and clandestine cutting has caused the destruction of many trees. Further precautionary measures are planned for the next few years, and there is an extensive propagation programme to replace the trees felled legally for commerce (or those struck by disease).

There are two state-owned factories in India which have the capacity to produce 60 – 70,000 kg (130 – 150,000 lb) of sandalwood oil and can cater for world-wide demand. When each tree is 40 – 50 years old, and has a girth of 60 – 62 cm (24 – 25 in), it is carefully felled. The dark brown trunk gives off a very strong scent at this stage, especially near the ground and the fragrant roots. A mature tree can yield up to 200 kg (440 lb) of oil, an enormous quantity. The yield of oil from the roots varies from 6 – 7 per cent, and in the heartwood from 2 – 5 per cent.

Sandalwood has a long history. It is mentioned in old Sanskrit and Chinese manuscripts: the oil was used in religious ritual, and many deities and temples were carved from its wood. The Ancient Egyptians imported the wood, and used it in medicine, embalming and ritual, burning it to venerate the gods; they also carved fine art objects from it. The Ayurveda, the ancient Indian system of holistic medicine, recommended sandalwood for its tonic, astringent and anti-febrile properties; a powder made into paste was used for skin inflammations, abscesses and tumours. (This usage, for skin ulcers particularly, was echoed by P H Guybert in 1636, in his treatise on *Medicine Charitable*.) In the Indian pharmacopoeia, sandalwood is deemed to promote perspiration, and mixed with milk it was said to help blennoragia – the discharge of mucus. Many remedies recommend its use in association with cardamom.

In Europe in 1868, a Glaswegian doctor, Dr Henderson, drew practitioners' attention to this wonderful remedy, particularly quoting his success in cases of blennoragia. Later, French doctors Panas, Laber and Bordier, confirmed these researches. In France at this time, sandalwood was given in capsules of 40 g four to five times a day: 40 minutes after swallowing, a strong sandalwood smell was recorded in the urine of the patients. Roughly speaking these are the areas in which sandalwood was used earlier this century, for the mucus of chronic bronchitis, and for all urinary problems (cystitis, bladder infections and inflammations). It was also considered a useful diuretic and helpful in cases of diarrhoea.

It seems that the future of sandalwood is precarious. The repeated demands of the perfume industry over the last five years have caused large scale destruction to the trees, with alarming results in some parts of India. I now only very recluctantly use sandalwood if at all, and have turned to other essential oils with similar curative properties, such as galbanum and incense.

THE ESSENTIAL OIL

Description: *Once the oil has been distilled it is kept in the distillery for about six months so that it can achieve the right maturity and perfume. It* *develops from a very pale yellow to a brownish-yellow; it is viscous with a heavy, sweet, woody and fruity aroma which is pungently balsamic.*

The principal constituents: *Santalol (90 per cent and more), which is a mixture of two primary sesquiterpenic alcohols.*

Dangers: *Sandalwood oil can be adulterated with diverse oils such as castor, palm and linseed. This can be detected easily by experts, but the public can be deceived. There are so many other oils with similar properties that if you are at all concerned by environmental issues, please avoid buying sandalwood and use alternatives instead.*

ITS USES

In illness

Sandalwood oil is still one of the main remedies used in the Ayurvedic system of medicine. Asians and Arabs use it in self-treatment for a great number of diseases. In Europe, it mostly features in perfumery and soap, and it once had a major role in aromatherapy. In therapy it was often associated with other oils such as *baumes de pérou* or *tolu*, or cajuput or chamomile, and applied externally to skin inflammations such as those caused by allergy or **eczema**, or to **abscesses** and **cracked and chapped skin**. It was also very relaxing, and could help meditation. (Sheets kept in a sandalwood coffer or chest will smell beautiful, and help you sleep for the same reason.) Now, however, I do not think we should use sandalwood as the demand for it is destroying vast plantations and has lead to the cutting of the trees before maturity when far too young.

(*See also* **cystitis**.)

In beauty

As a cosmetic ingredient, East Indian sandalwood is very important. No oriental perfume is complete without it, and its sweet, powerful, lasting odour makes it an excellent fixative in perfume. Almost 90 per cent of East Indian sandalwood oil is used in perfumes, cosmetics and soaps.

Other uses

Sanders, saunders or santal are ingredients which appear in many manuscripts and old books. These sometimes refer to true sandalwood, more often other fragrant trees such as *Pterocarpus santalinus*. Raspings or powder were used in perfumed powders and pot-pourris, and red and yellow sanders even appeared in medieval British cookery books, used as food colorant.

One of the principal uses of the wood is in fragrant carvings, such as those sold in India, and in some kinds of cabinet making. The wood is soft and therefore easy to carve.

SASSAFRAS *(Sassafras albidum/officinalis – Lauraceae)*

The sassafras is a well-known North American tree which can grow to 18 m (60 ft) in height. Yellowish flowers are followed by oval bluish fruit. The leaves, which are deciduous, can be plain, double lobed like maple, or lobed on one side only, like a mitten. The tree is related to the bay and camphor.

In America the sassafras is called the 'laurel of the Iroquois', after Indians of the eastern United States who held the tree sacred and esteemed it for its therapeutic values. French colonists and explorers in the mid-sixteenth century wrote of how the Indians would make an infusion of the tree bark and give it to those suffering from fever and many other diseases. It was the Spaniards, however, who took the new remedy back to Europe. Cuttings were brought to England in 1610, and trees were cultivated in glasshouses.

In the late seventeenth century, Nicolas Lemery listed the properties of sassafras as being an aperitif and sudorific, as fortifying the sight and the brain. He, and others, considered it good for gout, sciatica and catarrhal discharge.

At one time, the United States was the only country to produce essential oil of sassafras where it was used to flavour drinks such as root beer. Medicinal teas – one was known as 'saloop' – were made from the bark, leaves and buds. Soap was also made from the leaves. But because of the high wastage involved (the roots are the most oil-rich part of the tree) trees are not now felled for oil production in the United States. Also, since 1958, the use of sassafras oil has been forbidden in the North American food industry; the oil's main constituent, safrol, has been found to be carcinogenic.

Brazil has continued producing a sassafras essential oil, but from a tree called *Ocotea pretiosa* which, although a member of the *Lauraceae* family, is a quite different tree. It is even more rich in safrol than the American oil, and the industry has suffered considerably following the American ban. The production in Brazil is approximately 1500 – 2000 metric tonnes per year (1987 figures), and the principal importer is Japan, followed by the USA, Spain, Italy, France and Britain.

Sassafras was an early flavouring of chewing gum and young leaves are dried and ground to make filé powder, an important ingredient in Creole cookery. The essential oil is still used in the perfumery and soap industry. A substance called heliotropine, derived from safrol, was once used in food to reinforce the flavour and aroma of vanilla in cola, custard and biscuits, for example.

THE ESSENTIAL OIL

Description: *The inner part of the roots has a strong balsamic smell, and it is these, plus the wood, bark and rootlets that are used for the production of the essential oil. Leaves and flowers can be added which results in a more lemony, subtler oil. The oil is yellow or reddish-yellow with a special safrol smell, acrid and aromatic, reminiscent of anise, lemon and fennel.*

The principal constituents: *Approximately 80 per cent safrol and pinene, 8 – 10 per cent cadinene, camphene, eugenol, oleoresins, phellandrene, tannic acid and wax. The Brazilian sassafras oil contains some 90 per cent safrol.*

Dangers: *As the quality of the oil can vary so much, you must buy very carefully, if at all. As there are so many other oils which can benefit rheumatic pains and gout, I think that sassafras is dispensable, particularly in view of its carcinogenic reputation. In addition, because the entire tree needs to be destroyed, the greenhouse effect is continuously being worsened and so sassafras should be eliminated entirely from use in therapy and industry. Because of the susupected carcinogenicity, it's use is severely restricted (to 0.05% in products) by EC cosmetics laws and IFRA.*

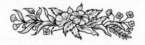

SAVORY
(Satureja hortensis [summer]/*Satureja montana* [winter] *– Labiatae)*

The two major savory varieties are very closely related. Summer savory is a bushy annual which grows to about 30 cm (12 in) in height; it has dark green, aromatic leaves, hairy stems, and tiny pink-lilac flowers. Winter savory is compact and erect, with small grey-green leaves and tiny rose-purple flowers; it grows to about the same height as its summer cousin. Both are plants of the Mediterranean *garrigue*, although they can thrive further north.

The Greeks called the herb *satureia* (which has now become *satureja*), from the word 'satyr', because it was reputed to be an aphrodisiac. Martial, Ovid and Virgil, for instance, all recounted tales of its efficacy. The Romans cooked meat dishes with savory and were responsible for its introduction to Britain. In the Middle Ages, St Hildegarde of Bingen advised savory for problems of gout, and it has been listed in the French and German pharmocopoeiae since 1582 as a stomachic and stimulant. A seventeenth century French surgeon, Pierre Argellata, claimed that he had managed to heal ulcers of the mouth and throat in over 100 of his patients with a decoction of savory; he boiled savory in very strong red wine and applied it to the ulcers. More recently, the essential oil of savory was used for toothache and rotting teeth, and Dr Cazin used it on people with earache.

Every 28th December since the Middle Ages, a special savory feast has been organized in Montpellier, France. The students elect one of their number as 'le petit évêque' (the little bishop), and crown him with a ring of savory. He leads the way through the city, followed by a noisy procession of students all banging drums and saucepans, and ringing bells. They gather in a sort of open-air pub where they drink a special savory wine (made much as the aphrodisiac wine below) – which is said to stimulate the brain as well as the body, and local people are always advised to keep their daughters in on that night!

THE ESSENTIAL OIL

Description: *This is steam-distilled from the leaves (the flowers too sometimes), and is pale orange. It is quite hot, like thyme, and a bit acrid.*
The principal constituents: *The oil is extraordinarily high in phenols (like oregano and thyme) and other constituents are 30 – 40 per cent carvacrol, 20 – 30 per cent thymol, and cineol, cymene and pinene.*

ITS USES

In illness

Because of the high phenol content, the oil is very strongly antiseptic, again like oregano and thyme, but it must always be used in dilution. It is very useful for hastening the **formation of scar tissue**, and for treating bites, **burns**, ulcers and **abscesses**.

For **cuts**, have ready a small bottle consisting of 70 per cent proof alcohol and 3 – 4 drops of savory essential oil. This will stop bleeding and stinging. Afterwards rub on an oil consiting of 10 ml (2 tsp) soya oil, 2–3 drops wheatgerm oil and 3 drops savory oil. This will help healing.

A herb tea made with fresh savory is a great tonic in the morning. Add a drop of honey.

To make an aphrodisiac wine similar to that of the ancients, add 5 g (¼ oz) savory leaves, 15 ml (1 tbsp) sugar or fructose, and 5 ml (1 tsp) Angostura bitters to a bottle of good port or Madeira. Steep for a while, then drink a glass when you need it.

(See also **acne, asthma, cold sores, flatulence, mouth ulcers** *and* **sexual problems***.)*

In cookery

Summer savory is considered better for cooking than winter, being less strong and coarse in flavour. Both are quite biting and more bitter than thyme. The herbs dry very well, and savory is then most reminiscent of thyme.

Use savory in meat stews and marinades, especially those for game; it is also good with grills of fish or chops. Use it with discretion though, as it can dominate.

Savory is called '*Bohnenkraut*' in German, meaning, 'bean herb', and has long been cooked with all kinds of beans to help their digestion and the assimilation of their vitamins and minerals, thus avoiding flatulence. The herb is also added to *sauerkraut*, sausages and salami, and was once used to form a wrapping for some French cheeses.

Other uses

The herb can be used in pot-pourris, and was once a popular antiseptic strewing herb. Soap perfumed with savory, especially if combined with lime, has antiseptic properties and it leaves the hands smelling fresh.

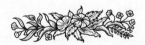

TARRAGON *(Artemisia dracunculus – Compositae)*

This small, bushy, perennial plant is thought to originate from Asia, but has now spread all over Europe. There are two varieties of tarragon: *A. dracunculus*, the 'true', 'French' tarragon, is the one valued in cooking and medicine; *A. dracunculoides*, 'false' or 'Russian' tarragon, has coarser leaves and a coarser flavour. Other members of the *Artemisia* family,

201

used in folk medicine, are *A. absinthium*, wormwood (used in the making of absinthe, now banned because of its thujone content), *A. vulgaris*, mugwort, and *A. abrotanum*, southernwood.

True tarragon has leaves which are bright green, narrow, lance-shaped and undivided (unlike other artemisias). They have a unique, pleasant, aromatic taste. The plant grows to a height of about 60 – 90 cm (2 – 3 ft), and is easily cultivated in a warm spot or in a sunny windowbox. It bears tiny, greenish-yellow flowers in August, but these rarely open in cool climates and as a result the plant rarely sets seed. It is propagated by cuttings, and if seeds *are* available, they are likely to be those of the prolific Russian tarragon. Tarragon is one of only three common herbal plants to come from the *Compositae*, the second largest family of flowering plants (along with calendula or marigold and chamomile).

The botanical names come from Greek and Latin: *artemisia* for Artemis, the Greek virgin goddess of the hunt and the moon; *dracunculus* from the Latin for 'little dragon' (probably derived from the Arabic *tarkhun* meaning little dragon as well). The French name *estragon* is derived from the Latin, and in fact the plant is referred to in old French texts as *herbe au dragon* and was used in the Middle Ages for bites and stings of mad dogs and other beasts. Another name at this time was *targon*.

The plant was thought to have been introduced to Europe by the Crusaders. Arab doctors had long recommended it for combating flatulence, and in the tenth century Avicenna advised its use for fermentation, bad digestion and flatulence. In 1548, Matthiole said it should be mixed with salad leaves (as did Gerard later), a practice which still exists in France. Tarragon gained a great reputation in the eighteenth century as a stomachic, stimulant and sudorific. In France, Dr Cazin had good results prescribing it for hiccoughs, dyspepsia, gout and rheumatism.

THE ESSENTIAL OIL

Description: *The oil is distilled from the leaves and is generally colourless, perhaps very slightly green. The smell is reminiscent of anise or fennel, and it has a wonderful, slightly spicy, taste.*

The principal constituents: *Phenol (up to 70 per cent estragol), with cymene, linalyl acetate, phellandrene and traces of aldehyde.*

Dangers: *As many react to estragol, also known as methyl-chavicol, the oil should be used very carefully.*

ITS USES

In illness

The oil is useful in massage oils to help **dysmenorrhoea, amenorrhoea, PMT** and **menopause**. The plant is digestive when eaten raw, and an infusion of chopped tarragon in 1 litre (1¾ pints) boiling water acts as a good diuretic.

(See also **constipation** *and* **menstrual cycle problems**.*)*

In cookery

Tarragon is considered one of the most important herbs in cookery, because of its wonderful flavour. It is particularly associated with chicken: place tarragon leaves under the skin of a chicken to be roasted, and put a whole halved lemon and a few more tarragon leaves inside the cavity before cooking. Tarragon also makes a wonderful vinegar: simply stuff some leaves into a bottle of white wine vinegar and leave for about 2 weeks before use (a good way of preserving tarragon, as dried it is virtually tasteless). Tarragon is used raw as garnish and in salads, in *bouquet garnis*, chopped in *fines herbes* (with parsley and chives), and in sauces like Béarnaise, Hollandaise and tartare. It also flavours mustard, pickled cucumbers or gherkins, and some local French liqueurs. In the Near East, the young tips or shoots are cooked and eaten as a vegetable.

One of the most significant characteristics of tarragon, apart from its subtle flavour, is its ability to season in place of salt which makes it very useful for those suffering from heart problems or obesity. This was appreciated very early on: a sixteenth-century botanist, Ruellius, said that 'it is one of the most agreeable of salads, which requires neither salt nor vinegar, for it possesses the taste of these two condiments.'

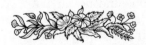

TEA TREE *(Melaleuca alternifolia – Myrtaceae)*

The tea tree is small, growing to 7 m (23 ft), with small, soft, narrow leaves and cream, showy, bottlebrush-like flowers which produce small, closely-set woody capsules on the branches. It is a paperbark tree closely related to the *M. leucadendron* which produces cajuput oil and *M. viridiflora*, which produces niaouli. The tea tree flourishes only in a relatively small area of New South Wales, one of some 34 species of *Melaleuca* unique to

Australia. Long used as a bush remedy by the early white settlers of the continent, it was not until after the First World War that any serious study of the oil and its application to orthodox medicine was begun, but from the 1920s until the Second World War, its fame grew. It was supplied to the Royal Australian Navy and to the Army in 1939 but after that, the output diminished. The tree grows in fairly dangerous environments for it thrives in dense thickets in marshes also greatly loved by spiders, snakes, mosquitoes and other biting and poisonous creatures. At this time chemical drugs, too, superseded the natural remedies until in the 1970s tea tree oil once again returned to the medical and commercial forefront. It has now become a major industry in Australia, and a major force in healing.

THE ESSENTIAL OIL

Description: *This is steam distilled from the leaves and terminal branchlets of the tree. A bush still of 1600 litres (350 gallons) capacity holds half a metric tonne of fresh leaves, takes 2 – 3 hours to distil, and yields 7 – 10 kg (15 – 22 lb) of oil.*

This is colourless to pale yellow, is clear and mobile, and smells firm and spicy, characteristically myristic or nutmeg-like, a masculine sort of smell.
The principal constituents: *Terpenes (50 – 60 per cent), cineol, sesquiterpenes and sesquiterpenic alcohols.*

ITS USES

In illness
In 1933 the *British Medical Journal* reported that the oil was a powerful disinfectant, non-poisonous and non-irritant, and in 1930 the *Australian Medical Journal* reported astounding results gained in general practice, ranging from rapid healing of septic wounds to scar regeneration:

> ' . . . a striking feature being that it dissolved pus and left the surfaces of infected wounds clear so that its germicidal action became more effective and without any apparent damage to the tissues. This was something new, as most germicides destroy tissue as well as bacteria.' (E.M. Humphrey)

In 1955, the United States Dispensatory reported that tea tree oil was actively germicidal – with an antiseptic action eleven to thirteen times that of carbolic acid.

As a germicide, it was tested in Australia in 1980 in a solution of only 4 parts essential oil to 1000 parts water. Against virulent organisms such as *Staphylococcus aureus* and *Candida albicans*, the results were, at 7, 21 and 35 days, no growth detected for any organism. (As a result of this, tests are now being carried out on the virus responsible for genital herpes and the potent typhoid bacillus.)

As a bacteriostat, results from a skin sterilization trial conducted in 1983 by and at the Associated Foodstuff Laboratories of Australia, were amazing. Using swabs, the bacteria count on unwashed hands was over 3,000 per 50 cm (20 in); the count on hands after washing in distilled water was over 2,000 per 50 cm (20 in); after washing in tea tree oil, the bacteria was less than 3 per 50 cm (20 in), the bacteria actually not detectable. Think how effective a single drop could be, simply added to dish washing-up water.

The oil also has an application in **burn treatment, gynaecological conditions** such as trichomonal vaginitis, **skin ailments** and **ear**, nose, **throat** and mouth **infections**. The potential use of tea tree oil could extend to baby care, hospital, dental and domestic products, and veterinary medicine, and indeed commerical companies are now exploring many of these avenues.

I have used the oil very successfully in curing a septic finger (see page vii), and it has proved very effective in inhalations for **colds and 'flu**, for **skin abrasions**, and for **acne**, applied on a cotton bud. As first aid, it is better than anything else I know.

(See also **abscesses and boils, anthrax, athlete's foot, bronchitis, chest infections, chilblains, cold sores, cuts and wounds, fever, folliculitis, hayfever, headaches, impetigo, mouth ulcers, neuralgia, pneumonia, sinusitis** *and* **stings and bites**.*)*

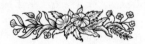

THUJA *(Thuja* spp. *– Cupressaceae)*

Thuja is a genus of five hardy, evergreen coniferous trees and shrubs native to North America and Canada (*T. occidentalis,* white cedar, and *T. plicata,* Western red cedar), Japan (*T. standishii*), China (*T. orientalis*) and Korea (*T. koraiensis*). The white cedar was the first American tree to be grown in France: it was introduced in 1526 from Canada and grew in the royal gardens at Fontainebleau.

The trees are cypress-like, and most are small and slow growing with the exception of the Western red cedar. The scale-like leaves are pressed closely to the stem, the flowers – both male and female on the same tree – are small and terminal, and the cones are small with scales and winged seeds. The foliage of all types, excepting only *T. orientalis*, are strongly aromatic, exuding an odour without being crushed and noticeable from several yards away.

The name *thuja* (or *thuya* in French) is a Latinized form of a Greek word meaning to fumigate, or *thuo* to sacrifice. Theophrastus described how trees of the genus were grown in ancient times in Cyrene near the temple of Jupiter-Ammon, and parts were burned in religious ceremonies to venerate the gods. The bark was often used to sculpt religious objects and statues. Another name for the tree is *arbor-vitae*, tree of life.

The American Indians used thuja, making the leaves and bark into a poultice for rheumatic joints and, because of the sudorific properties, decoctions to drink for virus infections.

Samuel Hahnemann (1755 – 1843), the father of homoeopathy, introduced the plant's medicinal properties to Europe, where it was used as a tincture. In Germany in 1875, doctors Mohnike and Brecher wrote a paper about the remarkable healing powers of thuja, particularly in cases of skin excrescences and tumours. They noted how quickly the skin repaired and healed itself after a twice-daily application of the tincture; the skin became pale and dry, inflammation reduced, and the tumours disappeared. Later, Dr Leclerc prescribed it for warts, skin abnormalities and as a stimulant of the urinary system because of the stimulant constituents (α-pinene, fenone and *d*-thujone).

THE ESSENTIAL OIL

Description: Thuja plicata, *or Western red cedar, is the variety recommended for its medicinal properties. The leafy young twigs, freshly cut and dried, are the parts used for distillation. There is more essential oil present in spring, very little in summer.*

The principal constituents: α-*pinene, borneol, bornyl acetate, d-thujone, fenchone and fenone. The properties of the oil are antirheumatic and antiseptic.*

Dangers: *I do not recommend the use of thuja essential oil in self treatment. It should only be used by a reputable practitioner as thujone is a dangerous constituent whether taken in large or small dosages. It should* never *be taken internally, and if precautions are not taken, even external application can be very toxic.*

ITS USES

In illness

In the hands of a professional aromatherapist Thuja essential oil gives very good results in treatment of **psoriasis** of the scalp, **skin** excrescences, skin rashes, and **alopecia**. Thuja can also be a remarkable ally in the fight against the bad abscesses of **acne**, and severe infection.

THYME (*Thymus* spp. – *Labiatae*)

Thyme belongs to a genus of over 300 species of hardy perennial herbaceous plants and sub-shrubs which are native to Europe, particularly around the Mediterranean. They have now spread all over the world, to America, and as far north as Iceland. Some are prostrate and mat-forming; others can grow up to 30 cm (12 in) in height, and these include *T. citriodorus*, lemon-scented thyme. *T. vulgaris*, or garden thyme, is that used mainly in cookery: it has narrow small leaves, which are dark green-grey, and clusters of tubular mauve flowers. (Other thyme flowers vary in colour from white through pale pink and lilac to deep red.) The leaves of all are aromatic, those of the cultivated generally more so than the wild; and those grown in warm climates are always more powerful than those of the chilly, damp north. *T. membranaceus*, a variety native to Spain, is the most fragrant, and there are caraway- and orange-scented thymes as well.

Thyme was said to have been used by the Sumerians as long ago as 3,500BC. The Ancient Egyptians called it *tham*, and used the plants in embalming. The Greeks knew of two types: Dioscorides talked of the white – used for medicinal purposes – and the black, which was not favoured as it 'corrupted the organism and provoked the secretion of bile'. Thyme was one of Hippocrates' 400 simples or remedies. Infusions of the herb were drunk at the end of banquets for digestive purposes, and offerings were made to Venus and other divinities. The name thyme actually comes from the Greek word *thumos*, or smell, because of the fragrance of the plant.

The Romans cooked with thyme and used it medicinally. Pliny recommended it as a remedy for epilepsy; he said that the herb should be made into a mattress and that after sleeping on it, the patient would be relaxed and calm. (Interestingly, thyme is reputed to have been added to the hay in the manger for the baby Jesus' bed.) Pliny also prescribed thyme boiled in vinegar as a headache remedy. Thyme was considered an antidote for snake bites; it was also burned outside houses to keep dangerous reptiles away. The Romans thought thyme dispelled melancholy and promoted bravery: soldiers would have a bath with thyme in it before going into battle, an idea still extant at the time of the Crusades, when ladies would embroider sprigs of thyme on their knights' scarves before they went to the East. In the Middle Ages, St Hildegarde prescribed thyme for plague and paralysis, leprosy and body lice. Thyme was a strewing herb in Britain, and was included in the posies carried by judges and kings to protect them from disease in public.

The respect for the properties of thyme has not diminished. Lemery, a seventeenth-century French physican and chemist, thought of it as a brain fortifier, and a stimulant of the digestive system. In 1719, Neumann isolated and discovered the thymol in thyme; later Cadéac and Meunier isolated carvacrol and pinene. During the eighteenth century, thyme was included in many preparations, one of them a *baume tranquille* for nervous disorders. In 1884, Camperdon, a scholar, studied the therapeutic properties and noticed that thyme had a direct action on the nervous system, and that it helped re-establish strength in convalescence. Dr Leclerc later prescribed it in cases of asthma, depression and respiratory infections, and for chronic coughs. Thyme oil was used, along with clove, lemon and chamomile essential oils, as a disinfectant and antiseptic in hospitals until the First World War. As it could kill yellow fever organisms, and was seven times stronger than carbolic, it was sprayed on the clothes of soldiers during the Crimean War to protect against disease and lice.

THE ESSENTIAL OIL

Description: *The oil is steam-distilled from the leaves and flower tops. It is fatty and thick, and the smell is pleasant, reminiscent of the fresh plant, but obviously more persistently.*

The colour can be red or white depending, it was once thought, on whether the plant used was white or red thyme. However, it has been proved that it is not the colour of the plant that influences the colour of the oil, it is the type of container in which the oil was distilled. In poorer countries, metallic containers are used, and these oxidate when in contact with the oil, turning it red. In other countries more expensive onyx containers are used, which do not react with the oil and so it retains its natural white colour. It is not known how the therapeutic value of the oil is affected by the oxidation.

The principal constituents: *25 – 40 per cent thymol and carvacrol, with borneol, cineol, linalool, menthone, p-cymene, pinene and triterpenic acid.*

Dangers: *Essential oil of thyme comes from the south of France, Spain, Israel and North Africa. Since the disaster at Chernobyl, I have used the white Israeli version because of fears about the radioactive content of thyme plants. Although many Western countries and many plants were affected by fallout, it seems to have 'fixed' more in thyme than other herbs. Despite this, many Western producers continue to sell oils for therapy, so it is doubly important to be sure of the provenance of any oil you buy. I also advise avoiding the red oil (see above).*

ITS USES

In illness

Thyme is a tonic and stimulant, and stomachic, digestive, antispasmodic, pectoral and balsamic. It can help **asthma, 'flu, colds, coughs, fever** and nervousness as well as aches and pains. It is also effective for **dermatitis**, for **skin infections** and irritations, for swellings provoked by **gout** or **rheumatic problems**, for **backache** and **sciatica**. I would not be without it.

(See also **abdominal pain, abscesses and boils, anorexia nervosa, anthrax, bruises, catarrh, cold sores, coughing, cuts and wounds, diarrhoea, gastritis, gum disease, halitosis, lumbago, muscular pains, pneumonia** and **stings and bites**.*)*

Aches and pains remedy

For **joint pains, backache** and **sciatica**, take a hot bath, mixing in 15 drops of essential oil of thyme, plus 2 tbsp bicarbonate of soda. To reinforce the oil's action, add a few drops of eucalyptus or cedarwood which work well together. After the bath, rub the affected areas with an oil made up of 15 ml (1 tbsp) soya oil, 2 drops wheatgerm oil, 10 drops of thyme oil and 5 drops of eucalyptus oil.

Tiredness and depression remedy

Take a warm bath, mixing in 5 drops of thyme oil and 3 drops of marjoram oil. Afterwards, rub the solar plexus and sacrum area with an oil made up with 15 ml (1 tbsp) almond oil, 2 drops wheatgerm oil, 7 drops thyme, 2 drops marjoram and 3 drops rose, mixed together very well. Follow with a tisane as below.

Thyme tisane

Infuse a good 15 ml (a heaped tbsp) fresh thyme leaves in 600 ml (1 pint) boiling water for 5 minutes. Drink hot, sweetened with honey. This is good for depression and tiredness, especially effective in the morning instead of tea or coffee, as well as when under stress or pressure at work. It is good too for **PMT, menopausal symptoms**, or for after **colds** or **'flu**. When applied externally, infused thyme can help reduce the swellings associated with **rheumatism** and **oedema**.

In beauty
For **acne**, a good astringent can be made by boiling a sprig of fresh thyme (or a pinch of dried) in 2 cups of water for 2 minutes, then leaving to infuse for 5 minutes. Add the juice of half a lemon and rinse the skin with this several times a day. Thyme oil can also be used in pre-shampooing lotions to combat **dandruff**: make as for the recipe on page 193, substituting thyme oil for the sage.

In cookery
Thyme is a major herb and is an essential part of a *bouquet garni* (together with bay and parsley). The plant dries very well, so its properties are always available for use in the kitchen. Thyme's fragrance also lasts in cooking, so it is good for long-cooking stews and casseroles; as thyme fixes the iron in meat, so it helps the digestion of stews and casseroles. These properties also make flatulence-inducing foods like beans easier to digest (as practised by the Ancient Egyptians). Its preservative properties make it a natural inclusion in things like pâtés, sausages, potted meats and pickles; fresh chopped leaves are also delicious added to bread doughs, omelettes and mushroom dishes. For its flavour, use thyme in marinades, under meats on barbecues, in stuffings, soups, stocks, *court-bouillons*, herb butters for grilled meat or oily fish, and the lemon-scented variety in sweet things like batters or syllabub. (In Iceland, they flavour sour milk with lemon thyme.)

Thyme can flavour herb vinegars and oils, and can make a savoury jelly. Thyme is one of the ingredients of the liqueur Benedictine: this was invented in 1510 as an elixir to revive tired monks, thereafter it was used to combat malarial diseases. Now it is a luxurious treat!

Other uses
Thyme oil is used in soaps and antiseptic preparations. Historically, lemon thyme has been included in pot-pourris, herb bags and pillows, and the garden type in anti-moth bags, on herb seats, and in lawns. Thyme is good for insect bites, and was once used as a medicinal snuff.

TURPENTINE
(Pinus, Larix, Pistacia spp. *– Coniferae, Anacardiaceae)*

Turpentine is a thin, volatile, essential oil, which is distilled from the resin of certain pine and other trees. It is used familiarly as a paint thinner and solvent, but it is also valuable medicinally. There are various qualities of medicinal turpentine: the most highly regarded, for instance, is called Venice turpentine, and is produced by the European larch (*Larix decidua, Coniferae*). The European maritime or cluster pine (*Pinus pinaster, Coniferae*) is a more frequent source, but the oil, Bordeaux turpentine, is less subtle. The tree that yields what is known as Indian turpentine, is the terebinth (*Pistacia terebinthus, Anacardiaceae*), of a family which includes the pistachio nut (*P. vera*), and *P. lentiscus* (a tree which produces mastic for chewing gum). These trees grow around the Mediterranean. Another tree from New Zealand, the *kauri* or *Agathis australis*, also produces oil and turpentine.

The properties of turpentine were known to the Greeks and Romans, Dioscorides saying the best was the white, clear variety. Pliny, Hippocrates and Galen favoured its properties, too. Venice turpentine was known during the Middle Ages, and the city became one of the principal markets for this medicinal drug. In the sixteenth century, methods of obtaining resin and distillation were recorded.

THE ESSENTIAL OIL

Description: *The resin runs naturally from the trees, but generally they are tapped, and then the resin is steam distilled to produce the oil. (Some turpentine-producing trees are sprayed with dilute sulphuric acid which causes the resin to exude.) The resin is yellow and fluid, translucent, slightly fluorescent, and does not harden when exposed to air. It has an agreeable smell and an acrid bitter taste.*

The principal constituents: *Borneol, resinic acid, sesquiterpene, terpenes (pinene, α and β) together with neutral substances.*

Dangers: *Turpentine should never be stored in a dropper bottle as the rubber will distintegrate.*

It is very often used to falsify other essential oils – eucalyptus, juniper, pine and rosemary, for instance, all of which are high in terpenes, the principal constituent of turpentine. Turpentine can also be adulterated, usually with white spirit or petroleum solvent (what is sold as turps substitute), and if this is used as an essential oil, it can cause terrible burns. As with all other essential oils, it is vital to be sure of the purity of turpentine.

Turpentine oil must never *be taken internally. Turpentine is a strong antiseptic and bactericide, but should only be used by a reputable practitioner. It must never be used neat, as even a small dosage can excite the nervous system; large doses can cause paralysis, exhaustion, cystitis, bladder infections and the need to pass water all the time. The oil should never be left where children or people who might be careless can abuse it.*

ITS USES

In illness
Despite the above, I use the oil in the practice, finding it good in cases of **rheumatism, sciatica** and **gout**.

Other uses
Another source of turpentine is the Aleppo pine (*Pinus halepensis*), the resin of which is also used in the Greek wine *retsina*.

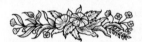

VERBENA (*Lippia citriodora* syn. *Aloysia citriodora* – *Verbeaceae*)

Lemon or lemon-scented verbena – not to be confused with its relative, vervein, *Verbena officinialis* – is a native of South America (Chile and Peru). It was introduced to North Africa, India, Australia, the Caribbean islands and the island of Réunion and reached Europe around 1760. It is a perennial, deciduous, slender shrub which reaches about 1.5 m (5 ft) in height, less in temperate regions. The leaves are long, pale green and pointed, and the flowers are tubular, purple and grow in terminal clusters. The entire plant smells strongly of lemon.

Lippia comes from Augustin Lippi, a seventeenth-century Italian naturalist. The plant is now more correctly defined as *Aloysia citriodora*, although it is also know as *Verbena* or *Lippia triphylla*.

In *Parte pratica de botanica* (1784), Palau y Verdera was one of the first to describe the plant, giving its therapeutic values as a fortifier, regularizer of the nervous system, and a stomachic; he said it helped with bad digestion and flatulence, nervous palpitations, dizziness and hysteria.

THE ESSENTIAL OIL

Description: *The leaves and stalks are steam distilled for the oil which is liquid, and a yellowish-green. It has a fresh lemony smell which is hot and bitter at the same time, so subtle that it has proved difficult to reproduce synthetically.*

The principal constituents: *30 – 45 per cent citral, with caryophyllene, cineol, geraniol, limonene, linalool, methylheptenone, nerol and terpineol.*

Dangers: *Real essential oil of lemon verbena is rare and rather expensive so it is often falsified or adultered with citronella or lemongrass. These make the fragrance considerably less subtle, so beware. (Sometimes lemongrass oil is called* verveine des Indes). *Verbena oil from* Lippia citriodora *is restricted by IFRA because of its skin sensitizing property in some people.*

ITS USES

In illness

Like lemongrass, verbena has a high citral content, which makes it a very good antiseptic and bactericide. Verbena is also a very good stomachic, tonic and antispasmodic. I find it has a sedative effect on the nervous system, too.

For a tonic tisane in the morning – much better for you than tea or coffee – infuse a large pinch of the dried leaves in 600 ml (1 pint) boiling water for 7 minutes maximum. Add a slice of lemon or some honey if you like, and you will feel much better, ready to face the day.

To cheer you up, whether you're simply low, or a little depressed, you could diffuse the fragrance of the oil throughout your home.

(See also **appetite, loss of** *and* **depression**.*)*

In beauty

Because of its strongly antiseptic properties, I recommend verbena for cases of **acne** with badly inflamed boils. Mix together 25 ml (1 fl oz) grapeseed oil, 1 drop wheatgerm oil, and 9 drops verbena oil: apply every night on the face after cleansing. Apply verbena oil neat, a few times a day, on cysts and whiteheads.

To avoid infection, never share your oil or lend it to anyone.

(See also **dermatitis**.*)*

213

In cookery

Use the leaves in anything that requires a lemon flavour – chopped in stuffings for fish or chicken, in sausages, in salads, or in fruit jellies and sweets. Leaves can be used instead of lemongrass in many South-East Asian recipes.

Other uses

The oil and plant play quite a considerable part in the food and drink industry for a flavour of lemon, and it has been used for centuries in the soap, perfumery and cosmetic industries. The dried leaves can also contribute their fragrance to pot-pourris and herb bags.

VETIVER
(Vetiveria zizanioides/Andropogon muricatus – Gramineae)

Vetiver oil comes from vetiver grass which is cultivated in tropical and sub-tropical climates. The grass, a close relative of other aromatic grasses such as lemongrass, is upright with narrow odourless leaves: it is the roots which has a strong scent, similar to sandalwood or violets. In India, vetiver is known as *khas-khas* or *khus-khus*.

The crop is approximately 1 tonne per hectare per year, and each crop yields about 2.7 – 3.2 (6 – 7 lb) of oil. In 1987, the worldwide production of vetiver was about 250 tonnes, with the majority coming from Haiti and Indonesia. In the 1970s, China started to cultivate the grass, and exported substantial quantities; however, most reputable perfumers said it was not of the quality of that from Réunion, generally considered the best.

THE ESSENTIAL OIL

Description: *The grass has to be at least two years old before the roots can be dried in the hot sun. These are then cut up very finely and the oil extracted by use of alcohol, cetone or benzene, or by distillation, the latter the only one for therapeutic use. The oil is a very dark brown with a warm, peppery, spicy, woody, earthy smell.*

The principal constituent: *An alcohol called vetiverol.*
Dangers: *It is an expensive oil as the roots yield so little oil and unfortunately this has led to its adulteration with synthetics. In fact, in the 1970s, vetiver oil acquired such a bad name because of the adulterated version's noxious effects on the skin, that its usage was restricted in many countries. For this reason, it is not now used in therapeutic practice.*

ITS USES

In beauty
Vetiver's main role has always been in perfumery, especially in the Orient. It is used principally as a fixative, and many aftershaves and eau de colognes incorporate vetiver in their formulae. It is also used in high-class soaps. The roots are used powdered in Indian scents.

In cookery
Khas-khas is used in India to flavour sherbets and sweetmeats, and *khas* syrup or water can be found occasionally in specialist Indian shops.

Other uses
Throughout the ages, in both the East and West, vetiver's fragrance has been used to keep insects away. In India, small bundles of roots were hung in wardrobes, and woven into mats, fans and the screens or 'tats' which overhang windows, doors and verandahs (these latter, when wet, cooled the interior of the house, at the same time emitting a wonderful fragrance). Cottons and muslins were impregnated with the oil to protect them, from moths especially. And in Russia, little sachets of essential oil of vetiver were attached to the lining of expensive fur coats. To make insect repellant for furs, wools and cashmeres, impregnate pieces of blotting paper with vetiver oil and leave them in wardrobes and drawers. It is much more effective and sweet-smelling than moth balls.

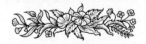

WINTERGREEN *(Gaultheria procumbens – Ericaceae)*

Wintergreen belongs to a genus of 200 species of evergreen flowering shrubs. It originates from the northern United States and Canada, and grows to about 30 cm (12 in) in height. Its habitat can be mountainous where it is often found protected by other trees and taller shrubs, or it also grows on sandy deserted plains. It has large, oval, glossy and toothed leaves, and drooping white or pink bell-shaped flowers, followed by bright red globose berries with a beautifully pronounced aroma.

In America, wintergreen is also known as the partridge berry and checkerberry, and has been used for centuries by the Indians for its remarkable therapeutic properties. They masticated the leaves when they had pain or fever, prepared refreshing drinks with them, and fed the berries to food animals such as poultry, partridge and deer. The leaves were classified in the American pharmacopoeia until recently, but now only the essential oil is mentioned. One early nineteenth-century remedy using wintergreen, called the Swain Panacea, was reputed to cure all sorts of problems. Earlier this century, a French pharmacist made his reputation and fortune by selling a wintergreen cure for all chronic forms of joint and muscle pains.

THE ESSENTIAL OIL

Description: *The leaves have to be macerated for up to 24 hours in hot water in order to produce the fermentation which releases the essentials from which the oil is distilled. The oil is colourless but when older becomes a reddish brown and should not be used.*

The principal constituents: *90 – 95 per cent methyl salicylate, ketone, secondary alcohol, and an ester, the latter two responsible for the characteristic smell – aromatic, reminiscent of camphor, with a note of vanillin and* baume de Pérou.

Dangers: *Unfortunately, commercial wintergreen oils are often made with an artificial base such as salicylic acid, or from distilling the bark of* Betula lenta, *a species of birch. Do obtain the oil from a reputable source otherwise results can be very disappointing.*

ITS USES

In illness
The oil is antiseptic, a diuretic, stimulant, emmenagogue and anti-rheumatic. It is for the latter problem that it is most famous, and most deserves it reputation, as it is very useful in many **rheumatic conditions**, for **gout**, and for **stiffness** due to old age. It also revitalizes and

gives energy following **muscular pains**, particularly good for athletes for instance. The leaves themselves were once warmed and pulped to make poultices for muscular and rheumatic swellings (and boils).

For any of the above conditions, take a hot bath and add 6 drops of the oil. After the bath, rub the affected parts with an oil made from 10 ml (2 tsp) soya oil and 5 drops wintergreen.

(See also **oedema**.*)*

In beauty
Wintergreen can be successful in treating **cellulite** used in conjunction with other essential oils.

YLANG-YLANG *(Cananga odorata – Anonaceae)*

The trees from which the essential oil is distilled – known as perfume trees – originated in the Philippines and have now spread throughout tropical Asia. They were introduced to the island of Réunion in 1884, then to Madagascar, nearby Mayotte and Tahiti; they can be found in the wild in Malaysia, India and Indochina. The trees are generally small, but can reach a height of about 30 m (100 ft). The bark is smooth, with shallow cracks, and the branches 'weep' like willow. The leaves are large, oval and shiny, as much as 20 cm (8 in) long, with a slightly hairy underside. The flowers form in axillary clusters, greenish to start with, then, about 20 days later, they become yellow and very highly perfumed. These flowers appear constantly, but are more abundant in the rainy season. A many-seeded, greenish fruit succeeds the flowers.

Many varieties of the tree are cultivated for their essential oil, the ones bearing the smallest flowers producing the most subtle perfume. (Strangely, the flowers of the wild trees have little perfume.) A young tree of about 5 years old yields about 5 kg (11 lb) flowers; when it reaches the age of 10 years, it can give as much as 10 – 15 kg (22 – 33 lb). In 1979, the world production of ylang-ylang was 100 tonnes, 70 tonnes of which came from the Philippines, considered to be the best oil. Recently, however, exports have diminished due to neglect of the plantations and a shortage of combustible wood for the process of distillation. In addition, pure ylang-ylang has been replaced by an oil from another variety of *Cananga, C. odorata* var. *macrophylla*, which grows abundantly in Java. This gives an essential oil of inferior quality used in cheap perfumes and the soap and cosmetic industries. This oil, called *cananga*, is very much cheaper to buy than the expensive and subtly scented ylang-ylang.

John Ray (1628–1705), an English botanist, was the first to mention the tree, describing it as *'Arbor sanguisant'*; later it was called *'Borga cananga'* and *'Unona odorata'*. In his *Histoire naturelle des drogues simples* (1866) Guibourt described the plant, and compared its scent to that of narcissus; he recorded an island recipe for a pommade made from the flowers of *Cananga* and those of *Curcuma* (turmeric) which the natives used as a body rub to prevent fever and contagion during the rainy season. In the islands, the natives also mixed the flowers with coconut oil to protect their hair from sea salt when they swam; called 'borri-borri', this mixture was also good for the health of the skin, and helped avoid the bites of snakes and insects. The essential oil of *cananga* later became part of the nineteenth-century hair oil known in Europe as Macassar.

A French physician, called Gal, looked into the therapeutic properties of the oil in 1873. Later, at the turn of the century, chemists Garnier and Rechler did some research in Réunion. They found the oil had a good result on malaria, typhus and other fevers. They recommended it as an antiseptic for intestinal infections, diarrhoea and flatulence. They recognized a regulatory heart action and a calming effect. Ylang-ylang has also been classified as a pulmonary and urinary system antiseptic, and a sexual stimulant, good in cases of frigidity. However, a story was reported fairly recently that a man suffering from impotence and knowing of ylang-ylang's aphrodisiac reputation, actually swallowed 5 ml (1 tsp) of the oil. He had a heart attack and later died.

THE ESSENTIAL OIL

Description: *This is produced by the distillation of the fresh flowers, a process which has to be completed very quickly. The oil is very liquid, clear and has an extraordinary fragrance, with high notes of hyacinth and narcissus.*
The principal constituents: *α-pinene, benzoic acid, cadinene, caryophyllene, cresol, eugenol, isoeugenol, 5–7 per cent linalyl acetate, 8–10 per cent linalyl benzoate and 30–32 per cent linalool, and geraniol.*
Dangers: *The oil is very often falsified with cocoa butter or coconut oil. To test, leave a sample in the freezer for a short while; if it has thickened and become cloudy, it is sure to have been adulterated. Sometimes the oil sold as ylang-ylang at a very inflated price is* cananga. *Unfortunately, because of the demand for the oil from the perfumery industry, particularly that of France, the distillers often ignore the use of the oil in therapy; if the oil is not of the very best quality, the therapeutic properties are of little value.*

ITS USES

In illness
Because of its wonderful scent, I have found ylang-ylang particularly useful as a stimulant – (put 5 drops in a warm bath) and as a soother and relaxer. Nervous or emotional people who tend to get palpitations or suffer from low blood pressure, should carry the oil in a small bottle; when nervous, a few drops on a handkerchief, inhaled deeply for a few minutes, will have a very beneficial effect.

(See also **sexual problems** *and* **stress.)**

In beauty
Ylang-ylang in an oil which helps the skin to tan. Mix together in a 60ml brown bottle, 10 ml (2 tsp) coconut oil, 5 ml (1 tsp) wheatgerm oil, 45 ml (3 tbsp) almond oil and 10 drops pure ylang-ylang. Rub into the skin. Use only if you tan easily. Never over-expose yourself, and avoid the sun at midday (the best time for acquiring a good healthy tan is around 4 pm).

(See also **dandruff** *and* **hair problems**.)

Part Three

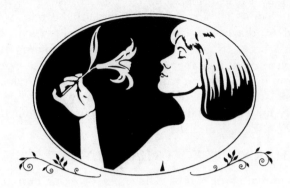

A-Z OF
AILMENTS

Plants and oils marked in bold appear in Part Two, the
A – Z of Aromatherapeutic Plants and Oils, where more
detailed information will be found.

ABDOMINAL PAIN

There are many causes of abdominal pain. Most of them are trivial, but some can point to more serious illness. If the pain is severe or is accompanied by diarrhoea, vomiting, fever or headache, it is best to seek medical advice. In general, pains can be symptoms of less serious disorders such as cystitis, of menstruation, and of digestive problems such as constipation or colic. Even eating hot, spicy or strong foods or eating too fast – the latter often associated with anxiety and stress – can cause discomfort. Some abdominal pains can be caused by pulled muscles.

AROMATHERAPEUTIC TREATMENTS

- Many abdominal pains can be relieved by drinking herb teas. **Chamomile** and **mint** are particularly good. Drink them slowly, and not too hot. After the tea, take ten minutes' rest, lying flat on your back, with feet slightly raised, and breathing slowly. Think about this breathing: hold your breath for a count of four, then relax. A hot water bottle held to the stomach can help.
- A clear vegetable soup with **thyme** and sea salt can help too.
- Put a drop of **chamomile** oil in a bowl of hot water and inhale, breathing as above.
- Gently massage the tummy with oil made from 5 ml (1 tsp) soya oil and 1 drop **chamomile** or **calendula** .

(See also **anaemia, colic, constipation, cystitis, diarrhoea, digestive system problems, indigestion** *and* **stress.***)*

ABSCESSES AND BOILS

An abscess is a pocket of pus that can occur in any part of the body, and is due to invasion of bacteria such as *staphylococci* or *streptococci*. A boil occurs around a hair follicle that has become similarly infected. Both are painful to the touch. White blood cells gather at the inflamed area to get rid of the infection, by absorbing the invaders and liquefying them, thus creating the thick yellow pus. As the white blood cells accumulate, so the liquid matter increases in volume: the boil or abscess then comes to a head, ruptures and the infected pus escapes.

Abscesses and boils tend to appear when someone is run-down, excessively tired, or on a poor diet; they are common, too, at times of hormonal upheaval – puberty, menstruation and menopause – or in those who suffer from acne, diabetes and some blood disorders. If abscesses or boils are large or many, or on the face or neck, a doctor should be consulted as septicaemia could develop. Antibiotics may be prescribed, or the abscess or boil may be lanced to drain it of pus.

If an abscess forms in a joint or gland in the chest or abdominal cavity, medical advice should be sought immediately. *Never* wait until an abscess or boil bursts, as this could lead to a serious general infection.

Many essential oils can be of help, primarily because of their antiseptic and antibiotic properties. There are as many different types and causes of abscesses and boils as there are kinds of skin, so you may have to experiment with different oils. Those which are particularly effective are **basil, chamomile, eucalyptus, geranium, juniper, lavender, oregano, palmarosa, rosemary, clary sage, thuja, thyme** and **wintergreen. Tea tree oil** is now being hailed as a wonder remedy, as it works on the pus without affecting the surrounding tissue. Chamomile and clary sage are the best for sensitive skins.

AROMATHERAPEUTIC TREATMENTS

(See also **baume de Pérou, galbanum, patchouli, sandalwood** *and* **savory**.*)*

- When pus starts to gather, at an early stage of abscess or boil – even when the area is simply inflamed – apply heat, then dab the area and spot gently with **tea tree** oil. Apply castor oil afterwards. This allows the pus to collect, and avoids the infection spreading.
- Local heat can also be applied to draw out pus and bring boils or abscesses to a head. Make up a poultice of crushed linseed or oatmeal (see pages 23–4), add a few drops of essential oil – **oregano** or **tea tree**, for instance – apply, and leave in place for the advised time.
- Whatever the cause, a change of diet, even if temporary, is indicated to help clean out the system. Fast for a day, drinking only mineral water, then eats lots of raw fruit and vegetables. Avoid stimulants like alcohol, tea and coffee, and eliminate fat and animal products for a short time. When you start cooking again, include lots of herbs, garlic and onions.
- Immaculate cleanliness is vital as infection can spread. The sufferers must always use separate towels, and these should ideally be washed and boiled frequently to avoid re-infection. Add a few drops of tea tree oil or oregano oil to the final rinsing water to disinfect the towels.
- To draw pus, boil face towels in water with a drop of the chosen oil, then apply as hot as possible to the affected area. This is particularly good for facial acne.
- In France, fresh chervil or **parsley** are crushed and applied to boils. This is also good for inflammation, bruising and broken capillaries.
- Apply an essential oil neat on a cotton wool bud to the boil or abscess.

- A few drops of an oil can be added to bath water.
- Boils on the back can be treated by a green clay mask (see page 24) once or twice a week. Using a cotton wool bud dab on an essential oil – **juniper, oregano** or **basil**, say – three times a day.
- If an abscess is caused by a thorn, a whitlow or similar, boil 600 ml (1 pint) water with 15 ml (1 tbsp) sea salt, and leave covered in a bowl to cool to a bearable heat. Meanwhile clean the finger or area as thoroughly as possible with some **chamomile, oregano** or **tea tree** oil. Dip the finger in the water for as long as you can stand it, then clean again with the essential oil, and cover with a thick plaster of clay (see page 24), containing 1 drop of the same oil. Leave as long as possible again and this will draw the pus and matter out. Clean off with boiled water and finish with essential oil once more.
- Cut a fresh fig in half and heat through briefly in the oven. When hot but still juicy, apply the cut side as hot as possible to an abscess. The heat and a property of the fig – perhaps simply its stickiness – will draw the abscess.

(See also **acne, anthrax, dental abscesses, follicultis** *and* **skin problems.)**

ABSCESSES, DENTAL

(See dental abscesses.)

ACNE

Acne is a very common skin condition, caused by over-production of oil in the glands of the skin particularly on the face, chest and back. It generally occurs at puberty or menopause and is due to hormonal imbalances. The excess oil blocks the pores, often forming blackheads, and if these become infected with bacteria, spots or boils can develop. Acne can be mild – such as the small pimples that many women develop before their periods – or it can be severe, causing cysts or boils, scarring and enlarged pores.

Stress and anxiety can play a part in acne, and many adolescents and young adults suffer particularly. Diet, exercise, fresh air and cleanliness are vital in acne treatments.

Essential oils can be very helpful in acne treatments. The oils suggested below have been working for me in my practice for some 26 years, but if

lavender, say, doesn't work after a month, then you should try another essential to see if that suits your skin better. You might also have to consider the source of your oil, checking that it is top quality, and it may be necessary to try a new shop or supplier. Once you have started with one oil, it is always best to use that oil for everything whether it be for cleansing, saunas, baths or poultices, for example.

Treating acne with essential oils is a slow process, so do not expect instant results. It may take up to a year, but healthy skin will be the result.

AROMATHERAPEUTIC TREATMENTS

- Make herbal teas with fresh **chamomile**, chervil or **rose petals**, which are all good for the skin. To combat the stress which so often accompanies as well as causes acne, drink teas made from **orange** blossom (bigaradier) and leaves, both of which are naturally antiseptic and tranquillizing.
- Meticulous cleansing is vital. An acne skin is very sensitive, and at the beginning should be looked after like a baby's skin! Wash gently with an unscented pH balanced soap in warm water, and rinse thoroughly in cold. Make an astringent by boiling a sprig of fresh thyme in 600 ml (1 pint) water, then leaving to infuse for 5 minutes. Add a little lemon juice when cool, then rinse the skin with this two to three times a day. You could use a pinch each of **mint** and **savory** for a stimulant astringent; or a pinch each of fresh chervil, **rosemary** and **savory**, for the natural and gentle antibiotic action of the chervil.
- Use morning and night after cleansing. Don't be afraid to put oils on your already oily skin: these natural essences contain substances which act on the skin oils, and will quickly be absorbed. Keep the oils in a small dark glass bottle. Some good essential oils for acne are **aspic, calendula, chamomile, juniper, lavender, mint, myrrh, myrtle, neroli, palmarosa, patchouli, petitgrain, tea tree,** and **thyme:**
- For a *normal* skin, mix together 50 ml (2 fl oz) soya oil, 6 drops wheatgerm oil and 10 drops of your chosen oil.
- For an *extra sensitive* skin, mix together 25 ml (1 fl oz) soya oil, 25 ml (1 fl oz) almond oil, 6 drops wheatgerm oil and 10 drops of your chosen oil.
- Apply these oils twice, the second application when the first has been absorbed: use hot compresses – pads of gauze dipped in boiled water – to aid the absorption.
- Men with acne need to be very careful when shaving. They must not use electric or battery shavers, but a razor with blades. These blades must be changed every time – an expensive business, but avoids re-infection if a spot or boil is nicked. Apply wet hot towels to the

face as the barber would do, containing a few drops of essential oil. Then use a facial oil instead of aftershave, as for the normal skin above, but using oils with more masculine smells such as **lavender** or **tea tree.**

- Pure essences can be applied neat to individual boils or abscesses, never anywhere else. Apply at night after cleansing, using cotton wool buds, and continue until the boil has completely disappeared.
- Have a facial sauna three or four times a week (see page 22), using a drop each of **lavender, chamomile** and **petitgrain**, or 2 – 3 drops of either **tea tree** or **lavender.**

OTHER TREATMENTS

- Eat a good diet, because eating badly can make the condition worse. If your diet contains too much sugar, for instance, this encourages bacteria. Ensure you have well-balanced meals containing foods rich in the skin vitamins A, B_6, B_{12}, E and F, plus plenty of fresh fruit and vegetables. Eat plenty of garlic and onions for their bactericidal properties, and celery for its blood-cleansing properties.
- Avoid fatty foods such as pork and lamb, as well as chocolate and sweets. Drink mineral water, diluted fruit juices and herbal tisanes instead of the stimulant tea, coffee and alcohol.
- If you are prone to eating snacks, replace them with dried almonds (which contain magnesium), walnuts, pumpkin and sunflower seeds.
- Take plenty of exercise, particularly out of doors. Sunlight can be very helpful, but does not produce a cure.

(See also **abscesses and boils, anxiety, constipation, menopause, skin problems** *and* **stress.***)*

AGEING SKIN

As the body ages, cell division slows down. This happens at different times in different people, and can be affected by many outside factors (see below). As far as the skin is concerned, the slowing down of cell division means that various organs in the skin work less efficiently. The inner dermis network of collagen and elastin fibres which gives skin its plump contours, suppleness and firmness, begins to alter, losing its tension and plumpness, and wrinkles form. The outer layer of skin cells, the epidermis, also becomes thinner resulting in the flat, lifeless appearance of an older skin.

Nothing can prevent this natural process, but essential oils can do more than most potions to slow down the effects. Essential oils encourage the skin cells to regenerate more efficiently, and help the skin to lubricate itself, keeping it supple and less prone to wrinkling, as long as you use them in moderation.

AGEING FACTORS

- Diet is of supreme importance, as the quality of the food you eat will make a difference as to how the organs of the body operate. The proper nutrients will make these work more efficiently, and the skin will directly benefit. The main dietary culprits as far as skin is concerned are excess alcohol, tea and coffee, which are all diuretic and stimulants.
- Illness and strong drugs affect the skin, too, hastening ageing, as does cigarette smoking.
- The sun is a major factor in premature ageing of the skin. The UV rays actually dry up the collagen and water in the skin, causing wrinkles, and make the skin feel leathery. Faces should always be shaded or sunblocked, whether swimming in Florida or ski-ing in the Alps. UV lamps are as dangerous to the ageing skin.
- Central heating can dry up some skins, as most rooms are not well ventilated. As the skin on the face is so exposed all the time, in and out, it must be very carefully looked after.
- Fresh air and moderate exercise are good for the circulation and thus the skin. Excess exercise, however, can be deleterious: many athletes and ballet dancers, for instance, age very early, as minerals and other nutrients required by the whole body, including the skin, have already been appropriated.
- Stress is also an ageing factor hastening the natural process, and the skin can suffer during times of major emotional upheaval, such as death of someone close, or a divorce.

AROMATHERAPEUTIC TREATMENTS

- Eat moderately of a good healthy diet, and drink a lot of mineral water and herbal teas (this also helps to minimize the drying effect of exposure to sun, wind and central heating).
- Relax as much as possible, try not to worry about things, and drink tisanes made from naturally tranquillizing ingredients such as orange blossom and orange leaves.
- Massage essential oils into the skin. The oils are of benefit, but so is the actual massage, encouraging the circulation and improving the muscle tone.

227

● Use 50 ml (2 fl oz) almond or hazelnut oil (for sensitive skins), or wheatgerm as a base. Add 8 drops of your chosen essential oil, for a six weeks' supply, and store in a dark bottle. Use morning and night.

> *Dry skin* **rose** or **galbanum**
> *Dry patches* **carrot**
> *Wrinkles* **rosemary** to start, then **rose** or **galbanum**
> *Blackheads* **juniper** or **neroli**
> *Broken capillaries* **rose** or **cypress**, with witch-hazel compresses

● A beauty mask once a week can help an ageing skin. Mix together 30 ml (2 tbsp) runny honey and 4 drops of your chosen oil. Apply with a spatula over the face, leave for 10 minutes, then remove with warm water. Apply some witch-hazel or rose water. If the skin feels very dry after one application, apply again.

(*See also* **orange, palmarosa, patchouli** *and* **rose**.)

(*See also* **anxiety, broken capillaries, depression, menopause** *and* **skin problems**.)

ALOPECIA

Alopecia is the medical word for loss of hair, and it can be partial or total. If the hair loss occurs in patches, it is known as alopecia areata; if loss is total, it is alopecia totalis. Alopecia includes what is called male pattern baldness. In men this is generally inherited, and varies with age. Women can suffer from age-related hair loss or hair thinning, but can also suffer during times of hormonal upheaval such as pregnancy and menopause. Hair loss can be caused by a number of different illnesses (typhoid, for instance), some treatments for major illnesses (chemotherapy and radiotherapy), and by bad diet or malnutrition. Stress can be a contributory factor, but by far the most common cause in women is maltreatment of the hair – repeated dyeing, bleaching, perming, etc.

In some cases of hair loss, broken skin can form scabs and scars; hair will not grow back through scarred skin.

AROMATHERAPEUTIC TREATMENTS

● Massage is very effective for the problem, stimulating the skin and underlying hair follicles. See the oils below.
● A strong nettle or watercress decoction rubbed in to the scalp can help

retain and encourage hair growth. This is an old French remedy. Bring 60 ml (4 tbsp) nettle leaves to the boil in 500 ml (18 fl oz) water. Boil for 7 minutes, then simmer for 20 minutes. Strain and pour into a bottle and add 45 ml (3 tbsp) cider vinegar. Rub some of this into the scalp twice a day.

Pimento massage oil

20 ml (4 tsp) coconut oil, warmed
3 drops wheatgerm oil
6 drops **pimento** *oil*

Mix these together, and rub your scalp with a little a few times per week.

Horseradish massage oil

Horseradish is the most important oil for the hair, and this should be used as soon as hair loss begins. If you can't find horseradish oil, the juice of the root could be used instead.

40 ml (1 ½ fl oz) grapeseed oil
10 ml (2 tsp) soya oil
2 drops wheatgerm oil
15 drops **horseradish** *oil*

Mix together. Apply to the scalp and massage very gently. Leave for a few hours, then wash off with a very mild shampoo.

Clary sage massage oil

Clary lotions and rubs can help prevent oiliness and dandruff as well as revitalize growth, helping alopecia and general hair loss.

20 ml (4 tsp) soya oil
5 drops **clary sage** *oil*
5 drops rum

Mix these together and apply twice a week, massaging in well. Leave overnight if possible, and shampoo off in the morning.

(See also **chamomile** *and* **tarragon**.*)*

OTHER TREATMENTS

- A major treatment to prevent hair loss, and reverse the loss once it has started, is dietary. Rather than taking pills, eat more foods which

229

contain vitamins and minerals that are good for the hair, capillaries and circulatory system. Cut down on stimulants such as tea and coffee, and drink calming tisanes such as savory, thyme, mint, bigaradier (orange leaves) and melissa.

Vitamins B, C and F are good for the hair; cobalt and iron are helpful in regulating the circulatory system; copper helps stop hair falling; iodine protects the capillaries; and magnesium is a general tonic.

- As stress can contribute to the problem, eat foods with the natural sedative bromine in them: asparagus, celery, cabbage, melon, leeks, radishes and raisins.

AMENORRHOEA

This is the absence of normal menstruation in women after puberty and before the menopause. It is not unusual for a girl to miss a few periods when she has recently started menstruating, but in later life, irregularity can be a symptom of something amiss. Pregnancy and breast-feeding are obvious times when bleeding does not occur; sometimes after stopping taking the contraceptive pill, periods may not be regular again for up to a year.

Women suffering from anorexia nervosa often stop menstruating because the body lacks the necessary nutrients to synthesize the hormones involved in the menstrual cycle. Shock or severe stress can also interfere with the cycle as can several illnesses. Long-distance air travel can disturb the cycle too: many air-hostesses, for instance, don't have regular periods because the body clock is in constant turmoil.

AROMATHERAPEUTIC TREATMENTS

- **Sage** leaves, which are highly oestrogenic, should be taken in tisane form (together with some chamomile). Drink **chamomile** in tisane form too.
- Rub the tummy with an oil made from 20 ml (4 tsp) soya oil, 2 drops wheatgerm oil, and 4 drops each of **clary sage** and **chamomile** oil. (You could use 8 drops of either instead, or 8 drops **parsley** or **cypress** oil.)
- Avoid stimulants like tea, coffee or alcohol. Drink herbal teas and tisanes instead.
- **Parsley** as a tisane or eaten raw is good too, regulating periods.

ANAEMIA

Anaemia, the most common of the blood diseases, is caused by a deficiency of haemoglobin, the chemical that carries oxygen in the blood. If haemoglobin is reduced, oxygen is less available to all body cells, including those of the brain, and this can cause dizziness, tiredness, pallor of skin, weakness, brittle nails, lack of appetite, abdominal pains and general malaise. There are several types, but the most common is iron-deficiency anaemia, due to a lack of iron, the trace element which produces haemoglobin. This anaemia can be caused by heavy menstrual bleeding, blood loss after an operation, dental or medical, and is common in pregnancy, when iron supplies are being utilized by the growing foetus.

To avoid the condition eat a diet rich in iron and the B vitamins, particularly B_6, B_{12} and folic acid, all needed for the blood.

AROMATHERAPEUTIC TREATMENTS

- Carrots are particularly valuable for anaemia because of the carotene, which helps fix iron in food. They must be eaten raw, or cooked very quickly (in a wok, say). Thyme used in cooking also fixes iron (add it to vegetable cooking water).
- Drink lots of fresh orange juice as vitamin C helps the body absorb iron. Blackcurrants are even more rich in vitamin C.
- Anaemics don't enjoy eating, so their appetites need to be stimulated. Good foods are cabbage, fennel, mint, ginseng, onion, apple, watercress, celery, rosemary, savory, parsley, thyme and horseradish. With the meal, a glass of port or red wine – claret or Burgundy – can help stimulate appetite too.
- To revitalize the body, mix together 50 ml (2 fl oz) soya oil, 2 drops wheatgerm oil and 3 drops each of **lavender** and **melissa** oils. Rub this in daily. For the same effect, rub neat lavender or melissa oils – you could alternate them – into the tops of the hands or soles of the feet every day.

Liver with spinach and mâche salad

This makes a really nice and revitalizing lunch, especially during menstruation. Use common sense about quantities! The liver and spinach are both high in iron, and the *mâche* – or lamb's lettuce – is high in chlorophyll, also revitalizing.

Leave lamb's or chicken liver in milk for 30 minutes to rid it of toxins, then pat dry, cut into small pieces and dip in wholemeal flour. Fry some chopped onions in a little olive oil until softened, then add the liver and some fresh sage leaves. Fry for a few minutes only, until just cooked.

231

Prepare a spinach and *mâche* salad, and dress with fresh lemon juice and a little freshly ground black pepper. Add the cooked liver and onion to this. (In season, a few sage flowers would be delicious.) Accompany with a glass of red wine which contains many minerals.

(*See also* **abdominal pains, appetite, loss of,** *and* **fatigue**.)

ANOREXIA NERVOSA

A complex disorder in which individuals – usually adolescent girls in western societies – show a strong aversion to food because they are scared of putting on weight. It is thought to have a variety of causes – among them social pressure and fashions which equate slimness with beauty, family pressures to succeed, or family disharmony. The girls fail to eat, or if they do eat, they purge themselves with laxatives or by self-induced vomiting. They lose weight at an astonishing rate and can become severely ill, requiring hospital and psychiatric treatment.

Even at quite early stages of the condition many of the vital organs and functions of the body can suffer. Anorexia nervosa can be fatal.

If you have a teenager at home who is anorexic, take great care of her/him, and seek sympathetic medical advice. A happy home atmosphere is vital for an anorexic. Reduce all pressures, have things as near normal as possible, and above all, do not lecture about food. No one should ever be forced to eat.

The food which you serve an anorexic must be appetizing, attractive, interesting and colourful to look at. Salads of mixed leaves, dark and light greens, are good, and you could add the bright colours of fruit such as bananas and apples, with nuts and raisins. Make the effort to cook what used to be the sufferer's favourite dishes and reassure them that the right food in small quantities will not fatten or result in weight gain. Offer small portions of food a few times a day. Some possibilities might be a meat consommé or light vegetable broth; a pudding made from milk with mixed cereals such as millet, rice and/or buckwheat; a lot of fruit juices, freshly squeezed.

AROMATHERAPEUTIC TREATMENTS

- For a suspected anorexic, cook foods containing lots of herbs and spices. The aroma of these can often restore an appetite. The culinary bay leaf and coriander are particularly good.
- Some herbal tisanes can help stimulate appetite. **Marjoram, melissa** and **thyme** are good, either a little of each together, or on their own.

Add 5 ml (1 tsp) leaves to 600 ml (1 pint) boiling water and infuse for 7 minutes. Drink between meals, sweetened with a little lavender, rosemary or acacia honey.

• The same essential oils can help stimulate appetite too. Use **marjoram, thyme** or **melissa** oils neat on the back of the hands, the soles and tops of the feet, and the solar plexus. Or you could add 3 drops of one of them to 10 ml (2 tsp) soya oil and 2 drops wheatgerm oil, for rubbing into the body.

(*See also* **appetite, loss of,** *and* **stress**.)

ANOSMIA

This means the complete loss of the sense of smell. It can be temporary, as during a cold, or it can be permanent, when the olfactory nerves are damaged by disease or injury. Some virus infections, brain injury or tumour, shock and some drugs can cause a permanent loss.

Whether temporary or permanent, this can be a very distressing problem, as the sense of smell gives so much pleasure and has so many beneficial aspects – helping digestion, for instance.

AROMATHERAPEUTIC TREATMENTS

• Put some sea salt and 1 drop of **chamomile** oil and/or **rosemary** oil in a bowl of hot water and inhale with a towel over your head. Do this a few times a week. If you can't find these oils, use a pinch each of **basil** and **chamomile** leaves in the hot water.

• Mix together a drop of **chamomile**, 10 ml (2 tsp) **grapeseed** oil and 2 drops wheatgerm oil. Massage this gently around the nose, paying particular attention to the curve of the bone and out as far as the cheek bones on either side.

OTHER TREATMENTS

• Often excessive dryness inside the nose can cause deficiences in the sense of smell. This must be corrected by putting some moisturizing oil in each nostril or spraying distilled water near the nostrils. Walking in the rain can help too. Turn off central heating in the bedroom – where you spend a major proportion of each 24 hours – or use a humidifier with a drop of essential oil added.

ANTHRAX

Anthrax is a disease of sheep and cattle, caused by the bacterium *Bacillum anthracis*, which can be transmitted to man. The meat, skin, hair and excreta of affected animals can carry the infection. Butchers, vets, farmers and woolworkers are the most vulnerable to the disease, which can pass through a skin abrasion or bite; woolworkers can inhale the organism which leads to a form of bronchopneumonia. The first symptom is normally a painful itching followed by a pimple or boil on the body, usually the face or neck; this becomes hard with a reddish purple centre under which pus collects. Many boils can lead to serious illness, with weakness, nausea and high fever; gangrene can develop in affected areas.

Anthrax in humans is extremely rare, but isolated outbreaks in animals do occur. Everyone dealing with infected animals should take very careful precautions, and should consult a doctor immediately if the condition is suspected. Preventive vaccines are available to farm workers, and large doses of antibiotics can treat the disease once developed.

AROMATHERAPEUTIC TREATMENT

- Anyone dealing with (sick) animals should clean their hands thoroughly afterwards, using 15 drops of **tea tree, thyme** or **geranium** oils to 600 ml (1 pint(distilled water.

(*See also* **abscesses** *and* **boils**.)

ANXIETY

(*See* **stress**.)

APPETITE, LOSS OF

An unwillingness or inability to eat can be a symptom of a wide variety of diseases. It can be serious, as in a teenage girl suffering from anorexia nervosa, or a baby or old person; but usually it is temporary, the result of a minor infection or disorder such as indigestion, gastroenteristis, colds or tonsillitis, or it could be that your body needs a rest from food. If a baby is not feeding, consult your doctor.

AROMATHERAPEUTIC TREATMENTS

- Herbal teas such as **fennel** or **anise** are good appetizers, mixed with **verbena** or **mint.**
- The smell of cooking is a major appetite enhancer. Microwave ovens are distinctly unhealthy in this way as there is no smell when food is cooked in them. The look of food is as important to an older, reluctant eater as it is to a child.
- Mix 3 drops of **rose** essential oil into 5 ml (1 tsp) wheatgerm oil, and massage into the solar plexus before meals.

(*See also* **chamomile** *and* **cloves.**)

OTHER TREATMENTS

- All children go through phases of not wanting to eat. One way of getting round this is to make food and eating fun for them. I remember forming faces on the plate for my son: a base of mashed potato with tomatoe wedge ears, pea or bean eyes, beetroot mouth and sticks of celery for the hair. Most children would respond to this 'game' and enjoy eating it!
- Dr Maury recommends a glass of Banyuls or Sauternes before meals as an appetizing aperitif.

(*See also* **anorexia nervosa.**)

ARTHRITIS

There are several forms of arthritis, the general term for inflammation of a joint. Osteoarthritis mainly affects the load-bearing hips, knees, spine and shoulders, and is to a certain extent the result of the natural wear and tear of ageing. Rheumatoid arthritis is a disease of the connective tissue which can appear – usually because of family history – in quite young people. Arthritis can also appear after injury, physical over-exertion or intense emotional stress, usually between the ages of 30 and 40. Wearing away of bone or loss of the synovial fluid which lubricates the joints, can cause intense pain and restrict movement.

The symptoms of rheumatoid arthritis include swelling and pain in the joints (particularly on movement), fatigue, weight loss, anaemia and fever, with skin over the affected part hot and shiny. These symptoms can disappear and recur at a later date.

AROMATHERAPEUTIC TREATMENTS

- Apply hot compresses to the affected areas morning and night. Dip a small towel in a basin containing very hot water, mixed with 15 ml (1 tbsp) cider vinegar, 2 drops each of **pine** and **cypress** oils, and 1 drop of **lavender** oil. Follow with an application of an olive or nut oil. Keep the area warm.
- Make up an emulsion with something like a mild shampoo, adding to it 1 drop each of **pine, juniper** and **cypress** oils. Add to a bath when running the hot water and lie in it as long as possible. Afterwards wrap yourself in a warm towelling dressing gown and rest on your bed for 10 minutes.

Pimento massage oil

The pimento oil is very warming, so can help relieve pain.

10 ml (2 tsp) soya oil
2 drops wheatgerm oil
3 drops pimento oil

Mix together and apply to the affected area. Massage in well, then cover with a hot compress or poultice. Apply soya oil neat to the skin afterwards, as it might be tender.

OTHER TREATMENTS

- Arthritis sufferers should watch their weight, as increased poundage leads to increased pressure on the joints. Follow a good reducing diet and eat healthily.
- During attacks, avoid meat, salt, coffee, alcohol, tobacco and fats. Eat a vegetarian diet for a while, re-introducing meat very slowly into the diet.
- Eat vegetables which are beneficial such as artichokes, asparagus, cucumber, cabbage, beans, endive, leeks, mâche or lamb's lettuce, radishes, sorrel and tomatoes. Eat fruits such as apples, bananas, blackcurrants, cherries, grapes, grapefruit and strawberries. All these detoxify, cleansing the system.
- Eat foods which contain calcium and magnesium – needed to form the lubricant synovial fluid – such as milk (goat's in particular), watercress, parsley, pulses such as lentil, nuts (but *not* salted ones as sodium or salt must be avoided), and proteins such as sardines and mackerel.
- Exercise is often good for the initial stages of osteoarthritis, because keeping the joints mobile prevents them seizing up.
- Drink a tea made from apple skins during attacks. Wash 2 apples well first, then boil the skins in 600 ml (1 pint) water for 15 minutes. Drink throughout the day.

(*See also* **backache, bursitis, inflammation, lumbago, muscular pains, rheumatism, sciatica, stiffness** *and* **stress**.)

ASTHMA .

Asthma is a disorder of the upper respiratory tract, in which the smooth muscles of the walls of the bronchi of the lungs contract in spasm, narrowing the air passage. This characteristically causes shortness of breath, wheezing, choking and coughing. It often goes hand in hand with bronchitis, nervous disorders and hayfever, and also tends to afflict people of a nervous disposition. However, almost half of the incidences of asthma are allergy-induced, starting in childhood (and often in relation to eczema). As with hayfever, pollen, dust, feathers and animal fur can be the allergens.

Asthma sufferers should avoid using essential oils as many can provoke allergic reactions. The adulteration and falsification of so many oils can make it difficult to rely totally on the oil and its source. You should consult your doctor or practitioner to have any oils tested. Inhalations of essential oils, for instance, may actually worsen an asthma attack.

Discover the allergen if you can – remove dust-harbouring curtains, carpets, cushions and feather pillows, and vacuum clean daily. Avoid pets if possible.

AROMATHERAPEUTIC TREATMENTS

- Avoid stimulants such as tea, chocolate and coffee, and replace with herbal tisanes: **eucalyptus** and **thyme** together; or *tilleul* (lime or linden flowers), **marjoram, thyme** and **savory**. Add 30 g (a good ounce) dried or fresh herb or flower to 1 litre (1 ¾ pints) boiling water. Infuse for 20 minutes, then drink two to three large cups per day. This is especially helpful during an asthma attack.

(*See also* **anise, basil, myssop, laurel, rosemary** *and* **clary sage**.)

- Take as much exercise as possible. Swimming is good because there are few irritants like dust or pollen.

(*See also* **hayfever** *and* **respiratory system problems**.)

ATHLETE'S FOOT

This is a fungal infection of the feet, known medically as *Tinea pedis*. It is a form of ringworm and the flesh between the toes becomes soggy and flaky, and it is very itchy. If the toenails are affected, they become brittle and discoloured. It is highly contagious and is commonly transmitted in places like gymnasium and swimming pool changing rooms and bathroom floors, as the fungus thrives in these moist conditions. At home, sufferers must use their own towels and wear protective footwear.

AROMATHERAPEUTIC TREATMENTS

- When going to places where the infection might be picked up, rub the feet before and after with neat **tea tree** or **geranium** oil.
- If you do pick up the infection, mix together 10 ml (2 tsp) soya oil and 2 drops each of wheatgerm, **tea tree** and **geranium** oils. Rub in between the toes, and around the nails every day.
- Bathe the feet often in a large bowl of salted water containing 5 drops of **tea tree** or **clary sage** oil. Soak for 10 minutes at least, then dry thoroughly.

(*See also* **lemongrass**.)

OTHER TREATMENTS

- Sweaty feet are most prone to the fungus. Feet which are enclosed in nylon socks will sweat more and encourage the fungus. Wear cotton socks when necessary, and open sandals as often as possible. Change socks daily and wash them very thoroughly.
- Foods rich in vitamin A are necessary for the general health of the skin. These include apricots, oily fish, and yellow and dark-green fruits and vegetables.

BACKACHE

Backache may originate from a multiplicity of complaints. The cause of any type of backache must be established before any treatment can be undertaken. In the case of a sudden pain such as that of lumbago, an awkward movement or lifting something heavy may be the origin of the pain: or prolonged standing can impose unusual strain which has a perceptible effect on the body and can be responsible for back pain. High heels can tilt the body off balance, as can the frontal bulk of a pregnancy. Flat feet or a slight difference between the length of legs can put the body off balance; this demands an abnormal effort from the back to maintain the correct position.

Occasionally an infection, like 'flu, can attack the back as it can affect the joints or the larger muscles involved.

AROMATHERAPEUTIC TREATMENTS

- Take hot to warm baths containing essential oils: a few drops of **aspic, juniper, lavender, nutmeg, pepper, pine** or **rosemary,** are all valuable oils.
- After the bath, lie on your bed or on a carpeted floor, and massage the painful area – or get someome else to do it for you. Put a small pillow under your stomach to keep the back supported. Use 5 drops of any of the above oils in 10 ml (2 tsp) soya or grapeseed oil.
- You could also fill a flannel glove with fresh **pine** needles, **rosemary** or **lavender**, dunk it in boiling water, and place it on the back.
- A poultice (see pages 23 – 4) made with one of the above oils can help alleviate pain very quickly.
- Backache not only loses the most working days in a year of *any* complaint, but it can also cause a great deal of stress and nervous tension. Put a few drops of a calming oil – **mandarin, neroli, petitgrain, rosemary** or **thyme** – on a piece of cotton wool and put on a lamp or radiator near you.

OTHER TREATMENTS

- Once the cause is established, treat appropriately. A new mattress which offers good support may be required.
- Gentle exercise, like swimming, is good for sore backs, as are stretching exercises. Often, weakened stomach muscles can contribute to back problems.

(*See also* **bursitis, lumbago, muscular pains, rheumatism, sciatica** *and* **stress**.)

BEDSORES

Also known as pressure sores, these are painful places which can become ulcerations, occurring on the body where there is constant pressure and irritation. They are most common on the buttocks, heels and elbows of bedridden patients.

AROMATHERAPEUTIC TREATMENTS

- The sores develop because of a lack of blood supply to the skin – particularly in old people, who already have a poor supply. One answer is massage, which assists the circulation, and **chamomile, geranium** and **patchouli** oils are particularly helpful.

Massage oil
This should be used before and after sores develop.

20 ml (4 tsp) castor oil
4 drops wheatgerm oil
3 drops **chamomile** *or* **geranium** *oil*

Mix together, and massage into vulnerable or affected areas.

OTHER TREATMENTS

- Turning the patient as often as possible can prevent the sores.
- Keep the skin dry and clean, and use protective padding.

BITES

(*See* **stings.**)

BLISTERS

A blister is an area of skin swollen by an accumulation of fluid – serum, the watery component of blood – underneath. Blisters can be the result of injuries, burning, scalding, chafing (from new shoes, or unaccustomed manual work), or insect stings, or can be caused by infections such as eczema, impetigo, herpes or chickenpox. When a blister bursts, the revealed tissue beneath may become infected, so it must be kept clean.

Treat as for **burns** or **cuts and wounds**.

BROKEN VEINS AND CAPILLARIES

Characterized by fine red spider veins in the cheeks, this is a circulatory problem that afflicts fair delicate skins which also tend to burn in the sun. The effect at a distance is that of ruddiness. Often the capillaries are not actually broken, just weak and transparent so that the blood shows through them.

AROMATHERAPEUTIC TREATMENTS

- Use cool compresses of **parsley** tea on the face daily, and massage with an oil containing parsley oil (see page 169).
- **Palmarosa** is effective too; mix 3 drops of palmarosa and wheatgerm into 5 ml (1 tsp) almond oil. Apply at night.
- **Rose** essential oil is very effective for capillaries, see page 183. Other good oils are **calendula, carrot, chamomile** and **cypress**.
- Avoid stimulants such as tea, coffee, alcohol and chocolate which cause the capillaries to dilate. Drink herbal teas such as rosehip, and freshly squeezed fruit juice.

OTHER TREATMENTS

- Eat foods rich in bioflaonoids and vitamin C, both vital for capillary strength and health: citrus fruit, fresh vegetables and buckwheat. Wheatgerm contains vitamin E which promotes better circulation.
- Protect the skin from sunlight and strong or icy winds. Use sun blocks and good barrier creams.
- Never wash your face in hot water or use facial saunas. Over-hot baths, saunas and Turkish baths should be avoided too.

(*See also* **ageing skin, circulatory problems, constipation, haemorrhoids** and **varicose veins**.)

BRONCHITIS

Bronchitis is an inflammation of the larger air passages – the bronchi – which lead to the lungs. There are two categories. Acute or sudden onset bronchitis can occur after a bacterial or viral infection such as a cold; this persists and leads to a chronic cough. Acute bronchitis can be particularly dangers in babies and old people because of the increased risk of pneumonia. Chronic bronchitis is caused by long-standing irritation of the lining of the bronchi, such as cigarette smoking or living or working in a damp, foggy, dusty or fume-laden atmosphere. Some people seem to be more prone than others to developing bronchitis. When the weather is changeable – as in spring or autumn – the tendency to develop the disease is greater. Bad posture, lack of exercise and nervous tension can all make one more suceptible to suffering from the disease because they reduce the ability of the lungs to work to full capacity.

The principal symptoms are coughing, phlegm production, fever and chest pains.

AROMATHERAPEUTIC TREATMENTS

- None of these remedies will work if you continue to smoke.
- Drink plenty of fluids, especially fresh pineapple and lemon juices and hot herbal tisanes. Use bay (**laurel**) leaves, **eucalyptus leaves, hyssop, lavender, mint, pine** buds or **rosemary**. Hyssop, eucalyptus and bay are expectorant. Boil 15 ml (1 tbsp) leaves in 600 ml (1 pint) water for 3 minutes, then infuse for 5 minutes. Drink, sweetened with honey, a few times per day.
- A good tea for acute bronchitis is made by boiling together 5 **cloves** and 6 **eucalyptus** leaves in 600 ml (1 pint) water for 2 minutes. Leave to steep for at least 5 minutes, then strain and add the juice of a ½ lemon.
- Teas made from marshmallow flowers and leaves, or olive leaves, are also thought by French phytotherapists to be beneficial.
- Always make sure that there is sufficient humidity in the sickroom or bedroom. If you do not have a humidifier, vaporize the room during the day and one hour before bedtime. Use a mixture of 600 ml (1 pint) warm water, 15 drops **eucalyptus** oil and 5 drops **oregano** oil (or 15 of **tea tree** plus 5 of **lavender**). Shake the vaporizer well before use.
- An alternative to using a humidifier is to have a bowl or large dish containing water and a few drops of oils, as above, beside the radiator.
- Apply a poultice of linseed or **mustard** seeds to chest and back (see page 24). Make up an oil with 15 ml (1 tbsp) soya oil, 2 drops wheatgerm oil, 5 drops **eucalyptus** oil and 2 drops **oregano** oil. Rub this into chest and back after the poultice has lost its heat.

OTHER TREATMENTS

- Nutritious food is essential in building up the body's defences. A poor diet which fails to supply the body with sufficient quantities of nutrients will mean an undernourished body less able to fight off infection. Vitamins A and C are important, as are proteins and plenty of fluids.
- For long-term prevention of bronchitis, eat lots of garlic and onions, raw when possible, for their antibacterial effect. Supplement with two to four garlic perles daily, especially during the winter months.

Other good foods are turnips, radishes, horseradish and seaweed, all lubrificant.

- During a bout of bronchitis, the patient must be kept in a constant temperature, a warm bed in a warm bedroom. Cold damp air can act as an irritant, as can direct heat – from an open fire, say, which also produces sulphur dioxide, one of the air pollutants which can cause chronic bronchitis.
- A turnip 'syrup' can be helpful. Peel and slice 900 g (2 lb) turnips and arrange on a flat dish. Cover with 450 g (1 lb) fructose, and leave for a few hours. The turnip juices will mix with the fructose, forming a liquid. Bottle this sweet liquid, and take 5 – 7 teaspoonfuls a day.

(*See also* **chest infections, coughing, fever** *and* **respiratory system problems**.)

BRUISES

A bruise is the result of an injury to skin tissue, and the coloration is caused by blood leaking from damaged blood vessels into surrounding body tissue. The fading of colour from blue, purple or black to yellow marks the breaking down and absorption of that blood. There can be pain, particularly when the injury is to skin immediately above a bone, when the blood-congested tissues will swell and stretch more tightly across the bone. Most bruises heal without attention.

Obese and anaemic people are most susceptible to bruising. Some women bruise more easily during menstruation.

AROMATHERAPEUTIC TREATMENTS

- Some essential oils can help – **aspic, calendula, cypress, geranium, lavender, marjoram, mint** and **parsley** among them. Mix 10 ml (2 tsp) grapeseed oil with 5 – 6 drops essential oil – particularly calendula, cypress or parsley – and rub gently and briefly on to the affected area. Do not massage a bruise.
- Fresh **chervil, hyssop, lavender, parsley** or **thyme** can be used as a poultice. Wash the plant, place in a bowl and pour hot water on top. Wrap in a fine handkerchief and then place on the bruise when the leaves have cooled a little.
- Arnica – a tincture made from flower heads. (*A. montana*, the mountain daisy) – is the sovereign homoeopathic remedy for bruising, often used in lotion form in conjunction with witch-hazel (*Hamamelis*

virginiana, a tree). The former should only be used on unbroken skin; the latter is available from chemists as a water distilled from the leaves and bark.

OTHER TREATMENTS

- If you bruise readily, avoid stimulants like tea and coffee and eat a diet rich in vitamin C and the bioflavonoids (see page 250). This will help strengthen the blood vessel walls.
- If the swelling and pain are severe, apply a cold compress. Crush ice cubes in a towel and apply it to the area of bruising. Elevating the limb (leg or arm) can be helpful too.

BUNIONS

This is a very painful and ugly inflammation of the joint between big toe and foot, which can develop into an actual deformity of the bones, with the big toe pushing towards and against the other toes. The joint swells, and the skin becomes shiny and red. Bunions are most common in middle-aged women and, in the majority of cases, are the result of shoes that do not fit properly – too narrow, too tight, too high. Children and young people should always wear shoes that are the correct size and width, as their bones are more easily deformed than those of adults.

AROMATHERAPEUTIC TREATMENTS

- After a long day, or a long walk, take time to massage your feet. This will activate circulation in the foot and relax the toes. Using an oil like **mint** or **spearmint** will also cool the feet and disperse any swelling. Mix 2 drops mint or spearmint with 5 ml (1 tsp) grapeseed or soya oil, and rub into the feet well. You could also have a footbath, in the basin or bidet: fill with warm water, and add a few drops of mint or spearmint.
- When the bunions have actually developed, many recommend rubbing garlic cloves on them. I find this rather an unpleasant idea and suggest a better solution is to rub in some cold cream containing a few drops of **baume de Tolu**.

OTHER TREATMENTS

- Comfortable shoes which support the feet well are the answer, whether you have bunions or not.

• In hot weather, do not forget that your feet can swell, therefore shoes must not be too tight. Sandals are best, as they also let the feet breathe. Fabric-topped shoes are good, too. Always try to wear natural fabrics like cotton on the feet. Go barefoot whenever possible, avoiding stockings and tights in summer.

BURNS

Burns are caused by dry heat (*e.g.* fire, electricity, the sun,), and by moist heat or scalds (*e.g.* boiling liquids and steam). The skin is damaged, superficially or more seriously, with considerable pain if nerve endings are still intact. Needless to say, all burns, except those which are quite obviously minor, require immediate professional attention. On your way to the doctor, cover the burn with a wet saline compress.

Thanks to their natural antibacterial and antiviral properties, essential oils are tremendously helpful for treating minor burns – or indeed any instance when the integrity of the skin is damaged. They not only reduce the possibility of infection, but also stimulate the regeneration of new skin cells and so encourage healing. Among the best are **benzoin, eucalyptus, lavender, patchouli** and **clary sage**.

(*See also* **aspic, galbonum, geranium, savory** *and* **tea tree**.)

AROMATHERAPEUTIC TREATMENTS

• For minor burns, immediately apply **lavender** essential oil neat to the burn, and cover well with a damp compress. This should preferably be of gauze or muslin so that the wound can breathe. Never use an adhesive dressing or plaster. Apply every 4 hours until better.
• Potato or carrot juice are useful alternatives, as is immersion in cold water.

BURSITIS

Bursitis is one of the most common rheumatic conditions. A bursa is a small sac containing lubricating fluid which is situated between moving joints. It can become inflamed through injury, infection, repeated use or unusual pressure when the liquid content increases, causing pain and limiting movement. If often affects shoulders, but is well known for its appearance in elbows and knees (tennis elbow and housemaid's knee).

The symptoms can include sharp pain, hot and tender skin, and swelling. Some types of bursitis may require surgery.

AROMATHERAPEUTIC TREATMENTS

- Essential oils can be helpful. Mix 5 drops of **rosemary, geranium, cajuput** or **eucalyptus** with 10 ml (2 tsp) soya and 2.5 ml (½ tsp) wheatgerm, and rub gently into the inflamed area.

(*See also* **camphor of Borneo.**)

OTHER TREATMENT

- Avoid using the joint until the inflammation has diminished.

(*See also* **oedema** *and* **rheumatism.**)

CATARRH

Catarrh is the term applied to excessive secretion of phlegm from the air passage of the lungs, the larynx, the nose and the sinuses. The most common causes are colds and 'flu; hayfever, bronchitis, sinusitis, and rhinitis may also be involved.

Many essential oils are decongestant and expectorant – helping to clear out the chest and lungs – and therefore can help catarrh considerably. Among them are **benzoin, chamomile, eucalyptus, frankincense, hyssop, mint, niaouli, pine** and **clary sage**.

AROMATHERAPEUTIC TREATMENTS

- To clear the nostrils, boil a large handful of fresh **thyme** in 600 ml (1 pint) water for 10 minutes. Leave until lukewarm, then dip a piece of cotton wool in the solution. With head back, squeeze the liquid into each nostril.
- If you are feeling strong, a wonderful remedy consists of putting a few drops of pure **lemon** juice in each nostril. It is painful, but very effective.
- Put a drop each of **thyme** and **eucalyptus** oils in a bowl of hot water and inhale, with a towel over your head, for 10 minutes.
- Essential oils of both **benzoin** and **niaouli** can be added to a bowl beside the bed while sleeping.
- Add **eucalyptus** oil to baths.
- Drink tisanes of **mint** and **eucalyptus** together, or **hyssop, sage** and **chamomile**.

(*See also* **pepper; bronchitis, chest infections, colds, hayfever** *and* **sinusitis.**)

CELLULITE

Cellulite is brought on by a hormonal change, invariably character-ized by high levels of oestrogen, which encourages the body tissues to retain water. When the fat cells become interspersed with this water, the skin takes on an 'orange peel' appearance if squeezed between the fingers, and often feels uneven and bumpy too. It usually appears on the thighs, buttocks and hips, but it can also manifest itself on stomach, upper arms and even on the back of the neck.

Although considered primarily a 'beauty' problem in Britain, in France doctors look upon cellulite as a medical condition. A researcher, Dr Balaiche, sees the cause as a dysfunction of the endocrine glands, excess quantities of folliculin or oestrogen being produced by the ovaries. These dysfunctions can be at their peak in puberty, and during preg-nancy or the menopause, when the body is trying to adjust to the change. They can also occur during the monthly ovulation and menstruation.

Digestive problems are very often a major cause of cellulite. Women who assimilate food badly – who eat too fast, or who don't chew food properly – can develop it. Constipation is another major factor: poor elimination means a build-up of waste and by-products of normal metabolism in the system, with no possibility of efficient release.

Other factors are nervous disorders and bad posture. Long-term stress not only interferes with digestion, assimilation and elimination, but can cause insomnia, restlessness and bad posture in its sufferers. Bad posture can encourage bad circulation and this results in cellulite in many places such as the ankles, legs and hips. (Flat feet can contribute to cellulite too.)

The contraceptive pill, excess of medication during illness, and smoking can all cause cellulite. Smoking, particularly, robs the system of vitamin C and the bioflavonoids which are essential for healthy collagen (the connective fibres that support muscles, skin and the vessels of the circulatory system). Nicotine also interferes with the circulation; with cellular exchange drastically slowed down, conditions are created for the formation of cellulite – which, once formed, tends to stay.

AROMATHERAPEUTIC TREATMENTS

- For a tea rich in vitamin C and citrin, boil the washed skin of a **lemon** in 500 ml (a scant pint) of water and leave overnight before adding the juice of the lemon. Drink first thing in the morning. For a diuretic tisane, infuse about 20 g (about ¾ oz) lettuce and 10 g (just under ½ oz) fresh chervil – a good herb for the circulation – in 500 ml (a scant pint) of boiling water.
- Drink mineral water, diluted fruit juice and herbal teas like **sage** or

cumin, avoiding ordinary tea, coffee and alcohol which, although diuretic, exacerbate cellulite.

- Baths containing essential oils are good, but these must always be warm, not hot. Rub the skin first with a loofah, to activate the circulation, then add 2 drops each of **cypress, lavender** and **lemon** oils. Finish with a cold shower, and then rub an oil made from mixing together 10ml (2 tsp) soya oil, 2 drops wheatgerm oil and 7 drops **cypress** oil into the affected areas.
- Massage with the oil is helpful. Always start off gently to prepare the skin and underlying tissue, then you can work on the affected areas as if you were kneading bread.

(*See also* **wintergreen**.)

OTHER TREATMENTS

- Take plenty of regular, sustained exercise to boost the circulation and lung efficiency, to galvanize a sluggish system into activity, and help with the elimination of cell wastes. Cellulite tends mostly to form in those who sit about all day. Swim, walk briskly, dance, cycle; these are all good forms of exercise.
- If you are stressed, learn a meditation technqiue or a method of deep relaxation. This plus exercise forms the foundation of any anti-cellulite lifestyle.
- A sensible diet is just as important. Put yourself on a spring-cleaning diet of fresh fruits and raw vegetables every few months, say, and chew them well to help assimilation, digestion and waste elimination. Avoid salty and smoked foods such as ham and bacon, sugar and refined carbohydrates – these encourage fluid retention. Bran is vital for elimination. Celery is a good vegetable for this, too, and can be mixed with carrots, cucumber or apple. One French doctor put his patients on a cure of pineapple which was juiced and eaten, for a period of 20 days per month for a few months. While I wouldn't advise anyone to try this for so long, it could be worth trying for a few days. The coriander soup on page 88 is good, too.
- Known detoxifying elements are vitamin C and the bioflavonoids which strengthen the circulatory system, so eat foods containing both, such as citrus fruits, blackcurrants and vegetables. Vitamin E has a stimulating effect on the circulation, so simply scatter some wheatgerm on cereals or yoghurt.
- The main function of the thyroid gland is to control the speed at which oxygen and food products are burned up to produce energy. The hormones produced by the thyroid are formed from compounds of iodine, normally obtained from food such as sea fish and some cereals

and vegetables. Boost this by taking some kelp (seaweed) tablets daily. If these keep you awake at night, dissolve a few in your bath water. Garlic is a rich source of iodine as well.

(*See also* **circulatory problems, digestive problems, menopause, menstrual problems** *and* **stress**.)

CHEST INFECTIONS

Chest infections can be due to or can be caused by colds or 'flu, and old and young people are particularly prone to them. They can cause difficulties in breathing, a build-up of catarrh or phlegm in the bronchis, sore throats, and coughing. Temperature can be high, and some infections can lead to bronchitis or pneumonia. If symptoms are at all worrying, do not hesitate to consult the doctor.

AROMATHERAPEUTIC TREATMENTS

- Preferably, you should rest in bed. The heat in the bedroom should not be too dry, though, as this can irritate and exacerbate a cough. Put a bowl of water near the source of heat; for even more effect, put in a few drops of an expectorant oil such as **eucalyptus, cajuput, niaouli, pepper, pine** or **tea tree** (these oils are valuable used in inhalations, too).
- For recurring chest infections in the winter, take a preventative drink every morning before the winter comes. Put 100 g (4 oz) **eucalyptus leaves**, some **juniper berries** and some ginseng in 500 ml (18 fl oz) vodka, and leave for about 2 – 3 weeks to macerate. Add 30 ml (2 tbsp) fructose, and mix. Dilute 10 ml (2 tsp) with water and drink every morning.
- Poultices for chest infections are well-known to be effective, both in traditional medicine and aromatherapy. Make up a poultice with fresh **mustard** seeds crushed into a paste, and apply very hot to the chest. Do not take it off when it starts to give off heat and feel burning on the skin, but leave for about 5 – 10 minutes (no longer than 20 though, as it can actually affect the skin). The skin can be very red, so apply some talcum powder, then wrap up very warmly – wrap two or three scarves around your chest – for a couple of hours. This brings phlegm up very quickly.
- Cabbage which had been boiled until very soft was once used *as* a poultice in France. A linseed poultice (see page 24) containing any of the above expectorant oils is very effective, too. Follow this with

249

the application of an oil made from 10 ml (2 tsp) grapeseed oil, a little wheatgerm oil and 3 – 4 drops of whichever oil was used in the poultice.

- An oil for the chest made with **eucalyptus** or **pine** oil is very helpful.

(*See also* **baume de Tolu** *and* **benzoin**.)

OTHER TREATMENTS

- Keep warm and stay indoors. Cold and damp air, car fumes, and fog, can make chest problems worse.
- Diet is important. You should eat lots of citrus fruit for their vitamin C content, and celeriac, garlic, onion, barely cooked greens and members of the cabbage family (for their sulphur content). Make a medicinal soup regularly from clear chicken stock, with 3 – 4 cloves, lots of pepper, juniper berries, and leeks, onions, celeriac, radishes, turnips, etc.
- Try to avoid eating things which might irritate a sore throat, such as nuts or toast.

(*See also* **bronchitis, catarrh, coughing, colds, pneumonia, respiratory system problems** *and* **throats, sore**.)

CHILBLAINS

These are the reddish-blue discolorations of the skin, accompanied by swelling, which affect parts of the body, particularly toes, fingers and backs of legs, exposed to cold. Children are particularly prone to them on their feet in winter. Poor circulation of the blood is a contributory factor.

AROMATHERAPEUTIC TREATMENTS

- Massage affected parts well once in the warm. **Lemon juice** is good for this, as it sterilizes and galvanizes at the same time.
- **Celery** water is a remarkable remedy for chilblains (see page 74), and eating celery will help as well.
- If the feet feel cold after a walk (or if shoes are constricting), massage the feet with an oil consisting of 10 ml (2 tsp) grapeseed oil and 5 drops **tea tree**.
- Rub neat **tea tree** oil on to the affected parts.

OTHER TREATMENTS

- Always dress yourself or children warmly in cold weather, with lined boots, thick trousers and good gloves.
- Drying the feet and hands well in cold weather will help prevent the condition developing.

CIRCULATORY PROBLEMS

The circulatory system of the body comprises the heart, arteries, and veins through which blood is carried to and from the body organs and tissues. The most serious problems of the circulatory system are those involving the heart – atheroma, angina pectoris, and coronary thrombosis – and to treat these is not within the competence of aromatherapy. What aromatherapeutic oils can do, though, is boost the circulation of the blood, helping a sluggish circulation, and thereby preventing the less serious circulatory problems such as haemorrhoids, cellulite and varicose veins on the legs. Stimulating the circulation of the blood is also extremely good for the skin, and strengthening the blood vessels can prevent things like broken facial veins or capillaries.

AROMATHERAPEUTIC TREATMENTS

- Massage stimulates the tissue, delivering fresh blood to the cells. Massage also facilitates the entry of essential oils, and using oils like **cypress, neroli, lemon** and **rose** will boost the circulation. Use a few drops in 10 ml (2 tsp) base oil.
- Avoid coffee, tea and alcohol, and drink tisanes made from herbs like chervil, **parsley** and **sage**.

OTHER TREATMENTS

- Diet is extremely important. Eat healthily of foods rich in vitamins C and E, and bioflavonoids which are very good for the circulatory system. Onions, garlic, citrus fruits, chestnuts, rye and wheatgerm are all good foods.
- Exercise regularly, walking and cycling briskly if you do not play a sport.

(*See also* **broken veins and capillaries, cellulite, constipation, haemorrhoids** *and* **varicose veins**.)

COLDS

The common cold – *coryza* is the medical term – is a highly contagious virus infection of the upper respiratory tract. It is caused by many different viruses, all of which are highly infectious, and are spread through the coughing and sneezing of, and the air breathed out by, the cold-afflicted person. Generally, the symptoms are sneezing, mild feverishness, aching limbs, heavy or prickly eyes, sore throat and catarrh. Colds are most common in winter, not necessarily because it is colder or wetter, but because the body's resistance to infection is lower – and illness, fatigue and depression can both be factors. Sometimes colds can lead to things like sinusitis or bronchitis, when bacteria invade the vulnerable system.

Despite being so common, there is as yet no cure, and although proprietary medicines and analgesics may help the symptoms, most colds have to run their course. Vitamin C is one of the substances believed by many to help prevent infection by building up the body's defences, but the medical establishment are very divided on the issue.

Aromatherapeutic oils can help keep cold germs at bay, prevent infection and ease symptoms. Many foods, including those which contain vitamin C, are useful, too, particularly the powerfully antibiotic onion and garlic.

AROMATHERAPEUTIC TREATMENTS

- To keep cold infections at bay, drink plenty of **lemon** and **mint** tisanes, and eat a healthy diet. Regular exercise is useful as well.
- To guard against infection, in the office, say, mix up an oil containing 50 ml (2 fl oz) soya or almond oil and 1 drop each of **cinnamon, clove, eucalyptus, niaouli** and **pine**. Sprinkle a few drops on a piece of dampened cotton wool and place on a radiator near you. Or mix the essences, minus the base oil, into water and put it in a spray bottle to spray your office.
- For added protection, you could add 1 drop of **clove, eucalyptus, niaouli** or **pine** to 50 ml (2 fl oz) soya or almond oil and rub it around your nose, or into your chest. This can be used, too, when the first symptoms of a cold appear.
- Gargle straightaway with warm boiled water containing 2 drops of **tea tree, geranium** or **thyme**, and a little fresh **lemon juice**.
- To relieve the stuffiness of a cold, use blends of essential oils in inhalations or in baths, rubbed on the chest, or sprinkled on to a handkerchief. **Cajuput, clove, eucalyptus, niaouli** and **pine** are useful for this. (*See also* **fever** for oils for the bath.)
- One of the most distressing symptoms of a cold (especially for an

aromatherapist!) is the loss of sense of smell. **Chervil, geranium** and **basil** are particularly useful for this, in the bath and in inhalations (see also **anosmia**).

- Rub **tea tree** (or **geranium** or **thyme**) under the nose, behind the ears and the back of the neck to help stiffness and recurring infection. If you wish to use it neat, check your reaction first with a skin test (see page 13).
- For a very severe cold, drink plenty of fluids, 1 large glass every hour. Or make a tisane – two-thirds **eucalyptus** leaves and one-third **lavender** flowers. Infuse in the normal way.
- A **thyme** tisane should be drunk several times a day after a cold to prevent it recurring (see page 209).

(*See also* **ginger, lavender, mustard** *and* **pepper.**)

OTHER TREATMENTS

- When you have a cold, keep warm and stay in bed. It will be more comfortable while you fight the symptoms, and you will not be spreading germs.
- If you have a fever – a good sign that your body is fighting off the virus – try to eat foods that are easy to digest so that the body's energies are not further sapped. You will not be too hungry anyway. Fresh fruit is good, as is yoghurt. The sweating of a fever means that you will lose liquid (particularly dangerous in a baby), so top the level up with diluted fruit juices and tisanes (see the **hyssop** tisane and syrup on page 114, and the spicy tisane on page 288).

(*See also* **anosmia, bronchitis, catarrh, chest infections, coughing, ear problems, fever, headaches, influenza, pneumonia, respiratory problems** *and* **sinusitis.**)

COLD SORES

There are several types of the virus herpes: herpes of the mouth and genitals are two types of the *H. simplex* virus; and *H. zoster* is shingles, caused by the chicken pox virus.

Herpes of the mouth – or cold sores – once contracted, can recur as it can be activated by exposure to cold or heat, by menstruation, fever or infections of the upper respiratory tract. The blister-like sores, announcing their arrival by tingling and itching, occur mostly around the mouth and can last for a week or more. There are several proprietary medicaments, but nothing can really prevent the virus erupting.

Aromatherapy has limited ways in which to alleviate cold sores. In France, Dr Belaiche recognized only a 20 per cent chance of success with plant essence applications. Dr Maury is more optimistic about homoeopathy, but still does not believe that all cases can be helped.

AROMATHERAPEUTIC TREATMENTS

- Applications of **chamomile** or **calendula** lotion (a strong decoction, see page 25), or either of the essential oils neat could relieve pain and swelling. **Tea tree** oil could be used too.
- Drink infusions of mixed **thyme, savory,** and **chamomile** several times a day instead of tea or coffee.

OTHER TREATMENTS

- To avoid triggering the virus in the sun, wear a reputable sun block.
- Take multi-mineral supplements and a homoeopathic remedy like oligo elements. Some people believe lysine, an amino acid good for the skin, can help as well.

(*See also* **shingles**.)

COLIC

Adult colic – a series of acute abdominal pains – is a symptom of a number of digestive system problems (see page 268). It usually occurs after eating, particularly fermented cheeses such as Brie, overripe melon or fruits which are not ripe enough. It can also occur during attacks of gastric 'flu.

Colic is very common in babies and young children when it is often caused by air or gas caught in the immature intestines. This causes pain, and a restless baby might draw up his legs in spasm, cry, then relax. Infantile colic can also be caused by an allergy to cow's milk.

ADULT COLIC – AROMATHERAPEUTIC TREATMENTS

- Drink a herb tea made from a pinch each of **fennel** and **anise** (herb or seeds), and **melissa**, and 300 ml (½ pint) boiling water. Infuse for 7 minutes then drink warm, sweetened with honey if desired.
- Mix 2 drops each of **melissa** and **chamomile** with 30 ml (2 tbsp) soya oil and 2 drops wheatgerm. Gently massage the tummy with

this in a clockwise direction. Afterwards apply a hot towel (dip in hot water and wring out) to the stomach. You will feel virtual instant relief.

INFANTILE COLIC – AROMATHERAPEUTIC TREATMENTS

- Fennel is an ingredient of commerical babies' gripewater. Boil a little **fennel** and **carrot** together until soft, then sweeten the cooled water with a little honey and give it to the baby. **Chamomile** tea will have the same effect.
- For an older child, a tisane of **orange** leaves can help.
- Massage the stomach of a colicky baby or child with an oil containing the digestive **caraway** (see page 64).
- Fill the baby's room with soothing vapours on a piece of cotton wool on the radiator. Use a drop of **pine** and **orange**, or **lavender** and **orange**.

(*See also* **neroli** *and* **petitgrain**.)

INFANTILE COLIC – OTHER TREATMENTS

- Cuddling, rocking and generally comforting – over the shoulder so that the baby can pass wind – should help.

COLITIS

Colitis is an inflammation of the colon and the symptoms are diarrhoea, sometimes with blood, and pain in the lower part of the abdomen. It could be caused by bacterial infection or by a number of other disorders. It is very often associated with a nervous disorder, anxiety or stress. Fever, loss of appetite and weight could also occur.

TREATMENTS

- Rest and something to help the diarrhoea is vital (*see* Diarrhoea).
- A simple and bland diet should be followed, avoiding raw fruits and vegetables (especially their skins and seeds), whole cereals, fresh bread, sugar, fried or fatty foods, and game meat. Do not eat dairy products as these can often be painful to digest. Give your intestines a rest by cutting out alcohol – spirits and cold beer especially – and sparkling or fizzy waters.

- Drink a lot of fluids – still mineral waters and herbal tisanes, especially **chamomile** (mauve if you can get it).
- Avoid large meals and eat very slowly, chewing each mouthful well. Do not talk too much while eating and never have an argument: stress and good digestion just don't go together!
- Eat boiled or steamed rice or barley (drink the cooking water of the latter). Cook fruits as a compote and sweeten with a little honey or fructose. A good dish is one of toasted bread and steamed vegetables cut up into small pieces and mixed.
- Gentle (rather than strenuous) exercise helps the body to relax, and you should practise meditation and relaxation techniques.

(*See also* **lemongrass**; **abdominal pain, diarrhoea, fever** *and* **stress**.)

CONJUNCTIVITIS

(*See* **eye problems**.)

CONSTIPATION

This is the condition in which defaecation is difficult and infrequent, and it can cause stomach pain and discomfort, tiredness and stress – the latter often exacerbating the original complaint. Defaecation is difficult because the waste matters of the body have become compacted and hard. Pre-menstrual and pregnant women and those on heavy medication can suffer, but the most common cause is a diet lacking in fibre or roughage. Fibre is present in vegetable foods – the cellulose which forms the main structure of grains, vegetable and fruit – and as these are unable to be digested by the body, they enable wastes to pass through the bowel relatively quickly.

Prolonged constipation can lead to or contribute to a number of problems, including general malaise, a greasy or unhealthy skin, cellulite and haemorrhoids.

AROMATHERAPEUTIC TREATMENT

- Mix together 10 ml (2 tsp) grapeseed oil and 5 drops of **rosemary** oil and massage this into the tummy in the morning. Lie on the floor and rub it in in a clockwise direction for 20 minutes, breathing deeply and contracting the abdominal muscles when exhaling.

OTHER TREATMENTS

- Eat a diet rich in fibre – fresh fruit and vegetables (including their skins), whole grains and pulses, and sprinkle some bran – oat or wheat – on to meals.
- **Fennel** and **tarragon** are both mild laxatives, so should be eaten often. **Carrot** is good too, as are cereals such as rye, millet and wheat.
- Avoid tea, coffee and chocolate and all refined foods.
- Drink 15 ml (1 tbsp) first-pressing olive oil first thing in the morning followed by a glass of warm water.
- Exercise is an important factor in constipation as it is in all circulatory problems.

(*See also* **abdominal pain, cellulite, circulatory problems, digestive system problems, haemorrhoids, pre-menstrual tension** *and* **varicose vains.**)

COUGHING

Coughing, a protective response helping to rid the lungs of irritants, can be a symptom of a wide variety of diseases. It can be associated with asthma, bronchitis, 'flu, hayfever, pneumonia, sore throat, tonsillitis and sinusitis, or with smoking. Its most common cause, though, is the common cold.

AROMATHERAPEUTIC TREATMENTS

- **Rose** is one of the most effective remedies, as it acts on the mucus, and helps alleviate the cough. Drink infusions of rose petals, and use to gargle as well (see page 182).
- **Hyssop** is good too, see the infusion and syrup on page 114.
- Drink lots of tisanes made with expectorant herbs like **lavender, melissa, mint, rosemary** or **thyme**. Tisanes made with tiny **pine** cones are helpful as well.
- **Cinnamon**-flavoured drinks relieve a cough, as does the **cure-all** on pages 80-1.
- Inhale **eucalyptus**, or have an infusion of leaves beside your bed to try to avoid bouts of midnight coughing.
- Rub a **geranium** oil (a few drops in a little base oil) on the torso daily, or add a few drops to the bath.
- Make up a linseed or other poultice for the chest (see pages 23–4), adding a few drops of any of the following oils – **baume de Canada,**

cajaput, carrot, frankincense, mustard, oregano or thyme. See baume de Tolu for an excellent rubbing oil for the chest.

(*See also* geranium, chamomile, cypress, ginger, oregano, pine *and* turpentine.)

OTHER TREATMENTS

- Stay warm and inside if you can; if you must go out, wrap up warmly and wear a scarf. Remember that every time you cough in public, you are probably spraying out the germs that caused the problem in the first place.
- Several foods can be eaten to prevent and alleviate coughs, among them lemon and ginger, the former with its vitamin C, the latter with its warmth. Garlic, turnips, leeks, radish and horseradish are all expectorant, helping to loosen mucus.

(*See also* asthma, bronchitis, hayfever, influenza, pneumonia, respiratory system problems, sinusitis *and* throat, sore.)

CRACKED SKIN

Many people suffer from cracked skin on their hands and feet, particularly in winter when it is associated with frostbite. It can be extremely painful, and looks unpleasant. Cracked skin can also be caused by skin diseases such as psoriasis.

AROMATHERAPEUTIC TREATMENTS

- Mix 4 drops tea tree oil or myrrh with 10 ml (2 tsp) castor oil which has been slightly warmed and a couple drops of wheatgerm oil. Apply thickly on the hands and fingers, wrap in gauze (two layers at least), and wear loose cotton gloves on top. Do this at night, and repeat the treatment for a shorter time in the morning. Do this for a week or more until the condition has really improved.
- If you don't have the above oils, use chamomile flowers. Place in a *bain-marie* (a double boiler or a bowl in a roasting pan of hot water) a heaped tbsp of chamomile heads, 100 ml (4 fl oz) almond oil and 10 ml (2 tsp) castor oil. Infuse the mixture gently for 1 hour. Allow it to cool, then strain the flowers from the oil. Plunge your hands in the perfumed oil for at least 20 minutes. You can do the same with the feet, but you must double or triple the recipe. The longer you can leave your hands (or feet) the better the result will be.

● See the *baume de Tolu* remedy on page 278.

(*See also* **patchouli** *and* **sandalwood**; **frostbite** *and* **psoriasis**.)

CRAMP

Cramp is the sudden involuntary contraction of a muscle or group of muscles, and can cause acute pain. Writer's cramp – literally caused by constant writing – is now a prescribed industrial disease and liable to state benefit in Britain. Many people suffer from cramps in the calf of the leg or foot during sleep, said to be particularly common in young anaemic women, when the leg is not receiving sufficient blood; pregnant women suffer too. Women suffering from dysmennorhoea are prone to debilitating stomach cramps, caused by the contraction of the muscles surrounding the uterus wall. Although all menstruating women have contractions, these can be up to four times as strong in women with dysmennorhoea.

AROMATHERAPEUTIC TREATMENTS

● Rub the leg vigorously until the pressure is relieved. Use an oil if you like – 5 ml (1 tsp) soya with 2 drops **geranium** could be good.
● For stomach cramps, apply heat – a hot water bottle or a hot poultice made of linseed with 2 – 3 drops of **chamomile**. A chamomile drink or an infusion of **melissa** and **mint** can also help.

(*See also* **coriander**.)

OTHER TREATMENTS

● Cramps in the leg can be relieved by bending the knee as far as it will go, or contracting the opposite muscle to that in contraction. If in bed, the flow of blood to the legs will be increased if you stand up until the pain departs.
● For those suffering from stomach cramps, eat a light diet: white rice and cooked salad vegetables and fruit are the best, avoiding coffee, tea and alcohol. Masticate your food very slowly and carefully to give your stomach and digestive system less work to do.
● Consult your doctor if the cramps are very severe.
● Yoga breathing is a great help.

(*See also* **muscular pains**.)

CUTS AND WOUNDS

Most cuts and scratches do not require medical attention unless infection sets in or they were caused by a dirty or rusty object (when a tetanus injection might be necessary). Obviously, if a wound is deep and a lot of blood is being lost, help should be sought.

The skin does a remarkable job of healing itself. The blood produces clotting factors which seal the wound in about two hours, and then a scab is formed to complete the sealing. In most cases, there will be no permanent scar.

Essential oils can help considerably in the sterilization of wounds, reducing the possibility of infection. They also stimulate the regeneration of the new skin cells, encouraging the wound to heal. Most essential oils have antibacterial properties, so virtually any oil can be useful for minor wounds.

If you pierce your finger or cut any part of your body while outside, do remember that the chlorophyll in green leaves can act as a natural antiseptic. Using dock leaves to soothe nettle stings is a well know remedy, but apply crushed herbal leaves immediately and bleeding and infection will be stopped. Use bay (**laurel**) leaves, **marjoram, parsley, rosemary,** or **thyme. Hyssop** is particularly effective.

(*See also* **acne, anthrax, dental abscesses, folliculitis** *and* **skin problems**.)

AROMATHERAPEUTIC TREATMENTS

- Wash the cut or wound carefully, swabbing away from the wound, and using clean swabs each time. A drop of **eucalyptus, geranium, clary sage** or **tea tree** essential oils in the water will cleanse and reduce the chances of infection.
- Another good swabbing medium is boiled water with some sea salt in it, plus a drop of one of the above oils. Bandage well. If the wound is fairly deep, change the bandage every two hours, swabbing each time with cotton wool dipped in the boiled water and sea salt.
- **Lemon juice** comes in handy to sterilize wounds. It stings though!
- If caught without oils, many green leaves containing chlorophyll can help sterilize minor wounds. Poultices of fresh **hyssop** or **rosemary**, for instance, are good for cleansing and healing.
- **Chamomile, eucalyptus, geranium, lavender** and **palmarosa** help healing, and properties in **chamomile, geranium** and **pepper** promote cicatrization of the wounds. All can help with the latter stages of post-operative scarring, or wound stitches, and **rose** is particularly effective for the face.

- When scabs form, let them dry and do not ever peel them off. Clean scabs twice a day. **Calendula** is particularly good although the oil is difficult to obtain; an infusion of the flowers would be an excellent alternative. A few drops of a very strong infusion added to some cold cream will help cicatrization and prevent scarring.

(*See also* **benzoin, galbanum** *and* **savory**.)

CYSTITIS

This is an infection of the bladder, and is caused by bacteria entering the bladder through the urethra. It is more common in women because the female urethra is shorter than in men and is closer to the anus. The condition causes frequent and usually very painful urination, and there may be a raised temperature. Any blood in the urine should be reported to your doctor.

Women on the pill are more prone to cystitis because the pill hormones alter the bacterial flora of the urethra as well as the vagina. Pregnant women are prone, too, because the enlargement of the womb can press on the bladder. Other illnesses such as bronchitis, a bad cold or constipation can provoke a urinary infection as well. Even smells such as that of fresh paint can cause cystitis attacks in some women. Honeymoon cystitis is so-called because it is frequent in newly married women, and indeed frequent sex can stimulate the proliferation of bacteria in the urethra of some women. (This condition could also be urethritis, an actual inflammation of the urethra itself.)

AROMATHERAPEUTIC TREATMENTS

- Bath or use the bidet frequently, adding a few drops of helpful oils – **cajuput, cedarwood, chamomile, eucalyptus, juniper, pine** or **sandalwood**. My favourites are **niaouli** and **parsley**. Although it may be inconvenient, washing is particularly useful after intercourse. Cold water is best in the bidet; never have water too hot, even in the bath, as heat can irritate the bladder.
- Make massage oils from 20 – 25 ml (¾ – 1 fl oz) soya oil and 5 drops of **cajuput, juniper, niaouli, parsley, pine** or **sandalwood**, and massage into the top of the hands and feet, the tummy, lower back and sacral region. Follow this with hot and cold compresses applied alternately.
- Diuretic herbal teas are very useful. One tea can be made from the wispy hairs off corn-on-the-cob; boil for 10 minutes, drink 5 – 6 large

glasses a day, and eat the corn as well. Another uses 3 pinches of cherry stalks boiled in 500 ml (a scant pint) of water for 2 minutes then steeped for 5. Infuse **pine** needles in much the same way (see page 179).

- Other foods and herbs useful for cystitis sufferers are chervil, celery, **fennel** and **parsley**. Eat all of them, the chervil and parsley as generous garnishes or in soups or teas; juice parsley and celery; eat celery and fennel, herb and vegetable.

(*See also* **celery, fennel** and **lavender**.)

OTHER TREATMENTS

- Keep warm and drink plenty of fluids – at least 4 litres (7 pints) every 24 hours.
- Empty the bladder well each time, for any urine left in the bladder can stagnate and become further infected. It is best for everyone, whether prone to cystitis or not, to pass urine frequently: the pressure of a full bladder – which can hold more than 800 ml (nearly 1 ½ pints) – can damage the pelvic floor muscles.
- Exercise, perhaps surprisingly, is also good for cystitis, because weak pelvic floor muscles will encourage the retention of urine in the bladder. A simple exercise, good for the prevention of cystitis (as well as for the muscles used in love-making), is to stop the flow of urine by contracting the muscles a couple of times each time you urinate.

NASTURTIUM AND MÂCHE SALAD
Serves 2 as a side salad or 4 as an hors d'oeuvre

This is an easy salad to prepare and may be served as a side salad or as an *hors d'oeuvre* and it is highly recommended for sufferers of cystitis. When it occurs, eat the salad three times daily. *Mâche* (corn salad or lamb's tongues) is one of the salad leaves richest in chlorophyll, and this has a revitalizing effect on the body. It is also an effective lubricant and very beneficial to the lungs, intestines and arteries. The flowers of the nasturtium stimulate the gastric and liver functions.

450 g (1 lb) mâche or lamb's lettuce (try to use the smallest and greenest leaves)
25 g (1 oz) nasturtium flowers
a little lemon juice or cider vinegar

DRESSING
1 tbsp lemon juice
a pinch of sea salt
30 ml (2 tbsp) first pressing virgin olive oil
freshly ground black pepper

Place the vinegar or lemon juice in water and carefully wash the salad leaves and petals. Pat dry gently as they bruise easily. Mix together the dressing ingredients and place in the salad bowl. Place the salad over the dressing and toss just before serving.

(If you cannot find nasturtium flowers, use rose petals, either white, pink or red. This will alter the therapeutic value slightly.)

DANDRUFF

This is a very common problem, caused by the shedding of scales of dead skin from the scalp. This in turn is caused by the sebaceous glands in the scalp and those with greasy skin or acne, with *over-active* glands, are particularly prone to dandruff. The condition, like alopecia, is often also linked to emotional upsets, hormonal imbalances, poor eating habits, and excessive use of, or an allergic reaction to, chemicals on the hair.

Aromatherapeutic oils are very effective for treating a number of hair problems, and a few are particularly useful for dandruff.

AROMATHERAPEUTIC TREATMENTS

- The night or two hours before shampooing, mix 2 drops **patchouli** into 10 ml (2 tsp) grapeseed or soya oil, and massage into the hair.
- Make very strong herb tea of fresh or dried **thyme** or **rosemary**, and infuse for 10 minutes. Rub the strained cooled tea on to the scalp. Do this between shampoos. You could also add the juice of quarter of a **lemon** to the teas; lemon is astringent, and can help with the excessive sebum associated with dandruff.
- If the problem is excessive dryness of the scalp and hair, massage the scalp with coconut oil. This is not too greasy and washes off easily. It comes in crystalline form, so needs to be warmed before use – on the radiator or under the hot tap. Spoon out 10 ml (2 tsp), warm until liquid and add 1 drop each of **chamomile** and **lemon** oils for fair hair, and 1 drop each of **patchouli** and **ylang-ylang** for dark hair. Massage for 5 minutes into the scalp, then cover with a hot towel for 20 minutes. Wash off.

  You could add a capsule of oil of evening primrose to the mix; this contains vitamin E.

(*See also* **cedarwood** *and* **clary sage**.)

263

OTHER TREATMENTS

- Shampoos that are too strong can cause dandruff, so if you are prone, choose the mildest 'frequent-wash' varieties, and rinse them off very well.
- Drying the hair with a hot hair dryer can also cause the problem. When possible, leave the hair to dry naturally.

(*See also* **alopecia, hair problems, menopause, pre-menstrual tension** *and* **stress.**)

DENTAL ABSCESS

This is caused by tooth decay, by bacteria eating through the enamel of the tooth, reaching the dentine, then the pulp, causing an abscess to form at the root of the tooth. If this is not treated quickly, the tooth could die. Infections so near to the brain are dangerous, too, so professional help should be sought as quickly as possible.

AROMATHERAPEUTIC TREATMENTS

- To help the pain until you get to the dentist, suck a **clove** for its antiseptic and analgesic effect, or dab a little clove oil on the tooth.
- To prevent the bacteria which cause tooth decay, keep the mouth clean with gargles containing a few drops of an antiseptic oil such as **chamomile, clove, geranium, lemongrass, niaouli** and **rose.**
- A cut garlic clove rubbed on the gums is antiseptic – if a little antisocial! Chewing fresh **sage** leaves would be pleasanter.

Antiseptic mouthwash

300 ml (½ pint) water
30 ml (2 tbsp) white wine vinegar
a few cloves
1 cinnamon stick
a little lemon juice

Boil these together for 10 minutes, then cool, and keep in the fridge for a few days. Use as a mouthwash and gargle twice a day.

(*See also* **toothache**.)

DEPRESSION

This is a condition which affects most of us at some time or another, but which can become an illness requiring treatment if unduly prolonged. There are many causes of depression, chief among them fairly obvious ones such as failure at work, loss of a lover, or death of a relative or friend. Unrelieved anxieties about work, money, health and living conditions can add up ultimately to a more acute depression. Sadness, general despondency and tearfulness are common symptoms, but if these 'take over', showing no signs of diminishing after a week or so, and the health of the sufferer and/or family are beginning to be affected, then proper treatment is required.

Many plants and plant oils have an effect on the nervous system. At its simplest, pleasant smells can always help lift the spirits. Oils can help balance the nervous system, relaxing and restoring imbalances, and galvanizing into action. Particularly effective are the citrus oils like **neroli**, and others like **basil, marjoram, melissa, thyme** and **verbena.**

AROMATHERAPEUTIC TREATMENTS

- The energizing herbs **marjoram** and **thyme** are good. Eat them in salads or cook them with other foods.
- Avoid the caffeine stimulants like tea and coffee and replace them with teas of **marjoram, mint, verbena** and **thyme**. Boil ginseng roots in a double boiler for a couple of hours and drink a glass of the liquid first thing in the morning.
- Diffuse a few drops of **marjoram** or **thyme** in your rooms. They will help cheer you up. When in season, cut **hyssop** and **thyme** flowers and have them on your table. They are happy flowers and their scent will slowly diffuse around you. A flowering lemon or orange tree will also be uplifting.
- A few drops of oils such as **basil, marjoram, neroli** and **thyme** can be mixed with some grapeseed oil and rubbed on to the back of the hand, the stomach and solar plexus. Also use them in your bath.

(*See also* **rose, rosemary** *and* **sage**.)

OTHER TREATMENTS

- Depressed people need to talk about themselves, so a sympathetic ear is always useful, as is reassurance of worth, effectiveness and that the bad times will pass. Cheerful companions can help bring a depressed person out of their low state.

- I think it is very important to eat well when even the slightest bit depressed. The vitamin content of most foods is vital in combating depression. Try to eat meat, and foods which contain vitamins A, B and E, and treat yourself to a glass of good red wine.
- Wheatgerm, which contains vitamin E, is a great energizer; sprinkle it on cereals and salads. Nuts, too, are good; and pears and apples are wonderful for the nervous system because of their bromine content.
- Exercise is a great booster for the spirit and the body, even if it is only a brisk walk with the dog.

(*See also* **stress**.)

DERMATITIS

Dermatitis is a skin condition roughly synonymous with eczema, both being characterized by inflammation, swelling and itchy rashes and which may lead to blisters and weeping scabs. The skin often thickens and flakes, and patches may be pigmented differently from the rest of the skin.

Many forms of dermatitis are associated with hereditary allergic tendences – such as food allergies to dairy products or gluten. Others are the contact form, the result of handling something against which the skin develops a reaction such as a substance in industry, a washing-up liquid, shaving foam or antiperspirant. One of the earliest and most common forms of dermatitis is in fact nappy rash, a reaction in babies to the acid in urine. Dermatitis and eczema can appear for the first time or worsen during periods of emotional stress, or when overtired or run down.

AROMATHERAPEUTIC TREATMENTS

- In both diseases, the skin is hot, itchy and dry, and many lotions bought over the chemist's counter can help (calamine, for instance). Some essential oils can be of use, but many types of eczema and dermatitis are not compatible with oils; check carefully first. A cold strong chamomile infusion can be dabbed on to the affected areas; or an oil made from 2 drops **chamomile**, 1 drop **carrot**, 15 ml (1 tbsp) almond oil and 5 drops wheatgerm oil can help.
- Other oils which might help are **aspic, cedarwood**, and **niaouli**.
- For contact reactions on the hands, after washing up say, a **calendula** tisane can be rubbed in. Another (curious) remedy is to rub your hands

with cold wet ground coffee after you have brewed a cup. It is very messy, but it's soothing and cheap.

• A cooling remedy for the face can be made by spraying warm mineral water from a spray bottle. The mineral water could be replaced by an infusion of **chamomile** or **calendula**.

• Dermatitis on the hands and neck is a prominent characteristic of the nutritional disease, pellagra. This is caused by a deficiency of vitamin B$_3$, nicotinic acid or niacin. The disease is seen in populations whose diet consists mainly of maize, and little protein. For the skin, apply compresses of **verbena** or **thyme** tea, or an oil made from 5 ml (1 tsp) castor oil, 3 drops wheatgerm and 1 drop of **galbanum** or **frankincense**.

(*See also* **lavender, myrrh, orange** *and* **pepper**.)

OTHER TREATMENTS

• A priority should be to find out the cause for the appearance of the dermatitis or eczema. If it's stress, deal with that as far as possible; if it is a contact form, avoid or change the suspected product, wear gloves when washing up, etc. See your doctor about more specific medical tests to find the cause.

• People who suffer from rashes often have a sensitive digestive system, so diet can play a great part in the treatment of disorders like dermatitis and eczema. Eat foods rich in minerals like sulphur, and vitamins: artichokes, lettuce, cucumber, celeriac, radishes, watercress and nuts. Make soups with lots of leeks, onions, potatoes and carrots in them – these are good blood cleansers. *Fromage frais, Petit Suisse*, yoghurts, nuts and fruit like grapes, **lemons**, grapefruit and pineapple are also helpful.

(*See also* **eczema, skin problems** *and* **stress**.)

DIARRHOEA

Frequent loose or liquid bowel movements, which may or may not be accompanied by stomach pain, can be caused by many factors – by stress or fear, by taking laxatives, or certain drugs. Holiday diarrhoea is caused by exposure to bacteria the body has no immunity against, and many 'flu viruses cause diarrhoea as well. If more than one person is affected, the diarrhoea may be the result of food poisoning by such bacteria as salmonella. Occasionally, diarrhoea may be the symptom of a more serious complaint.

AROMATHERAPEUTIC TREATMENTS

- If the diarrhoea causes lots of flatulence and is very painful, a linseed poultice (see page 23 – 4) with a few drops of **thyme** or **oregano** oils mixed in can provide comfort very quickly. Alternatively, dip a thick towel in very hot water containing some of the same essences and apply to the stomach.
- Include lots of bay (**laurel**) leaves and **thyme** in your cooking for a week or so after an attack to counteract any lurking bacteria.

(*See also* **chamomile** *and* **marjoram**.)

OTHER TREATMENTS

- Diarrhoea is especially serious in babies and old people, as it causes dehydration. Make them drink plenty of natural fluids.
- Keep warm, especially the feet, and a hot water bottle on the stomach can soothe any pain.
- Avoid food for a couple of days, especially fresh fruits, bran, dry biscuits and dairy produce.
- Carrots or pumpkins are good, as they are decongestant and have bulk, so cook them when you feel ready to eat again: added to a broth, mashed, or drunk as juice are the best options. Cooked apples and pears can also be good.
- White rice, especially pudding rice, has lots of starch, and can help stop diarrhoea.
- Quince jam is another food that could be useful – but too much and you will be constipated!

(*See also* **abdominal pain, colitis, digestive system problems** *and* **stress**.)

DIGESTIVE SYSTEM PROBLEMS

For the body to stay alive, it needs a constant supply of energy which comes from the food that we eat. This is broken down by the body so that the energy-rich nutrients can be absorbed properly. This digestive process starts as soon as food is taken into the mouth, if not before as a mouth-watering smell of food cooking can make saliva form in the mouth, so starting digestion before any food is tasted.

Between that initial saliva to final defaecation, lies a system of great complexity which can break down in major or minor ways. Common symptons of digestive disorders are abdominal pain, constipation, diarrhoea, flatulence, indigestion, nausea, weight gain and loss; more serious problems could include appendicitis, liver disease, cancer of stomach or colon, pancreatitis and ulcers.

Most digestive problems are caused by the wrong sort of diet, – basically too little fibre – but often lack of exercise, stress, inherited tendencies and a combination of factors may contribute as well. The application of aromatherapy principles can help prevent many digestive problems for many plant foods contain essential oils which stimulate the digestive system, so encouraging good digestion by galvanizing sluggish organs into activity. The smells of herbs while cooking foods can start the first part of the process – the production of saliva – and those same herbal oils can help break down the foods when in the gut. For no matter how wholesome and vitamin-packed various foods may be, the nutrients sealed in them are of little value if they are not released and assimilated properly. The essential oils of aromatic herbs, fruits, vegetables and spices should be incorporated in cooking and diet whenever possible.

AROMATHERAPEUTIC TREATMENTS

- If prone to digestive problems, always cook with herbs and spices which will help – **basil**, bay (**laurel**) leaves, **caraway, ginger, marjoram, mint, oregano, pepper, savory** and **thyme** are all valuable. Use bay and thyme in marinades; marjoram and oregano with cabbage, and savory with beans.

(*See also* **angelica, anise, cardamom, chamomile, cinnamon, cloves, fennel, horseradish, lavender** *and* **lemongrass**.)

OTHER TREATMENTS

- Avoid over-eating, particularly of rich, fatty and fried foods. Do not drink in excess, and do not smoke.
- Do not eat too late at night or the digestion will be working overtime causing indigestion and insomnia.
- Do not eat too fast, as this taxes the system.
- After an attack, you could fast for a day, drinking only water with added lemon juice. This will clean out the system and give your overtaxed body a rest. Go back to a light diet thereafter, which includes plenty of fibre.
- Drinking milk or taking antacids can help. Half a teaspoon of bicarbonate of soda in a glass of water is an old and successful remedy.

269

● Avoid cooking in aluminium or copper pans. Aluminium salts from pans can leach out into the food and interfere with the secretion of digestive juices.

(*See also* **colic, constipation, dyspepsia, flatulence, gastritis, heartburn, nausea, PMT** *and* **stress**.)

DYSMENORRHOEA

Many women experience minor or quite considerable discomfort when their menstrual flow begins each month. This is commonest in young girls who have just begun to menstruate, and can involve headaches, lower abdominal cramps and low backache. These discomforts usually disappear when and if the contraceptive pill is taken and the sufferer has had a baby. Some women in later life begin to suffer painful periods after years of normal periods; this can be the symptom of several physical disorders and requires medical attention.

AROMATHERAPEUTIC TREATMENTS

● Herbal teas can help to relieve the pain. Try **aniseed, caraway, chamomile, fennel, melissa** and **parsley**.
● Warm, not hot, baths containing a few drops of an oil like **cypress** are good, and you could also apply poultices to the stomach as for diarrhoea. **Calendula** and **chamomile** are good.

(*See also* **marjoram** *and* **tarragon**.)

OTHER TREATMENTS

● Simple proprietary painkillers may help, as will lying in a darkened room with a hot water bottle on the stomach.
● A glass of port or brandy, or a brandy with hot water and honey can help.
● Foods that are rich in calcium and magnesium – dairy products, canned fish and nuts and seeds – should be eaten before a period starts as they are needed for muscle relaxation. The iron provided by liver, parsley and spinach can help as well.

ONION TART   *Serves 4 – 6*

This dish is tasty and therapeutic at the same time. Onions not only contain vitamins A, B and C, bu also valuable minerals and trace elements such as sulphur, phosphorus, silica, iodine, potassium and calcium. The tart is good for those suffering from menstrual problems, but the sulphur in the onions is also good for the nervous system, and skin and rheumatic conditions.

6 – 6½ lb (2.7 – 3 kg) white onions, peeled (or red onions)
15 ml (1 tbsp) first pressing virgin olive oil
1 sprig each of thyme and rosemary
a pinch of sea salt.

PASTRY
250 g (9 oz) white or wholemeal flour
150 g (5 oz) cold butter, diced
20 ml (1¼ tbsp) each of olive oil and water
a pinch of sea salt

Slice the onion thinly, and place in a large, heavy-bottomed saucepan or wok. Add the olive oil together with the herbs and sea salt. Cover and simmer over a very low heat until the onions are thoroughly cooked, about 20 minutes. Do not allow them to brown.

Meanwhile, to make the pastry, quickly combine the flour, butter, olive oil, water and salt (a blender or processor is handy). The speed at which you work will ensure the success of the pastry. Roll the pastry out and place on an oiled 25 cm (10 in) tart dish. Prick the bottom of the pastry with a fork, and chill for a few minutes. Cover with foil and baking beans and bake blind in the oven preheated to 325°F (160°C) Gas 3 for 10 minutes. Take out of the oven and remove the beans and foil.

Pick out and discard the rosemary and thyme sprigs from the onions, and spoon the onion evenly over the pastry. Bake in a hot oven – at 375°F (190°C) Gas 5 – for 15 – 20 minutes, and serve either hot or cold.

To garnish, you may use black olives, anchovies or tomato, or serve simply as it is.

(*See also* **abdominal pains, cramp, diarrhoea** *and* **menstrual problems**.)

DYSPEPSIA

This is a general medical term used to describe a group of symptoms that are more commonly known as indigestion. Dyspepsia can cause several problems of the digestive system – among them pain and discomfort in the stomach, nausea, flatulence and heartburn. It can be caused by nervous tension, and many young women experience digestive problems before menstruation. But most commonly the symptoms are the result of gastritis.

Helpful herbs and spices to use in tisanes, and oils to use for massage are **basil,** bay leaves (see **laurel**), **caraway, ginger,** and **mint**.

(*See also* **digestive system problems**.)

EAR PROBLEMS

The ear is a very delicate organ, and may cause problems in a number of ways. Earache is particularly common in young children, and this is usually due to an infection spreading from the nose or throat and can be experienced during or after a cold or 'flu, or some other infection such as sinusitis. Feverishness and partial loss of hearing are quire commonly experienced as well. Earache can also be a symptom of dental decay, teething in a young child, or an abscess or boil in the ear canal. It could herald the onset of mumps which can be serious in an adult. If the pain is very severe, and there is neck stiffness and raised temperature, it is important to see a doctor.

AROMATHERAPEUTIC TREATMENTS

- If the earache is thought to be caused by a throat infection, gargle with a glass of boiled water containing 2 drops of **tea tree** oil Repeat every two hours. Warm lemon drinks can help too.
- Dip a cotton wool bud in warm almond oil and insert gently into the affected ear. A drop of warm **chamomile** or **calendula** tisane could also be inserted.
- Mix 1 drop **clove** oil in 5 ml (1 tsp) soya or grapeseed oil, and massage around the neck and ear.

(*See also* **marjoram**.)

OTHER TREATMENTS

- The main thing is to keep warm, and a covered hot water bottle held against the affected ear may help. If going out, wrap the head warmly, covering the ears well, as wind can cause and exacerbate earache.
- If dental problems are thought to be the cause – and even badly fitting false teeth, or bad jawbone alignment can cause earaches and headaches – see the dentist. Try to chew on the side opposite the pain, and if it is all very tender, liquidize any food first.

(*See also* **colds, influenza sinusitis, teething pains** *and* **toothache**.)

ECZEMA

Also known as dermatitis, eczema comes in several forms, all involving inflammation, swelling, rashes and itchiness.

Contact eczema is the same as contact dermatitis, in which the skin reacts to an irritant substance. Atopic eczema is the type which affects people with a family history of other disorders such as asthma or hayfever, and is the type most commonly seen in babies and young children. Stress and fatigue can cause or exacerbate eczema. Helpful remedies include **benzoin, cedarwood, chamomile, geranium, juniper, orange, oregano, patchouli, rose, clary sage** and **sandalwood**. See **dermatitis** for suggested treatments.

EYE PROBLEMS

The eye is a very sensitive organ, and anything affecting it should be reported to a doctor. Symptoms can include redness, irritation, sudden pain and blurred vision, and causes can range from allergic reaction, migraine or hayfever, to a foreign body in the eye or sheer tiredness. Occasionally, eye problems can be the symptoms of more serious disease. However, very many minor eye problems can be treated effectively at home.

Conjunctivitis is one of the commonest eye infections. It is inflammation of mucous membrane which can be caused by bacteria, virus, allergy or a foreign body. The eyes are red and irritated, and there is sticky matter in them in the morning. It can easily be cured by prescription creams, but will also benefit from many of the remedies below.

AROMATHERAPEUTIC TREATMENTS

- To treat sore itchy eyes, cover them with compresses soaked in either cornflower, **chamomile** or **marigold** infusions.
- **Fennel** is good for inflamed puffy eyes, or for conjunctivitis.
- **Parsley** juice and **lemon** juice are good for eye problems, as are **rose** infusions which are very soothing.
- For tired eyes, simply cover with cooling **rose** petals or slices of fresh cucumber, lie down and relax for 1 minute.

(*See also* **jasmine; headaches**.)

FATIGUE

Fatigue or tiredness comes in many forms, most of which are obvious, such as the muscular fatigue after strenuous physical exercise. Fatigue can also display itself in the form of headaches and listlessness after a late or an insomniac night, after a heavy session of mental work or emotional stress. Hormonal changes can bring about fatigue, so children undergoing puberty and pregnant and menopausal women often suffer. Lassitude can be the symptom of something more serious.

AROMATHERAPEUTIC TREATMENTS

- Relaxing oils are often the answer to fatigue. Mix 3 – 4 drops of **basil, lavender, neroli**, or **petitgrain** with 10 ml (2 tsp) soya oil and 2 drops wheatgerm. Massage into the temple, around the neck, and on the chest. You could also put a few drops in the bath.
- For fatigue due to emotional stress, turn to the oils of the citrus family such as **lemon, neroli, orange** and **petitgrain** (but do be careful about **bergamot**, which I never use on the skin). Use as above.
- For fatigue because of hormonal changes (such as those of puberty or menopause), oils such as **chamomile, cypress, geranium** and **clary sage** can help. Use as above.

(*See also* **nutmeg; headaches, insomnia, menopause, menstrual problems, muscular pains, pre-menstrual tension** *and* **stress**.)

FEVER

Strictly speaking, fever is an abnormally high body temperature, anything two degrees or more over the normal body temperature of 37°C(98.6°F). Many bouts of feverishness in both children and adults can be the result of physical over-exertion, or a reaction to high weather temperature; they can also mark the onset of a childhood disease such as measles. In adults, a fever is usually associated with a bacterial or viral infection such as bronchitis, cold, 'flu or tonsillitis.

Symptoms other than raised temperature are shivering, chills and feeling hot, and all this is actually a good thing, for it means the body is fighting the infection.

AROMATHERAPEUTIC TREATMENTS

- Herb teas are useful. Infuse 15 ml (1 tsp) **chamomile, eucalyptus, rosemary** or **thyme** (or mix them) in 600 ml (1 pint) boiling water for 7 minutes. Drink warm, sweetened with honey if you like.
- Mix 10 drops of essential oil into a small bottle of mild shampoo, and add a little to a warm bath while it is running. Lie in the bath, then go back to bed. My favourite oils for this are **eucalyptus, lavender lemongrass, rosemary** and **tea tree**, but you could also use **aspic, baume de Tolu, chamomile, clove, coriander, cypress, niaouli** and **thyme**.
- Massage the temples, back of neck, top of hands and soles of feet with an oil consisting of 5 drops of one of the above bath oils with 5 ml (1 tsp) wheatgerm oil.
- Stay in bed in the dark and cover your eyes with cold herbal compresses over your eyes. Use **rose** petals, **parsley** or chervil.

OTHER TREATMENTS

- Drink a lot of fresh juices and mineral water to replace lost liquid.
- Rice cooked with fresh **thyme** or **rosemary** is nutritious and easy to digest.

(*See also* **bronchitis, colds, influenza, pneumonia** *and* **throat, sore.**)

FLATULENCE

This is the distension of the stomach and intestines by gas which can be caused by inhaled air, or by bacterial activity. This gas has to escape, thus the flatulence which can be so embarrassing.

We all swallow a certain amount of oxygen and nitrogen from the air, and this has to be dispelled; when we are stressed or nervous, we speak faster and gasp, and this explains why we can be more flatulent or gaseous when anxious.

Other gases can be formed in the intestines by bacterial action and fermentation of some foods. Many people do not possess the enzymes to digest certain foods (lactose in milk or gluten in wheat, for instance), and this causes flatulence. Other foods encourage flatulence because of the amount of sugar they contain, which tends to ferment in the intestines. These foods include beans, salad vegetables such as radishes, green peppers and cucumbers, and members of the cabbage family.

Helpful herbs and spices to use in cooking and tisanes, and oils to use in massage oils for the tummy are **anise, basil, cardamom,**

cloves, horseradish, laurel, lemongrass, marjoram, nutmeg, oregano, pimento and **savory. Angelica** stems chewed after meals prevent flatulence.

(*See also* **digestive system problems.**)

'FLU

(*See* **influenza.**)

FOLLICULITIS

Folliculitis is similar to impetigo, but the infection is in the hair follicle rather than on the surface of the skin. It seems that *staphylococcus* or *streptococcus* penetrates the deeper parts of the skin, usually through the mouth of the hair follicle, and the infection spreads rapidly from one hair follicle to the other. The skin surrounding becomes inflamed and tender, with a discharge of pus.

The infection is sometimes transmitted by unclean hair-removing instruments. If you have a problem with surplus hair, ensure you go to a specialist with a good reputation. The instruments and needles need to be properly disinfected after each patient. Hygiene is terribly important in cosmetic work of this nature.

See **abscesses** and **boils** for ways of treating the condition. Wash the face each time with clean cotton wool dampened with warm water with a few drops of **tea tree** oil.

(*See also* **impetigo.**)

FRACTURES

A fracture is a break in a bone, usually the result of a fall or accident, and it can cause pain, bruising, swelling and, occasionally, deformity. In young people, a fracture usually involves the clavicle, wrist or ankle; in older people, particularly women, who may be suffering from osteoporosis (a condition in which bone substance is lost), fractures often involve the hip.

If a fracture is suspected, emergency medical help must be sought. An x-ray will be taken, and if a fracture is confirmed, a plaster cast for several weeks, followed possibly by physiotherapy, will be necessary in the majority of cases.

Aromatherapy can help, but obviously only in the most general of ways.

AROMATHERAPEUTIC TREATMENT

- Some plants and plant oils can activate the circulation gently after the plaster cast has been removed. **Elemi** is particularly good. Warm a base oil, put a little elemi in it, and apply gently to the area of the healed fracture.

OTHER TREATMENT

- To help the bones, eat foods that are rich in calcium, such as milk, cheese, nuts and leafy green vegetables. This is particularly effective for older people and menopausal women. Foods containing phosphorus, potassium and the vitamins A, C and D are good as well.

FRIGIDITY

(See **sexual problems**.*)*

FROSTBITE

This is damage to areas of the skin and underlying tissue usually at the tip of the nose, ear lobes, cheeks and chin and is caused by prolonged exposure to freezing temperatures. Hands and feet are very vulnerable, even if enclosed in gloves or boots. The blood vessels near the cold surface contract, cutting off the supply of blood to the area. The symptoms are intense pain followed by numbness, and the skin becomes white and hard. If immediate steps are not taken, severe cases may develop into gangrene and result in amputation.

Much was discovered about frostbite following the two World Wars, from the experiences of pilots whose hands had frozen at high altitudes, and also from those soldiers who suffered trench foot due to exposure of the feet to cold and wet for weeks at a time. The old belief that massaging snow into the skin would help has now been disproved; massaging these almost brittle areas of skin can actually lead to a gangrenous condition. At present, treatment for frostbite includes gradual increase of the skin temperature by putting the patients into a cold room at first, thus allowing the frozen parts to thaw out slowly. Any rapid increase in the skin temperature could result in death of skin cells and gangrene of the tissue.

AROMATHERAPEUTIC TREATMENTS

- Many essential oils are good for the circulation and can be used in massage oils, primarily those of the pine family such as **pine** and **cypress**. **Baume de Tolu, lavender** and **aspic** are effective too. Gently apply lavender neat to patches of affected skin; this helps the pain of the 'burning'.
- If out in snow for a long time, rub a little grapeseed oil with a few drops of **pine** added to it on your feet at the end of the day.
- Mix a little cold cream with 1 drop of your chosen essence and apply to the frostbite. Wrap the area warmly afterwards.

Frostbite and cracked skin remedy
Warm up the *baume de Tolu* by placing the bottle under a hot tap.

> 10 ml (2 tsp) almond oil
> 2 drops **baume de Tolu**
> 2 drops **chamomile oil**

Mix together and apply gently to the affected parts three times a day until much better, then once a day until completely healed. Wear cotton socks or gloves, or protect with gauze.

- After the frostbite, apply some **baume de Tolu, calendula, lavender** or **lavandin** daily for several weeks.

(*See also* **benzoin** *and* **geranium**.)

OTHER TREATMENT

- Hot stimulating drinks are good. Heat up a red wine with some **cinnamon, cloves** and honey.

(*See also* **cracked skin**.)

GASTRITIS

This is an inflammation and irritation of the stomach lining due normally to eating or drinking to excess. It is exacerbated by smoking, can be caused by taking aspirin, and can lead to ulcers. A hangover is an attack of acute gastritis, and chronic gastritis is the breakdown of the stomach lining in old age.

A particularly helpful herb is **thyme**.

(*See also* **digestive system problems**.)

GINGIVITIS

(*See* **gum disease**.)

GOUT

This is a disease of the joints which is caused by a build-up of uric acid, one of the body's waste-products. When this cannot be excreted properly by the kidneys, the crystals collect in the joints, inflaming them and limiting their movement. Symptoms usually reveal themselves as a severe pain in the big toe, but may affect other joints, and it is associated with men rather than women. Gout is not necessarily caused by high living and over-indulgence in food and alcohol, but it is a well-known fact that many suffer from gout in January after the excesses of Christmas! Stress can also play a part.

AROMATHERAPEUTIC TREATMENTS

- Put a drop of **pine**, or **rosemary, juniper, cajuput, niaouli**, or **tea tree** in hot water in a bidet and keep the feet in this bath for 10 minutes. Rub with the neat oil afterwards.
- A drop each of **lavender** and **frankincense** mixed in a little grapeseed oil can also be used as a massage oil.
- A **rosemary** poultice is good for gout.

(*See also* **chamomile, lovage, thyme** *and* **wintergreen**.)

OTHER TREATMENTS

- Do not wear tight or high shoes if the gout affects the toes. Soft slippers would be best.
- Diet is important in the treatment of gout. Eat foods like artichokes, carrots, celery, tomatoes, radishes and dandelion leaves. Avoid fat and red meats, and eat lots of raw vegetables and fruit and soups containing leeks and onions.

279

- Wine, especially port (which is a mixture of wine and brandy) is bad in excess, causing calcium deposits in the joints. But the French use wine as medicine, believing that a glass of one wine specific to the disease can actually benefit. For gout, Dr Maury advised Sancerre, Champagne, Savoie Blanc and *rosé* de Provence. He believed that the mineral content of the wines produces an alkaline reaction, at the same time helping to get rid of the deposits. But no more than one glass a day!
- A tisane of apples works well. Cut the flesh and skin into small pieces and leave to infuse for 30 minutes. Drink 2 – 3 cups between meals, warming the pot and the tisane each time by placing the pot in a pan of boiling water.
- Strong nettle tea is another French remedy. Blackcurrants and liquorice are good too.

(*See also* **rheumatism**.)

GUM DISEASE

Disease of the gums (or pyorrhoea) is more commonplace than the common cold, and is the principal cause of tooth loss in people over the age of twenty-five. It is more serious than tooth decay as disease in the gums threatens the bone in which the teeth are set, the very foundation of the teeth. The gum acts as a protective wrapping between tooth and bone, preventing infection reaching the bone. When the tightness of the join line between tooth and gum is loosened, gum disease is occurring.

The main factor in gum disease is plaque, the tooth coating formed by bacteria in the mouth. This is soft at first, and produces acid which can eat into soft gum tissue and into the hard enamel and other layers of the teeth. Within 24 hours, plaque on the gum line can cause gingivitis, an inflammation of the gum tissue which marks the beginnings of gum disease. Unless it is brushed away regularly, plaque can go hard, when it is known as tartar or dental calculus; this affects the gums too, leading to disease, and once it has been allowed to build up, can only be removed by a dentist.

The first signs of gum disease are bleeding gums, and any bleeding when brushing should be reported to the dentist. Red, swollen or tender gums follow, with recession of the gums, bad breath, and discomfort. The end results of untreated gum disease are loose, separating or lost teeth.

Although the main cause of gum disease is poor mouth hygiene, pubescent children and pregnant or menopausal women can suffer too (there is a hormonal association), as can those taking the contraceptive pill and smokers. Some diseases (diabetes, for instance) and blood disorders can make the gums react.

AROMATHERAPEUTIC TREATMENTS

- Mix 1 drop of **clove** oil and 2 of **thyme** with 75 ml (3 fl oz) cooled boiled water. Using a clean index finger or a cotton wool bud, gently rub the mixture on to the gums.
- Mix 2 drops of **clove** oil and 1 drop of **clary sage** or **thyme** into 300 ml (½ pint) cooled boiled water. Gargle with this.
- Every day, slowly chew some fresh **tarragon, thyme, sage,** or **mint**.

(*See also* **horseradish, marjoram, mint** and **myrrh**.)

OTHER TREATMENTS

- The primary factors in the prevention of gum disease are good mouth hygiene – regular and effective brushing and flossing, plus visits to the dentist – and good diet. The bacteria in the mouth love sugars particularly, which enable them to produce more destructive acid, so sugars in all forms should be avoided.
- Vitamin C is a vital aid to skin health and gum health in particular. One of the major symptoms of scurvy is bleeding gums which need to be 'cured' by the supply of vitamin C-rich lemons.

(*See also* **toothache**.)

HAEMORRHOIDS

Haemorrhoids, or piles, are swollen or varicose veins in the wall of the anus. The most common cause is strain exerted on the abdominal muscles by heavy or improper lifting, or by pressure exerted during defaecation and/or when constipated. Many overweight or sedentary people suffer from piles too, as do some women during pregnancy.

Haemorrhoids can form internally or externally, and are itchy, may bleed or cause pain in the area or in the abdomen. Medical advice should always be sought if blood issues from the anus, as this can be the sign of more serious disease. There are simple conventional remedies for haemorrhoids, but surgery may be required for severe cases.

AROMATHERAPEUTIC TREATMENTS

- Once haemorrhoids have been diagnosed, eating fresh myrtle berries or a myrtle jam can help. Essential oil of **myrtle** can be applied externally.
- To relieve the discomfort, witchhazel can be used, or a **geranium** cream (see page 106).

(*See also* **cypress** *and* **patchouli**.)

281

OTHER TREATMENTS

- To prevent haemorrhoids forming, eat a healthy diet rich in fibre and drink plenty of fluids. Avoid tea, coffee, alcohol and spicy foods. Include plenty of fresh garlic in the diet, as well as melons and chestnuts (freshly cooked or a purée).
- Exercise can keep haemorrhoids at bay, particularly any that strengthen the abdominal muscles. Yoga breathing and fast walking help too.
- Boil leeks in water and then make ice-cubes from the water. Rubbed on the inflammation, these give instant relief.

(*See also* **cellulite, constipation, circulatory problems** *and* **varicose veins**.)

HAIR PROBLEMS

Most of us tend to think of hair in terms of colour, condition and style, and forget that it also serves a useful purpose in protecting the scalp from extremes of temperature and in regulating the loss of body heat from the head. Approximately 100,000 individual hairs grow from hair follicles in the scalp, and they do so at a rate of about 1 cm (½ in) a month, although this varies slightly from person to person.

In many respects, hair is similar to skin because it reflects inner health. Each hair is made of the tough, stretchable protein material called keratin, manufactured by the hair follicle. The condition of the developing hair is largely dependent upon a good supply of blood carrying adequate quantities of amino acids, vitamins A, B, C and E, and minerals like calcium, zinc, iron and copper, to the hair follicle. Poor health can be responsible for hair that lacks lustre and life.

While the hair is being formed, different pigment molecules are laid down which determine the colour of the hair. Hair can turn grey early, following illness or a period of intense emotional distress, because such things interfere with the production of the pigment. A nutritionally inadequate diet is capable of doing the same thing.

Hair is formed from living material, but the actual hair itself is dead, and after a period each one is shed and replaced by another. Its condition depends on good health and nutrition as above, but also on how it is treated. Many problems such as unmanageability and split ends are caused by abusing the hair through using the wrong shampoos and overdoing the styling.

It is important to know your hair, to recognize whether it is normal, or whether it has a tendency to oiliness or dryness. Alongside each hair lies a sebaceous gland which secretes sebum to lubricate the hair and lend it a degree of protection. If the glands are overactive, and produce more sebum than is needed, the hair becomes oily and will need more frequent washing to take away the excess. Do not resort to a more concentrated, oil-stripping shampoo, as this will only stimulate the glands into producing even more oil to compensate. If, on the other hand, the glands are sluggish, the hair will become dehydrated and dry, so you should avoid moisture-robbing hair driers, heated curlers and exposure to sunlight, wind and sea water. Most hair problems not directly caused by illness can be traced back to excessive use of heating appliances, misuse of chemical treatments such as perming and colouring, and washing with over-strong detergent shampoos. These constitute one of the major causes of hair loss and they can contribute to dandruff, perhaps the most common hair problem.

Essential oils are extremely helpful in hair care as they influence the sebaceous glands and normalize their functions. They are beneficial to all hair types, and leave hair smelling good too (particularly **patchouli** and **ylang-ylang**).

AROMATHERAPEUTIC TREATMENTS

- Make an infusion using **chamomile,** nettle, **rosemary** or **clary sage**, and add a cupful to your shampoo to dilute it. Wash in warm water, then for the final rinse use cold distilled or purified water.
- If you have greasy hair, add 6 drops **patchouli** oil to 150 ml (5 fl oz) mild shampoo.
- Twice a month, treat dry hair to a massage, using the pre-shampoo conditioner on page 193. Massage into your hair for a few minutes and then wrap your head in a warm towel to aid the penetration of the oils and leave for an hour. When washing out the oil, use a gentle shampoo, not diluted this time, and afterwards rinse through with either fresh lemon juice for fair hair or cider vinegar for dark to help restore manageability and shine. This treatment is particularly good for dull hair and hair that suffers from split ends.

(*See also* **bay, cade, cedarwood, horseradish, laurel** *and* **sage.**)

OTHER TREATMENTS

- A good diet, as with virtually everything else, is essential for shiny healthy hair. Protein is particularly important, as are vitamins A, B and C. (Hereditary factors such as early greying and balding cannot, however, be completely prevented by nutritional means.)
- Good hygiene is also necessary for healthy hair. When washing, use a mild or gentle shampoo to wash as frequently as you want.

283

- If you have dark hair, make a leek rinse to keep the natural colour and lustre. Boil four medium leeks for 20 minutes in water, throw away the leeks and keep the water. Use as the final rinse.

(*See also* **alopecia, dandruff** *and* **skin problems**.)

HALITOSIS

Bad breath is often one of the first signs that something might be amiss in the body. It can be caused by many things, among them liver trouble, inadequate or poor digestion of food, lung and respiratory problems, infections of the throat or sinus trouble. Many dentists, however, believe that bad breath is mainly caused by conditions in the mouth, by saliva and mouth bacteria, and by tooth decay and gum infections.

Any sudden noticeable attack of bad breath should be discussed with doctor or dentist, in case something is wrong. Careful mouth hygiene will help in most cases.

AROMATHERAPEUTIC TREATMENTS

- Chew herbs like **parsley, thyme, mint** or **tarragon,** or a **cinnamon** stick, a couple of coffee beans, or **fennel** or **anise** seeds.
- For a mouthwash and gargle, add 1 drop of **myrrh** essential oil to a cup of cooled, boiled water. Other good oils to use in a gargle are **chamomile, fennel, mint,** and **thyme**.

(*See also* **clove** *and* **orange**.)

OTHER TREATMENT

- In many Indian restaurants *paan* is offered after a meal. This is a mixture of seeds which sweeten the breath, among them cardamom, caraway and coriander.

(*See also* **digestive system problems, gum disease, respiratory system problems** *and* **toothache**.)

HAYFEVER

Hayfever – the disease that afflicts many people during the spring and summer months – is an allergic form of rhinitis. Rhinitis is an inflammation of the lining of the nose, and it occurs in acute form (the common cold) and chronic (caused by dust, chemicals, smoke). Hayfever is a reaction to the wind-borne pollens from plants present in the air during spring and summer (other allergic reactions are to animal fur and household dust). The symptoms are much the same as those of the common cold – stinging and watering eyes, blocked and runny nose, and sneezing.

Several solutions are offered by conventional medicine. Antihistamine preparations may be offered, but these often cause drowsiness. Steroid injections can help severe cases, but are disliked because of side effects. Many people opt for the desensitization techniques, which familiarize the antibodies in the blood to the allergen.

AROMATHERAPEUTIC TREATMENTS

- Drink tisanes made from **pine** needles, **eucalyptus** leaves or rose-hips.
- For the throat, gargle with **lemon** juice or boiled water containing a drop of **tea tree** oil.
- Make inhalations containing a few drops of **cajuput, eucalyptus, niaouli,** or **tea tree**.
- Rub an oil made from soya or grapeseed and a drop of one of the above oils on the chest, and around the nose and sinus area.
- Put a few drops of one of the above oils on a handkerchief, and carry it with you when you fear an attack may occur.
- Boil some **eucalyptus** leaves in water and spray this liquid throughout the house, especially in the bedroom before you go to sleep.
- Cool sore itchy and congested eyes by applying compresses soaked in **calendula, chamomile** or **parsley** infusions.

(*See also* **basil** *and* **pepper**.)

OTHER TREATMENTS

- A good diet can help hayfever sufferers overcome the tiredness and depression the disease can cause: eat lots of raw vegetables and fresh fruit which contain vitamin C. Such a diet can also help prevent the constipation which many hayfever sufferers experience, and which may also contribute to the disease.
- Avoid milk and other dairy products. These encourage the formation of catarrh and mucus in the alimentary tract.
- Although they can't cure hayfever, pollen granules – (¼ tsp per day) and garlic perles can help.

(*See also* **respiratory system problems**.)

285

HEADACHES

Headaches can have many causes – 'flus, colds, stress, sunstroke, sinusitis, neuralgia, too much TV, or bright or bad light causing eyestrain. Your common sense should tell you which it is, and what might be the remedy. Many women suffer headaches when pre-menstrual, and often digestive problems can be a causative factor. Many headaches can be caused by something as simple as a cold wind, but a headache that persists should never be taken lightly.

AROMATHERAPEUTIC TREATMENTS

- Massage around the back of the neck, on the temples, and around the eyes can be most soothing. Essential oils which are good are **basil, chamomile, coriander** (in very small doses only), **lavender, melissa, rosemary** and **clary sage**. Mix 1 drop oil into 5 ml (1 tsp) grapeseed oil, and massage. **Juniper** is especially good as it gives off a tiny amount of heat.
- Covering the eyes with the palms of your hands can relieve eyestrain headaches, as can merely lying in a darkened room with your eyes closed. Eye compresses using **chamomile, rosemary** or **parsley** are good too.
- Inhalations are good for many congestive headaches, because if the catarrh in the sinuses is cleared, so the headache will go. Use **cajuput, geranium, niaouli** and **tea tree** essential oils.
- If you have a hangover headache, take a nice long hot bath with a few drops of an enlivening oil like **pepper** or **juniper** to wake you up.

OTHER TREATMENTS

- Acupressure, pushing the index fingers into the eye sockets near the nose, can help.
- If the headache is caused by digestive problems, fast, drinking only water with lemon juice added for a day.
- In general eat very little until the headache goes.

(*See also* **colds, eye problems, fatigue, influenza, migraine, neuralgia, sinusitis** *and* **stress**.)

HEARTBURN

This is a severe burning pain behind the breastbone, and is known also as pyrosis. It is a digestive problem, and is also linked with acid regurgitation, a condition in which the contents of the stomach flow back from the oesophagus and cause discomfort right up to the mouth due to stomach acids.

(*See* **digestive system problems**.)

HERPES

(*See* **cold sores** *and* **shingles**.)

IMPETIGO

This is a highly infectious skin disease, usually caused by *streptococcus* or *staphylococcus* which mainly affects children. Inflamed puffy patches or spots appear – usually on the face, scalp and neck, but sometimes on the hands and knees – which blister, then crust over. It is spread to other parts of the body – or to other people – by scratching and then touching unaffected areas of skin. It can be treated successfully by antibiotics, but aromatherapy can help too.

Strict hygiene is essential to prevent spread of the infection to other parts of the body or indeed to other people. Neglected impetigo can become serious in adults, with boils, ulcers, conjunctivitis and further complications. Impetigo on the scalp can lead to patchy hair loss.

AROMATHERAPEUTIC TREATMENT

- Oils which can help impetigo are **benzoin, calendula** (particularly good for the scalp), **carrot, chamomile, patchouli** and **tea tree**. Mix a few drops of your chosen oil with 5 ml (1 tsp) of grapeseed oil and 5 ml (1 tsp) wheatgerm oil, and apply to infected areas once a day.

OTHER TREATMENTS

- Vitamin A in the diet is vital for a healthy skin, so take plenty of carrots, yellow fleshed fruits and cod or halibut liver oil. Vitamins B and C are good too.
- Clean the face twice a day with fresh cabbage juice mixed with an acid soap.
- An old folk remedy is to dab the areas of infection at least ten times a day with cider vinegar, using a clean pad each time.

(*See also* **abscesses and boils, acne, alopecia** *and* **folliculitis**.)

IMPOTENCE

(*See* **sexual problems**.)

INDIGESTION

(*See* **digestive system problems** *and* **dyspepsia**.)

INFLUENZA

Influenza is a virus infection which often occurs in epidemics, mainly in winter. 'Flu is uncomfortable and highly contagious, but it is not dangerous except to the elderly or those with heart or lung disorders. Vaccines are available each year.

The major symptoms of 'flu are headache, aching muscles and back, high temperature, shivering, sweating, weakness, cough, sore throat, chest pains, catarrh and sneezing. The worst of the illness is over within two to three days, but other symptoms may last longer, for up to a week.

AROMATHERAPEUTIC TREATMENTS

- Drink plenty of fluids to replace losses caused by fever. The minerals sodium and potassium will be lost through sweating, so replace them by drinking the following spicy tisane: boil 1 stick of **cinnamon**, 2 **cloves**, 2 sprigs fresh **thyme** (or 3 pinches dried) in 1 litre (1¾ pints) water for 2 minutes, then infuse for 5 minutes. Strain and drink throughout the day.
- Drink tisanes made from plants which benefit colds and 'flu such as **chamomile, eucalyptus, hyssop, laurel** and **thyme**. Syrups made from **eucalyptus** and **hyssop** are also good as are inhalations of such oils as **eucalyptus, niaouli** and **tea tree**.
- To protect against infection, and for when the first symptoms appear, do as for a cold (see page 252). See also **palmarosa** and **pine** for anti-bacterial spray mixtures.

(*See also* **cinnamon, coriander, cumin, lavender** *and* **pepper**.)

OTHER TREATMENTS

- When you develop 'flu, stay in bed and keep warm. Do not attempt to go to work as the virus will spread.

• Eat foods which are easy to digest as for a cold.

(*See also* **chest infections, colds, diarrhoea, ear problems, fever, headaches, nausea** *and* **respiratory system problems**.)

INSOMNIA

Insomnia means that one is unable to sleep. It can occur during illness (although usually the body *creates* sleep in order that it may heal itself), but mostly it occurs when the insomniac is in a state of stress or anxiety. Insomnia can also be caused by physical states such as pre-menstrual tension and the menopause. Older people, too, very often suffer from insomnia although the older one gets, the less sleep is needed.

Very often the inability to sleep is caused by such easily remediable factors as lack of exercise, too many stimulants like alcohol or cigarettes, or eating too late in the evening. Chemical solutions like tranquillizers and sleeping pills are not the answer either. Many of these can be addictive, and they can cause anxieties, so are best avoided. The milder hypnotics can induce sleep quickly, and the stronger narcotics will probably guarantee sleep, but the speed at which a dependence on them builds up is horrifying, and can be very dangerous.

AROMATHERAPEUTIC TREATMENTS

• **Lavender** is a gentle narcotic, recommended for mental and physical strain. Drink as a tea, using 5 – 10 g (¼ – ½ oz) infused as below. You could also keep a sachet of dried lavender nearby when sleeping, perhaps in your pillowcase. Put some sachets of dried lavender in the cupboard where you keep your sheets, and add 10 drops of essential oil of lavender to your clothes softener when washing your sheets and bedclothes.
• Have a warm bath with essential oils half an hour before going to bed. Use **lavender, neroli** or **petitgrain**. Inhale the fumes and breathe in, relax for ten minutes in the water, then dry yourself and go straight to bed.
• A massage with essential oil – 2 drops **neroli, lavender, basil, melissa** or **petitgrain** mixed with 10 ml (2 tsp) of a carrier oil – can be useful. The massage should be gentle and relaxing.
• Stop taking stimulants like tea, coffee, cigarettes, alcohol or cola drinks after 5pm. Replace them with herbal teas. Some are sedative, such as linden flowers, which will be particularly good for people suffering from emotional shock and trauma. Infuse a full handful of dried

linden flowers in 1 litre (2 ¼ pints) boiling water, and drink two large cups an hour before going to bed, sweetened with a little honey if you like. Passiflora, too, is a natural sedative, useful for nervous depression and mental exhaustion. Infuse 40 g (1 ½ oz) as above.

(*See also* **lemon, mandarin, marjoram** *and* **rose**.)

OTHER TREATMENTS

- Trying to sleep in a room or bed that is too warm, cold or airless can cause sleeplessness. Switch off the central heating during the night (unless it is very cold); wear cotton or linen and use cotton or linen sheets, and open the bedroom windows during the day, or at least half an hour before going to bed, to allow fresh air into the room.
- Eat early, making your evening meal the lightest, with breakfast the main meal of the day. Salads, fresh vegetables and fruit are best. Mandarin oranges contain a substance which acts on the nervous sytem. Lettuce, too, is a natural soporific and it has a calming effect on the nervous system, is good for palpitations in menopause, for premenstrual tension, and for nervous disorders of all kinds. Eat it in soups, steamed as a vegetable, raw in salads, and in tisanes: infuse 50g (2 oz) lettuce in 1 litre (2 pints) boiling water for 10 minutes, then drink two large cups, sweetened with a small spoon of honey, 1 hour before going to bed.
- Exercise is important. Try to have a good hour's brisk walk during the day, and take a walk after your evening meal. Do some gentle stretching exercises – yoga is particularly beneficial – to help relieve some of the tensions of the day. And do some relaxation exercises when lying down in bed if you think you won't get off to sleep. In turn, press your head, shoulders, back, arms, bottom, legs into the mattress, then release. Stretch your arms, fingers, legs and toes out as far as you can, then relax. Pull your shoulders down towards your feet, releasing your neck, then relax. Feel the mattress taking your weight, with your muscles gradually relaxing.

(*See also* **menopause** *and* **stress**.)

JETLAG

Anyone who has taken a long flight will know the 'symptoms' of jetlag: fatigue, sleep disturbances, nausea and aching or swollen limbs. That the body is so affected is not surprising as by crossing several time-zones you apparently disrupt some 50 physiological and psychological rhythms in your body. The actual *process* of the flying itself – being enclosed in a pressurized plane for hours at a time, and the height at which the plane flies – also plays a part in jetlag. Frequent long haul travellers can have more long-lasting problems: air stewardesses, for instance, experience great irregularity in their menstrual cycles.

AROMATHERAPEUTIC TREATMENTS

- To avoid swollen ankles, put a small suitcase under your feet to elevate them and to prevent the thighs being pressed against the edge of the seat. Walk up the aisle occasionally to keep the circulation going; and massage your feet with a relevant oil (see **oedema**). Do foot exercises as well. Squeeze the toes together, hold for a count of five, and then release. Do this ten or fifteen times at a time.
- When you arrive at your destination, if you want to stay alert, put 10 drops of **lavender** in your hand and rub on the torso, followed immediately by a shower. If you want to sleep, take a bath with 3 drops of **geranium** added.

OTHER TREATMENTS

- On the actual flight, wear comfortable, loose clothes.
- Avoid eating anything on the flight other than citrus fruit.
- Dehydration is a major factor because of the low moisture content of the plane. To counter this, drink plenty of still mineral water (very important for children), and avoid alcohol (which dehydrates you even further).
- Take a moisturizing cream with you to counter skin dehydration.

(*See also* **oedema**.)

LARYNGITIS

(*See* **throat, sore**.)

LEUCORRHOEA

This is an inflammation of the vagina often caused by the proliferation of unwanted bacteria or even a kind of fungus which gives rise to a thick white or yellow discharge. It often occurs if women have been taking a course of antibiotics. Women who are most susceptible are those using the contraceptive pill, those who are pregnant, or those suffering from the metabolic disorder, diabetes.

AROMATHERAPEUTIC TREATMENTS

- Add to your bath 2 drops of **juniper** or **lavender**, or 1 drop of either of these in the bidet.

(*See also* **niaouli**.)

OTHER TREATMENTS

- To prevent leucorrhoea, a good diet is essential, one which is particularly rich in foods containing vitamins A and B.
- Avoid wearing underwear made from synthetic fibres such as polyester or nylon, as well as tightly fitting jeans.
- Never use harsh detergents, bubble baths or similar products as these can aggravate the condition.

(*See also* **thrush.**)

LUMBAGO

This is the term for a severe pain in the lumbar region of the spine, the lower back. It is caused by lifting heavy objects incorrectly, or by twisting the spine in an awkward position. It can appear in pregnancy. Some sufferers cannot stand upright again for some moments after stooping. Often lumbar pains are followed by sciatica but they may also be the early signs of a prolapsed or slipped vertebral disc.

Bed rest, heat and massage are ways in which the pain and the pressures can be relieved.

AROMATHERAPEUTIC TREATMENTS

- Lie in hot baths. Mix 6 drops **mustard** and **rosemary** oils or **oregano** and **thyme** into a little mild shampoo and add while the bath is running.
- Make a linseed poultice using about 45 ml (3 tbsp) linseed with 5 drops of **juniper, mustard, oregano, pine, rosemary** or **thyme**. Leave for at least 10 minutes and repeat a few times a day. You should feel immediate relief.
- Make an oil to massage in after the poultice. Mix 6 drops of one of the above oils into 10 ml (2 tsp) almond oil with 2 drops wheatgerm oil.

OTHER TREATMENTS

- It is essential to stay in bed for a few days. Put a large cushion under the knees to rest the back.
- Keep the back warm by wearing warm clothing. Cut up an old lambswool or cashmere sweater and wear a band of this around the back.

(*See also* **backache** *and* **sciatica**.)

MELANOSIS

Melanosis is a browning of the pigmentation of the skin, which can occur anywhere on the body. Melanin is the natural dark pigment that colours the skin, hair and eyes; it is melanin that is responsible for the protective darkening of the skin in suntanning, and it is a lack of melanin that is responsible for albinism. In melanosis, the brown appears in patches, and there could be a number of reasons for this. It could be too much sun, or it could be a liver deficiency. As many women develop brown spots when pregnant and around the time of the menopause, there could also be a hormonal link. The inclusion of **bergamot** oil in cosmetics and perfumes can cause brown patches as well.

AROMATHERAPEUTIC TREATMENTS

- Drink **parsley** and **chervil** tisanes as they seem to have a fading effect on the marks of melanosis.
- Apply these tisanes *to* the marks; you could also use essential oil of **lemon** or lemon juice, both of which are slightly bleaching. **Benzoin** too is very good.

OTHER TREATMENTS

- To prevent interference with the workings of melanin, always protect the skin in strong sunlight with sun block. Sunbathing is not very good for us, however pleasant it may be; it is one of the major factors in ageing skin. Do not forget to protect your hands in the sun.
- Eat plenty of foods containing vitamins A and E, which are good for the skin.

(*See also* **ageing skin, skin problems** *and* **sunburn**.)

MENOPAUSE

Because menopause is so rarely mentioned in medical books of even a generation ago, we might be forgiven for thinking that our grandmothers were more stoic than us or simply accepted more readily one of the most natural processes of the female cycle. But today, in an age when women have been liberated sexually, when they are more in control of their bodies, women are enslaved by the concept of beauty and youth. The media and the beauty industry have worked in tandem in the last few years, bombarded us with images of youth, and there is an ever-growing emphasis on regenerative products, treatments and cosmetic surgery. No wonder then that the menopause has become the villain, the ultimate threat to youth, the onset of age.

But menopause is a natural process which every women must undergo at some time, and the misinformation has generated a great deal of unnecessary fear. It is merely a new phase of the cycle, and although it may cause temporary discomfort, it passes. Generally occurring between the ages of 45 and 50, it essentially means the gradual or abrupt cessation of menstruation and the secretion of certain glands. What it does not mean is the concomitant cessation of sexuality, desire or youthfulness. Rather than becoming ugly ducklings overnight, many women acquire a new maturity, a new beauty and a new self-awareness and confidence, feeling more relaxed in general about their careers, lives and bodies.

The manner in which menopausal changes occur is subject to tremendous variation. For some, menopause is quick and relatively trouble-free; for others, it can be more disturbing, lasting a couple of years. Some symptoms are minor mental depression, irritability, excitability, hot flushes and itching skin. Dizziness, palpitations and insomnia may occur if the process is regarded with fear. And it is this attitude to menopause which is more damaging than anything. Relax, follow a few simple guidelines, and this phase can be undergone without too much *angst*. Accept it instead, and deal with it in the most natural way. You might gain from it, acquiring a new beauty and a new wisdom.

AROMATHERAPEUTIC TREATMENTS

- Drink **sage** and nettle teas, which are rich in substances akin to the female hormones.
- For mental depression, replace stimulant drinks by **thyme** and **rosemary** teas. Use these herbs in your cooking. Take some gentle exercise – walking, cycling, swimming. Use essences of **rosemary**, **lavender** and **thyme** in your bath (2 drops of each), and have a massage once a week with these essences added to 20 ml (4 teaspoons) almond oil.

- For irritability and excitability, replace stimulants such as coffee, tea, chocolate and alcohol, with herb teas which have a calming effect – **basil**, linden flowers, **orange** leaves, **chamomile** and passiflora. Avoid stimulants, especially after 5pm, and always eat early – salad and fresh vegetables are best. East slowly and in a calm atmosphere.
- Hot flushes can be embarrassing at times, and you might wake up at night feeling unpleasantly sticky and wet. Avoid eating spicy food and stimulants. **Sage** tea is good at this time. Wear cotton and linen. Apply an infusion of **chamomile** tea gently to the face with cotton wool. This stops the hot feeling, and helps the redness and itchiness. Avoid strong cosmetics and replace heavy make-up with a more natural one (heavy make-up makes one look older anyway). If the skin feels especially dry, apply almond oil on a damp cotton wool pad. Rinse it off with chamomile tea.
- For dizziness and headaches, massage the nape of your neck and your temples for a few minutes with neat essential oil of **lavender**, but always test for a reaction first. Lie down with your legs raised, and close your eyes.
- For palpitations, avoid stimulant drinks and replace with herbal teas (a mixture of **rose** petals and **sage** is good) or freshly squeezed fruit juices. When it is in season, have some lily-of-the-valley flowers near you. Close your eyes, inhale slowly, and repeat a few times. Lily of the valley contains digitalis, and its perfume regulates the heartbeat.

(*See also* **angelica, anise, cardamon, cypress, melissa** *and* **tarragon; depression, headaches, insomnia, melanosis, palpitations** *and* **stress.**)

MENSTRUAL CYCLE PROBLEMS

The menstrual cycle begins at puberty and continues through a woman's life until menopause, unless of course it is interrupted by pregnancy and lactation. This cycle involves the participation of several different hormones, which interact to bring about the maturation of ova within the woman's reproductive organs, the ovaries. Presiding over this process is a region of the brain called the hypothalamus.

In young women, puberty usually takes place between the ages of about ten and fourteen, although it can begin earlier or later. During this time, the hypothalamus starts to send signals to the pituitary gland, which appears to orchestrate the activities of all the other hormone-producing glands in the body. The pituitary responds by releasing hormones into the bloodstream. One of these is the follicle-stimulating hormone (FSH), which travels to the ovaries and instigates the maturation of an ovum within its own little capsule or follicle. As the ovum develops, the follicle starts to produce the ovarian hormone oestrogen. By the time the ovum is fully matured, the pituitary has released another of its secretions, what is called the luteinizing hormone. When this hormone reaches the ovaries it triggers the release of the ovum from the follicle in a process known as ovulation.

The empty follicle starts to produce the hormone progesterone. Meanwhile, the mature ovum, which is now highly receptive to the presence of any male sperm, begins its journey along the fallopian tube towards the uterus. If no sperm are available, and the ovum is not fertilized, it is lost from the body along with the lining of the uterus; this, which has been proliferating since the time of ovulation, is shed as blood in the process known as menstruation. On average, this menstrual flow usually lasts from four to five days, although it may be shorter or longer.

The whole cycle usually takes about 28 days, although it is not abnormal to find it can be up to seven days longer or shorter. The first day marks the beginning of the menstruation with ovulation taking place around the fourteenth day, but again this varies from one individual to another.

Most women suffer upsets in their menstrual cycles at some time during their life, and these can usually be traced back to some kind of hormonal imbalance. The sort of symptoms that accompany such upsets are diverse and are likely to be of an emotional as well as physical nature. Sometimes, women are given prescriptions for drugs such as diuretics or tranquillizers to relieve the symptoms, and perhaps even hormones in the form of the contraceptive pill or implants in an attempt to redress the balance.

The trouble with such remedies is that they fail to get to the heart of the problem. Because the hypothalamus, pituitary gland and ovaries are all involved in the menstrual cycle, it is likely that the imbalance comes from one of them being either under- or over-active. One of the reasons why stress is such a problem for women is because it affects the hypothalamus, which in turn transmits its disturbances to the ovaries and other glands, so disrupting the finely-tuned balance. The sex glands not only play a role as organs of reproduction, but also relate to a general well-being; when they are not functioning properly, tiredness and listlessness set in.

Essential oils provide a safe and effective means of treating menstrual disturbances because they appear to stimulate the endocrine glands and work toward normalizing the hormone secretions. Fabrice Bardeau, a French pharmacist, and doctors Valnet and Belaiche classify certain essential plants as being emmenagogues – acting to normalize and promote the menstrual cycles. Such plants and plant oils are **cypress, nutmeg, parsley** and **tarragon**. A possible explanation for their influence is that certain essences contained in the plants closely resemble the female hormones. Cypress, for example, is believed to have a chemical structure akin to one of the ovarian hormones. They can be used in the bath, as inhalations or for massaging the stomach and solar plexus.

(*See also* **anise, basil, horseradish, juniper, oregano, clary sage** *and* **tea tree; amenorrhoea, anorexia nervosa, cellulite, dysmenorrhoea, menopause, oedema** *and* **pre-menstrual tension.**)

MIGRAINE

A migraine is a severe recurrent headache, one of the commonest diseases of the nervous system. As many as 5 per cent of the population suffer from it, more women then men. It can be hereditary. It can involve visual abnormality and tingling or numbness in a limb before the attack, followed by a throbbing headache and nausea. It can last from a few hours to several days, and many people are severely incapacitated by it.

Migraines are caused by a sudden narrowing of the arteries leading to one side of the head, followed by a headache when the same blood vessels enlarge again. They are common in energetic, stressed people, have been linked to the contraceptive pill, and may be triggered by an accident or trauma, by certain smells, or certain foods such as cheese, chocolate, or red and white wines.

AROMATHERAPEUTIC TREATMENTS

- Feverfew (*Tanacetum parthenium*) is a herb that has recently come to prominence because of its effectiveness in treating migraine. Although not quite accepted by traditional medicine, research tests have shown that eating four leaves a day – in a sandwich, say, or a salad with other leaves like young dandelions or nettles – can help control incidence and severity of attacks. You could also make a feverfew tisane.
- As soon as the first symptoms appear, infuse **basil** leaves in hot water and drink as a herb tea. Mix 1 drop basil oil with 5 ml (1 tsp) soya oil and massage into the temples, nape of the neck and solar plexus in a clockwise direction – and relax on a bed for a few minutes. Repeat this a few times until the symptoms cease.
- Other plants and oils which could help are **chamomile, fennel, lemongrass, marjoram, melissa** and **oregano.**
- Some fish oils are said to be good for migraines too.

(*See also* **headaches, nausea** *and* **neuralgia.**)

MOUTH ULCERS

Called aphthous ulcers, these are tiny open sores which develop inside the mouth – on the tongue or roof of the mouth, on the mucous membrane inside the lips and cheeks, and in the groove between gums and cheeks. The ulcers are heralded by a burning and tingling sensation, and a slight swelling of the site. The centre of each is white, surrounded by an inflamed red border which is tender to the touch. The specific cause is unknown, although some believe it is a mild virus infection, thus the common recurrences of the problem. However, most research has shown that mouth ulcers are brought on by a state of anxiety or emotional stress, or by a sensitivity to certain foods and substances which produce allergic-type reactions. Ulcers can last for from two days to three weeks; they heal spontaneously leaving no scar.

AROMATHERAPEUTIC TREATMENTS

- Dip a cotton wood bud in **tea tree** oil and apply neat to the mouth ulcers for immediate relief. Do this a few times a day.
- Wash your mouth out with 600 ml (1 pint) warm boiled water containing 1 tbsp sea salt and 2 drops **tea tree** oil.
- Boil a handful of **carrot** leaves in 300 ml (10 fl oz) water for 5 minutes, then cool slightly. Use as a gargle.
- Avoid lemon juice and anything acidic. Use **rose, savory** or **clary sage** in a mouthwash. 1 drop to a tumbler of water.

(*See also* **cloves, marjoram** *and* **mint**.)

OTHER TREATMENTS

- As with all skin problems, a well-balanced diet, one rich in Vitamin A, would help prevent and cure mouth ulcers.
- Avoid eating acid and spicy foods, both of which can cause pain. Also avoid coffee. Do not eat hard bread, biscuits and salted nuts or other salty foods but try cream caramel and rice pudding, containing milk which is alkaline and can provide relief from the pain.
- Avoid smoking and alcohol.

MUSCULAR PAINS

Pains in the muscles can be caused by a variety of problems – by influenza, by rheumatism, by diarrhoea, or by being sick, by standing or sitting too long, by too little or too much exercise. Once you think you have discovered the cause, turn to the appropriate section for some more specific remedies.

AROMATHERAPEUTIC TREATMENTS

- **Wintergreen** is good for rheumatic muscular pain. Use 5 drops of it in the bath, and then massage with an oil consisting of 4 – 5 drops wintergreen, 1 – 2 drops wheatgerm and 10 ml (2 teaspoons) soya oil.
- **Rosemary**, used in the same way, is effective for muscular pains caused by too much exercise. Also good are **fennel, pine** and **thyme**.

(*See also* **backache, diarrhoea, influenza** *and* **rheumatism.**)

NAILS

Fingernails and toenails are made of the protein keratin, which is contained in the skin cells, so nails are modified skin tissue. Like skin, nails can benefit from aromatherapy. Also, like skin, they benefit from a good, well-balanced diet; protein and vitamins A and E are particularly important.

AROMATHERAPEUTIC TREATMENTS

- Make up an oil consisting of 10 ml (2 tsp) linseed or walnut oil, with 2 drops wheatgerm and 2 drops of a resinous oil such as **frankincense, galbanum** or **myrrh**. Rub gently on to each nail once a week to strengthen brittle nails. You could also take a winter or summer 'cure': rub on two or three times per week for two months.

OTHER TREATMENT

- Avoid nail lacquer and detergents (wear rubber gloves when washing up or using cleaning solvents).

NAUSEA

Nausea has many causes, both physiological and psychological. Psychological causes include disgusting sights and smells, and physiological causes include early pregnancy. Bad digestion, tonsillitis, 'flu, a hangover, migraine or food poisoning can also cause nausea and sickness.

Some food allergies can cause nausea as well, as can travel motion.

AROMATHERAPEUTIC TREATMENTS

- Do not try to take any food when feeling nauseous. A cup of herbal tea might help a digestive nausea – try **mint, fennel** or **anise.**
- To cope with the nausea of shock, lie down and drink some warm, watery herbal tea such as **melissa, bigardier** or lime flowers.
- If you have been sick, a light **mint** tea could help alleviate the nasty taste in your mouth.

OTHER TREATMENTS

- Well-browned toasted bread or well cooked and carbonized onion could calm pain and help digestion.
- Fresh air is often the answer – especially for those who suffer from motion sickness.

(*See also* **mint; digestive system problems, influenza, jetlag, migraine, stress** *and* **throat, sore.**)

NEURALGIA

Neuralgia, a symptom rather than a disease, is the pain felt when a nerve is irritated or compressed. Any inflammation or infection can cause it, shingles (or *Herpes zoster*) being one of the commonest; other causes are fractured bones or slipped discs pressing on nerves. Headaches, toothaches and sinusitis can trigger neuralgia. Often, though, a facial neuralgia, for instance, can be triggered by simply going out in a cold wind. Sciatica and migraine are types of neuralgia. Facial neuralgia can be successfully treated with aromatherapeutic remedies.

AROMATHERAPEUTIC TREATMENTS

- Make an oil to massage into the spot, with 5 ml (1 tsp) grapeseed oil, 2 drops wheatgerm oil, and 3 drops **mustard** or **pepper** oils.
- Prepare an inhalation using 1 drop of **eucalyptus, niaouli** or **tea tree**.
- Make up a linseed poultice using any of the above oils. Do not make it too hot for the face.

(*See also* **chamomile, coriander** *and* **oregano.**)

OTHER TREATMENTS

- If a particular nerve or set of nerves is vulnerable, always cover warmly when going out in cold weather. Wrap the neck and head well, particularly if the hair is thin.
- A very tight hat or headband can cause neuralgia in the face.

(*See also* **headaches, migraine, sciatica, sinusitis** *and* **toothache**.)

OEDEMA

Oedema is a condition in which excess fluid is retained by the body, causing swelling or puffiness of the tissues. It usually affects the hands, feet or around the eyes, but can be found in any part of the body. It was once known as dropsy.

There are many possible causes, the most serious being some form of kidney disease. Pregnancy, oral contraception, premenstrual tension, allergic reaction (to such as an insect bite), standing or sitting for too long, and injury can all cause the body to retain fluid. It is most commonly seen in the ankles, where the fluid arrives by gravity.

AROMATHERAPEUTIC TREATMENTS

- If the swelling appears in the face, apply witch hazel mixed with an equal quantity of mineral water. Make a herbal tea by infusing 1 tbsp **chamomile, chervil, parsley** or **rose petals**, in 600 ml (1 pint) boiling water for 7 minutes. Strain and cool, then apply compresses to the face. Repeat every hour.
- If the eye lids swell, leave the compresses on the eyes for 10 – 15 minutes. The best herbs to use are **chervil** and **parsley**.
- Warm baths containing a few drops of **lemon, mandarin, neroli, orange** or **petitgrain** can help. Baths or showers must always be warm, not hot.
- Massage the soles of the feet vigorously with an oil consisting of 15 ml (1 tbsp) grapeseed or soya oil, and 2 – 3 drops of **cypress** or **rosemary** oil.
- Massage the legs with an oil consisting of a base of 50 ml (2 fl oz) soya oil and 5 drops wheatgerm, plus 6 drops each of **cypress** and **lemon**.
- Morning and night, friction the top of the hands, soles of the feet, the abdomen and solar plexus with an oil made from the soya and wheatgerm base above, plus 8 – 12 drops of **aspic, basil, cedarwood, cypress, lavender** or **wintergreen**.

(*See also* **thyme**.)

OTHER TREATMENTS

- A good diet rich in vitamin B, particularly B_1, can help. This is contained in whole grains, organ meats, eggs, vegetables, nuts, onion and garlic. Also good in the diet are parsley, tarragon, leeks, celery, celeriac and juniper berries.
- Vitamin C has a mild diuretic action, so increase the intake of C-rich fruits in the diet.
- A watercress soup is wonderfully diuretic, especially for the bloating caused by PMT.
- Many wines can help fluid retention. Dr Maury recommends Chablis, Muscadet, Sylvaner, Pouilly Fuissé and Sancerre for their diuretic effect.
- Drink between meals, not with meals.
- If the swelling is in the ankles, avoid too hot baths, and tight shoes or socks or nylon tights or stockings. Sleep at night with the end of the bed higher then the head – or put a cushion under your knees. This is particularly useful if the swelling is caused by standing too long.
- Take lots of exercise to prevent fluid retention.

(*See also* **bursitis, jetlag** *and* **pre-menstrual tension**.)

PALPITATIONS

This is a general term used to describe the sensation of an irregular heartbeat – either the 'missing' of a beat, or a speeding up of the rate of beats. This is usually quite normal after exercise, say, or when stressed or frightened, or when stimulants such as caffeine or nicotine have been taken. Many women experience palpitations during menopause.

Palpitations may, however, be the symptom of some underlying heart disorder, and if recurrent should be checked by a doctor.

AROMATHERAPEUTIC TREATMENTS

- Drink tisanes of calming plants like **orange** leaves, lime (tilleul), bigaradier, **basil** and **melissa**, or a mix of **rose** petals and **sage**. A liquorice herb tea is good too, as is a tea made from boiled artichoke leaves. A **rosemary** tea at night helps men particularly.
- Garlic juice and perles can be taken daily as a preventative.
- Mix 2 drops each of **neroli** and **melissa** in 5 ml (1 tsp) soya or grapeseed oil, and rub clockwise on the solar plexus, on the back of the neck, top of the hands and soles of the feet.

(*See also* **anise**.)

OTHER TREATMENTS

- Avoid coffee, tea, cola drinks, chocolate, alcohol and cigarettes. Do not eat too much either.
- During an 'attack', dip the hands and arms up to the elbow in cold water for at least 10 seconds.
- Dip a sugar lump in cider vinegar and crunch it when you experience palpitations.

(*See also* **menopause** *and* **stress**.)

PEDICULOSIS

This is the medical term for infestation of the head or body with lice. There are three types which affect human beings: body lice, head lice (their eggs are known as nits), and pubic lice, or crabs. They all suck blood through the skin; these areas become itchy and scratching can lead to infections similar to impetigo. Lice are spread by close physical contact – nits spread like wildfire in schools, for instance – and crabs through sexual intercourse.

AROMATHERAPEUTIC TREATMENTS

- For head lice (*Pediculus capitis*), treat the scalp with an alcohol rub. Use a little tumbler of vodka, and mix into it 10 drops of a suitable oil – the nicest are **geranium, juniper** or **lavender**. Rub this into the scalp at night and wash off in the morning. Comb with a special head lice comb, and repeat treatment as necessary.
- Body lice (*Pediculus corporis*) can be picked up through mattresses and close contact with humans and/or animals. First rub the whole body with neat **lavender** oil, then follow every day until better with a rubbing mixture of 20 ml (4 tsp) vodka and 10 drops **lavender, aspic** or **juniper**. Change all bedding and clothes and wash thoroughly. Rub essential oil on the mattress and protect it (and you) with a thick, dry-cleaned cover. Cat or dog fleas can be treated in the same way, as can scabies.
- To get rid of pubic lice (*Phthiris pubis*), cut the hair very short and rub with neat oil as above. Be very careful not to allow the oil inside the body. Bathe often and always wear clean underwear.
- To stop the bites burning and itching, buy a good cold cream, add 2 drops of any of the above oils, and apply.

(*See also* **laurel; scabies**.)

PNEUMONIA

Pneumonia is an infection of the lung where the tiny air sacs in the lungs become inflamed and filled with mucus and pus. The primary causes are bacteria or viruses which enter the lungs via the upper respiratory tract. Chemical irritants and allergens can also cause pneumonia. Other infections such as bronchitis can lead to pneumonia; and the number of cases of pneumonia increase rapidly when there are epidemics of influenza.

The symptoms of the disease vary and can be mild or severe. They can include sharp pains in the chest, chill and fever, fast respiration, spitting blood and a persistent dry cough. The disease may be countered by the appropriate antibiotics, but it can be extremely serious in vulnerable people, and in the very old and young. A doctor should always be consulted, and hospitalization may be necessary.

AROMATHERAPEUTIC TREATMENTS

- The fluid intake should be high. Make tisanes with **eucalyptus, oregano** or **thyme** (5 ml [1 tsp]), or **cloves** or **juniper** berries (3 – 4), or a stick of **cinnamon**. Boil for 1 minute, infuse for 5 – 7 minutes, and drink with honey.
- Inhalations can be helpful, particularly when made with oils from the pine family – **pine** and **cypress**. Pine needles could be used in an inhalation.
- Because the disease is infectious, avoid close contact with a sufferer. Protect your family and friends by diffusing aromas in the patient's bedroom and other rooms of the house. Two to three drops of **cajuput, eucalyptus** or **tea tree** oil should be put in a bowl of hot water. Repeat every few hours.
- Poultices are good for lung problems. A mustard or linseed poultice with 2 drops each of **oregano** and **mustard** essential oils is good for pneumonia. Leave in place for 10 minutes, then rub the chest with an oil made from 15 ml (1 tbsp) soya, 2 drops of wheatgerm, plus 5 drops **baume de Canada** and 2 of **niaouli**, or 2 each of **cedarwood** and **cajuput** and 3 drops of **eucalyptus**. Cover the chest warmly afterwards. (See also **baume de Tolu**.)

OTHER TREATMENTS

- Stay indoors, keep warm and dry, and avoid cold and damp.
- A healthy and sensible diet is necessary to help increase resistance to any sort of respiratory disease, particularly foods rich in vitamins A and B.

- With high fever there is a loss of protein, and as this is needed for the repair of body tissue, its intake should be increased after a bout of pneumonia.
- Pineapple is excellent for congestive problems.
- Avoid alcohol, cigarettes and smoky public places.

(*See also* **bronchitis, chest infections, colds, coughing, influenza** *and* **respiratory system problems.**)

PRE-MENSTRUAL TENSION

Many women suffer from diverse physical and emotional upsets for some days before their periods begin: swollen ankles and hands, distended stomach, tender breasts, weight gain, constipation, greasy skin and hair, insomnia, headaches and mood swings. The precise hormonal disturbances that bring about such symptoms are still a bit of a mystery, but scientists now believe that the problem lies with an imbalance between the hormones oestrogen and progesterone. It is possible that during the week before a period, oestrogen levels in the blood remain unusually high, while progesterone falls too low, creating an imbalance between the two.

The secretion of both these ovarian hormones is under the control of the pituitary gland, so a deficiency here could certainly upset the balance. In turn, the pituitary is greatly influenced by the hypothalamus, in the brain, and this controlling centre also responds to stress and other psychological disturbances. This helps to explain why pre-menstrual tension can vary in severity from month to month.

AROMATHERAPEUTIC TREATMENTS

- Drink plenty of herb teas containing such plants as **calendula, mint** and **parsley**, and **chamomile** mixed with **orange** flowers.
- When cooking, season your food with **sage, basil** and **thyme**, as they make food easier to digest. Indigestion is often a problem before menstruation.
- Take two warm baths a day, and add 6 drops **parsley** and 2 drops of **neroli**, or 4 drops of **pine**, 2 drops of **parsley** and 3 drops of **neroli**. Afterwards, lie down on your bed for 10 minutes in a darkened room, placing a pillow beneath your knees.
- Make an oil by adding 4 drops of **parsley** and 3 drops of **neroli** to 25 ml (1 fl oz) soya oil. Massage this into your abdomen, lower back and the back of your neck.

(*See also* **baume de Tolu, cardamom, lemon, melissa, rose** *and* **tarragon.**)

OTHER TREATMENTS

- Sufferers from PMT should eat small, regular meals, choosing foods rich in the B vitamins, particularly vitamin B_6. Wholegrains, meat and offal are rich sources of vitamin B_6. Eating regularly is essential, for it keeps the blood sugar at a constant level and staves off cravings for undesirables like coffee. Eat early in the evening to avoid insomnia.
- Sufferers should avoid tea, coffee and alcohol and they should never resort to diuretics to banish excess fluid-related weight. This would bring about the loss of potassium and other important minerals in the urine, and result in feelings of even greater depression and fatigue.
- The mineral magnesium is very useful as it has a tranquillizing action. Rich sources are: nuts, dried fruit, whole grains, dark green vegetables, seafood.
- Evening primrose oil can be beneficial.
- Take plenty of gentle exercise.

(*See also* **constipation, digestive system problems, headaches, insomnia, oedema** *and* **menstrual problems.**)

PSORIASIS

Psoriasis is a common skin condition characterized by circular patches of red or pink dry and flaky skin. These patches can appear anywhere on the body, but predominantly on the knees and elbows and sometimes on the scalp and top of the forehead. Steroids are used in conventional medicine to treat psoriasis, but these can sometimes worsen the condition. The skin can become so dry that it cracks and becomes infected.

The specific cause of the disease is not known, but it can be hereditary, and it can be exacerbated by cold and damp and by stress.

Although psoriasis is difficult to cure, it can be treated with aromatherapeutic oils.

AROMATHERAPEUTIC TREATMENTS

- Wheatgerm oil can be applied to patches of psoriasis on the face; it should also be used as a cleansing oil.

- Or mix together 10 ml (2 tsp) wheatgerm oil and 2 – 3 drops of **benzoin** oil (or **thuja** or **cajuput**), and apply to the skin morning and evening. If this does not have much effect at first, slightly increase the amount of essential oil. If there is no result after about 2 months, try the remedy using another essential oil.
- Use compresses of **rose** water with **parsley** and **chervil** to remove excess oil.
- For psoriasis of the scalp, mix together 5 ml (1 tsp) castor oil, 4 drops **benzoin** (or **thuja** or **cajuput**) and 2 drops wheatgerm, and massage gently into the scalp. Wrap the head in a warm towel to help the oil penetrate, then wash off a couple of hours later, using a very mild shampoo (diluted perhaps with some **chamomile** tea). Never dry the hair with a drier, as direct heat will irritate the condition.
- Before shampooing, massage the scalp with an infusion of marigold flowers (4 flower heads to 600 ml/1 pint water) with the added juice of half a lemon.

(*See also* **calendula, lemon, oregano** *and* **thyme.**)

OTHER TREATMENTS

- As with all skin disorders, psoriasis can point to some deep-rooted ailment and so anything which is detrimental to health like smoking or drinking alcohol should be avoided.
- Diet is very important. Look for foods rich in vitamin A and lecithin and reduce the amount of animal protein and fat ingested.
- Research has shown that vitamin E could be effective in treating psoriasis. Take capsules of this daily together with cod liver oil and oil of evening primrose which are good, too.
- Eat lots of wheatgerm which is a good source of vitamins B_1 and B_2. Sprinkle it on salads, cereals, gravies and sauces, desserts and yoghurt.

(*See also* **cracked skin** *and* **hair problems.**)

PYORRHOEA

(*See* **gum disease.**)

RESPIRATORY SYSTEM PROBLEMS

Problems of the respiratory system include asthma, bronchitis, coughs, colds, laryngitis, pneumonia and more serious diseases like emphysema and lung cancer. The system itself is very sophisticated, specifically designed to exchange oxygen for carbon dioxide, but it is also very sensitive, and any problem, especially in the old or very young, should be taken seriously.

AROMATHERAPEUTIC TREATMENTS

(*See* **baume de Canada, baume de Tolu, cajuput, eucalyptus, frankincense, niaouli, pine, rose, rosemary** *and* **tea tree**.)

OTHER TREATMENTS

- To prevent problems, avoid polluted atmospheres as much as possible and do not smoke.
- Diet is very important to prevent infections. One rich in protein and the vitamins A and B in particular can help. Vitamin A maintains the health of the respiratory passages and a deficiency increases susceptibility to infections. The body's content of B can be depleted during respiratory illnesses like pneumonia, so B-rich foods are particularly important; research has suggested that there is a correlation between a B-deficiency and lung disease.
- Make a **mustard** poultice to relieve chest tightness (see page 24). Leave on the upper chest for 15 – 30 minutes until the skin becomes quite red.
- Look after any sort of respiratory infection, however minor. Cold and damp exacerbate, so stay inside in a warm but not too dry atmosphere. If you can, stay in bed for a couple of days to give the body time to recover, so avoiding secondary complications of bronchitis or pneumonia.

RHEUMATISM

Rheumatism is a general word for inflammation and pain with or without stiffness, which affects the soft tissue, ligaments, tendons and muscles that surround and are attached to the joints. It is a word used more by lay people than by the medical profession, and encompasses many other recognized diseases such as arthritis, bursitis and fibrositis.

AROMATHERAPEUTIC TREATMENTS

- Massage the affected area with an oil made by adding 2 drops **cajuput** oil to 10 ml (2 tsp) soya oil; also good is 1 drop **pine** with 1 drop **lemon** or **juniper** in 10 ml (2 tsp) soya oil.

- An old herbal recommends a **rosemary** poultice for rheumatism. Mix 100 g (4 oz) linseed and 10 drops rosemary oil. Apply to the inflamed area and cover the poultice with a towel to keep the heat in as long as possible. Leave for 10 minutes. Repeat twice a day for a few days until a little better, then continue once a day.

(*See also* **angelica, baume de Canada, baume de Tolu, carrots, citronella, cloves, coriander, eleni, eucalyptus, ginger, horseradish, laurel, lavender, lovage, mustard, oregano, parsley, pepper, pimento, sage, thyme** *and* **wintergreen**.)

OTHER TREATMENTS

- Diet can play a part in rheumatic problems, particularly one lacking in calcium and magnesium. These minerals are needed to form the synovial fluid which lubricates the joints. Rich sources of calcium include milk and milk products, green leafy vegetables, nuts and seeds and pulses. Foods rich in magnesium include nuts, whole grains, dark green vegetables and seafood.
- Warmth, warm clothing and bed rest are frequently necessary.

(*See also* **arthritis, backache, bursitis, lumbago, stiffness** *and* **sciatica**.)

RHINITIS

(*See* **colds** *and* **hayfever**.)

SCABIES

A skin disease caused by the burrowing of the mite *Sarcoptes scabiei*. The female lays her eggs under the skin, they hatch in three to four days, then reach adulthood in a few weeks when the whole cycle begins again. They are highly contagious, and can be passed on by less than close physical contact – one common cause of infection is thought to be coins, for instance, as the initial burrowing is often between the fingers. Intense itching – worst at night – can lead to infection of the pimples.

The conventional medical treatment for scabies is a top-to-toe application of a solution of benzyl benzoate.

AROMATHERAPEUTIC TREATMENT

Treat as for body lice – *see* **pediculosis.**

(*See also* **laurel**.)

SCARS

(*See* **cuts and wounds**.)

SCIATICA

This is an intense pain in the lower back sometimes also accompanied by pain in the buttocks and on the outside of the leg. This denotes pressure on the sciatic nerve, which runs from the lower back to the foot. Sciatica is often accompanied or preceded by lumbago, and may also be the first warning of a prolapsed or slipped vertebral disc. It is caused by lifting badly or bending awkwardly; it often appears after childbirth.

AROMATHERAPEUTIC TREATMENTS

- Bed rest, heat and massage are ways in which the pain and pressure can be relieved.
- Mix 2 drops of an appropriate oil such as **juniper, mustard, pepper,** and **turpentine** with 15 ml (1 tbsp) soya or grapeseed oil. Rub this gently on the affected areas. Wrap warmly afterwards, wearing something like leggings.
- A few drops of one of these oils can be added to your bath when it is running. Do not forget to wrap yourself up warmly afterwards.

See also **oregano** *and* **thyme**.)

OTHER TREATMENT

- There are some exercises which could gently stretch and strengthen the sciatic nerve. Lie on the back with one knee placed over the other and pull the knees gently towards you using your hands. You will feel the stretch in your buttock. Change knees around to stretch the other side.

(*See also* **backache, bursitis, lumbago, neuralgia, rheumatism, sciatica** *and* **stiffness**.)

SEXUAL PROBLEMS

Many sexual problems are minor and short-lived, and can be treated by aromatherapeutic principles. Aromatherapy can be very effective in alleviating the symptoms of things like depression, stress and anxiety; often psychological disorders like these contribute to a lack of sexual drive or response or to an inability to make love.

There are also many essential oils which are reputed to be aphrodisiac; if these properties cannot be actually proved, there is never any harm in trying them out!

AROMATHERAPEUTIC TREATMENTS

- Massaging the body with a wonderfully perfumed oil such as **rose** can help women particularly.
- A bath perfumed with an oil such as **ylang-ylang** (perhaps mixed with **savory**) can be very stimulating.

(*See also* **cedarwood, celery, clove, ginger** and **lavender**.)

OTHER TREATMENTS

- Avoid drugs such as sleeping pills and an excess of alcohol, as both depress the central nervous system and reduce desire.
- There is nothing like good old romance. Try a little candlelight, soft music and sweet perfumes.
- Dr Maury recommends the aphrodisiac properties of a glass of Médoc, Pouilly Fuissé or Champagne Brut. Or how about oysters and caviar. The Turks swear by a rose jam called *gul*; spread it on toast as a sexual stimulant.
- Mix up elixirs with wine, and have a little when needed – see **basil, celery** and, particularly, **savory**.
- Drink ginseng tea or very strong mint tea at the right time (or take the ginseng in tablet form).

(*See also* **depression, menopause** *and* **stress**.)

SHINGLES

Shingles, or *Herpes zoster*, is caused by a species of virus closely related to those that cause facial or genital herpes. It is also closely related to the virus that causes chickenpox, and only people who have had chickenpox get shingles. The virus infects part of a nerve, and after a few days of

311

fever, skin eruptions appear along the course of a set of nerves usually running across one side of the body, from under the ribs to under the armpit and on to the back (it can also spread from the face, infecting the shoulders). Because it is nerves that are infectd, the eruptions cause severe neuralgia, and this is extermely painful, lasting quite a while after the rash has gone. The doctor should be consulted quickly if shingles is suspected, especially for relief of this pain.

The rash consists of small blisters which gradually dry, forming scabs. If on the face, the blisters can leave terrible scars, and the blisters of some forms of shingles can actually be damaging to sight if near the eyes.

AROMATHERAPEUTIC TREATMENTS

- To soothe angry areas of skin, apply an infusion of **chervil, rose** or lime or linden flowers (*tilleul*).
- Apply three times a day an oil made from 15 ml (1 tbsp) soya or grapeseed, 2 drops wheatgerm, and 2 drops each of **geranium, lavender, myrtle** and **rosemary** (or simply 8 drops of one essential oil).

(*See also* **coriander** *and* **oregano**.)

OTHER TREATMENTS

- Wear loose comfortable clothing, and take analgesics.
- To avoid irritating the blisters, especially those on the face, do not use strong soaps to wash with, or use any other beauty products.

(*See also* **cold sores, cuts and wounds** *and* **neuralgia**.)

SINUSITIS

Sinusitis is a bacterial infection and inflammation of one or more of the sinus passages which are located in the bones surrounding the eyes and nose. Symptoms include nasal congestion, nose bleeds, fatigue headaches, ear pain, pain around the eyes, a mild fever or cough. It could be caused by the common cold, by 'flu, tonsillitis, or poor mouth hygiene. Recent research has suggested a connection with a deficiency in vitamin A. Cold and damp weather are contributory.

AROMATHERAPEUTIC TREATMENTS

- Treat yourself to inhalations containing a few drops of **baumes de Canada** or **Tolu, benzoin, cajuput, eucalyptus, niaouli** or **tea tree**.

- After the inhalation, mix together 10 ml (2 tsp) soya oil, and 4 drops of any of the above, and rub gently on the inside and outside of the nose.

(*See also* **chamomile** *and* **myrrh**.)

OTHER TREATMENTS

- As always, a good diet is very important taking plenty of vitamin A. Protein is important too, but avoid dairy products.
- Yellow and orange fruits and vegetables are a source of vitamin A, as are the yolks of eggs, dark green vegetables, hazelnut and walnut oils, and millet.
- Cod liver oil capsules taken daily act as a preventative.
- Avoid smoking, and do not eat spicy foods or drink tea, coffee or alcohol.

(*See also* **colds, ear problems, headaches, influenza, neuralgia** *and* **toothache**.)

SKIN PROBLEMS

The outer epidermis of the skin consists of many layers of skin cells. New cells are produced at the basal layer and travel towards the surface of the skin, losing their moisture and becoming flatter all the time, until they are shed as dead skin cells. By the time they are ready to be shed, these cells are rich in a protein called keratin, the same substance of which fingernails are composed, so they are quite brittle and scaly.

The epidermis rests on the inner dermis, which acts rather like a cushion, giving strength and support as well as contour to the skin. Within the dermis, there is an ordered network of tough collagen fibres lying within connective tissue. Also present are elastin fibres which give skin pliancy and make it pliable rather than strong. A young healthy skin has the capacity to increase its size by 50 per cent due to these elastic properties, but this function diminishes with age.

The dermis is richly supplied by many small capillaries bringing oxygen and other vital nutrients to the skin cells and carrying away the toxic waste products. It is also well endowed with nerve endings which transmit messages from the skin surface to the brain concerning temperature, touch and pain. Sebaceous glands are also present in the dermis, but they open to the surface at pores located in the epidermis.

These glands produce the oily substance called sebum, whose function is to lubricate the skin and to seal moisture in the cells. Their activity determines whether your skin is normal, oily or dry.

The skin is an organ with many different functions. It helps to maintain constant body temperature by shedding excess heat in the form of water, as sweat that cools as it evaporates on the surface of the skin. In this way it also eliminates toxins or unwanted waste products from the body. By blocking these channels with anti-perspirants and heavy face make-up the toxins can build up in layers within the skin, and may eventually be expelled as spots and pimples. Their appearance is often a sign that the cleansing organs of the body, primarily the liver and kidneys, are not working properly and the skin is called upon to act as a sort of dumping ground. Invariably, once the liver and kidneys are back to normal, the condition of the skin rapidly improves.

Sometimes, too, conditions such as eczema are a symptom of an internal illness or disorder, and act as a means through which the body can discharge its afflictions. If this eczema is treated with drugs, this eliminative pathway is removed, so the problem builds up inside and may erupt years later.

The skin is a mirror of body health, and its nature is greatly influenced by changes that take place from within, far more so than by any cream applied to the surface. For this reason any skin problem should be regarded as an indication that your health is not what it could be, and if treatment is to be successful, you have to consider the body as a whole. A skin problem may be the result of acute emotional anxiety, of biochemical disorders such as hypoglycaemia or diabetes, or of a reaction to aerosol sprays, antibiotics or other drugs – even to skin-care products.

But by far the greatest causative factor is diet. This is one of the major ways in which the health of the body in general and the skin in particular can be assured. Vitamins have a definite relationship with the skin. Very often blisters and cracking of the corners of the mouth are attributable to a deficiency of vitamin B_2 (riboflavin); a vitamin C deficiency leads to scurvy and gum disease; a lack of vitamin A results in excess dryness of the skin and hair, and vitamin E has recently been associated with the skin disease psoriasis. Many skin rashes and forms of eczema are allergies to certain proteins and so are related to diet.

Practically every skin disease has at some time or another been treated by some kind of diet. Acne and minor skin problems such as blackheads and pimples are treated with diets omitting meat, sugar or fats. At present a low-fat diet is recommended; in many cases of acne, for instance, an overactivity of the oil glands in the skin is responsible, and this could be related to ingestion of nuts, fried foods and too many stimulants such as alcohol, chocolate, pork and pork products, dairy products and tobacco.

Aromatherapy can benefit many skin problems, but the skin must always be respected, as must the potency of the oils. The oils should be applied in dilution or, occasionally, neat to skin, but be careful to avoid the eyes and the inside of the mouth and nose as the mucus membrane could be burned, become inflamed and swell. Please be very careful.

(*See also* **benzoin, bois de rose, cade, cajuput, calendula, carrots, cedarwood, cubeb, gaiac, galbanum, geranium, juniper, lavender, lemongrass, lovage, myrrh, rose, tea tree, thuja** *and* **thyme; abscesses and boils, acne, ageing skin, anthrax, athlete's foot, bed sores, blisters, broken veins and capillaries, bruises, burns, cold sores, cracked skin, cuts and wounds, dermatitis, eczema, frostbite, psoriasis, scabies, shingles, stings and bites, sunburn** *and* **wrinkles.**)

STIFFNESS

Stiffness in the joints can be caused by a variety of problems: rheumatic conditions, emotional problems and stress, lack of exercise, draughts, damp and cold, and old age. Stiffness could also herald a virus infection.

AROMATHERAPEUTIC TREATMENTS

- Have hot baths containing 2 drops each of **cajuput, niaouli** and **pine**, or 3 each of **eucalyptus** and **rosemary**. Rub your body energetically with a hot towel, and then rub an oil made from the essentials used in the bath in to the stiff joints: 15 ml (1 tbsp) soya oil, 2 drops wheatgerm, plus 4 drops of the oil combination already used. Wrap yourself in a hot towelling gown and rest or go to bed for 10 minutes to help absorption of the oils.

(*See also* **camphor of Borneo** *and* **wintergreen.**)

OTHER TREATMENTS

- A brisk walk or a few laps of the local swimming pool can restore suppleness to the joints.

(*See also* **arthritis, backache, bursitis, muscular pains, rheumatism, sciatica** *and* **stress.**)

STINGS AND BITES

The stings and bites of insects can be very painful, and should never be ignored.

AROMATHERAPEUTIC TREATMENTS

- When a bee stings, the sting is left in the flesh, and this can be removed by tweezers. Apply a drop of neat **geranium, oregano, tea tree** or **thyme**, followed by a cold compress to relieve the pain. Wasp stings and flea bites can be treated in the same way.
- The sting of a centipede or spider can be more severe. Bleeding is often encouraged so that any material deposited by the sting can be washed out. Apply neat oil as above – or tincture of iodine – followed by a cold compress.
- Other oils used neat on the affected part are good for relieving pain, such as **citronella** and **melissa**. Alternatively apply melissa or balm leaves directly on a bite to sooth it.
- Aromatherapeutic plants and oils can help prevent the appearance of biters and stingers in the first place. Buy a 1-litre (¾-pint) plastic spray bottle, fill with water and add 5 ml (1 tsp of mixed essential oils such as **mint** and **camphor** or **eucalyptus** and **camphor**). Vaporize the rooms, around curtains, windows, on chairs, in the corners of fitted carpets where fleas and moths might breed. Put some of the essentials in a bowl of water in each room.
- Other plants and oils can chase away insects: **basil, citronella, geranium, lavender, myrtle** and **niaouli**.

STRESS

Stress is a problem that is becoming increasingly common in today's technological society. Although it is difficult to measure, it is known to be the result of excessive demands on energy, mental or physical, and can lead to illness. It is important, therefore, that it is dealt with swiftly and efficiently before the body is too seriously affected.

Everyone has a different level of tolerance to demands made on their mental energy: some can cope well with high demands; others quickly reach their stress level limit. We all need a certain degree of stress, after all it is a natural function of the body. The hormone adrenaline is manufactured by the body during times of stress; but the almost continual stress of city life, worries about money, children, health, etc, is not natural, and a constant presence of adrenaline takes its toll, leading to hypertension, an increase in blood pressure, and a number of other major and minor body ills. Balance is the key.

Just as people cope differently with stress, so the body reacts differently: many people have stress headaches, or cannot sleep; just as many suffer stress-related digestive problems. Stress is known to reduce the body's general resistance to infection, and so people under stress can become susceptible to things like bronchitis. Stress also affects the skin; acne for instance can be exacerbated by it. Stress interferes with the levels of and interaction of hormones in the body, so it can lead to menstrual problems in women; it also interferes with the digestive system.

AROMATHERAPEUTIC TREATMENTS

- Allow time in the evening to unwind after a stressful day. Take a warm to hot bath with a few drops of a relaxing essence such as **basil, lavender, mandarin, marjoram, melissa, neroli, orange, petitgrain, clary sage** or **ylang-ylang**. After your bath, ensure you relax for a while, reading the paper or a novel, or watching television.
- Diffuse some calming vapours around the rooms where you live or work. Use those mentioned above. Or put drops on a handkerchief, on a blotter, or rub into your chest at some point during the day.
- To avoid insomnia, drink malted milky drinks before going to bed – the calcium of milk is a great tranquillizer and sleep inducer. Or take a calming herbal tea using **melissa, orange blossom** or **mint**, for example.

OTHER TREATMENTS

- The best way to deal with stress is to remove the stressor(s). That is easier said than done, but a realistic overview of the situation, perhaps helped by an adviser of some sort – financial, psychological, even just a good listening friend – can help.
- Try not to turn to chemical answers such as anti-depressants and tranquillizers. Many of these can help in the short term, but they do not cure the problem, only disguise it and a lot of people can quickly become psychologically and physically dependent on them.
- Try to avoid resorting to things like alcohol or tobacco. These are undeniably relaxing, but they are dangerous in excess, and can also become addictive.
- Meditation and yoga can help as can breathing exercises.
- Exercise is always good for someone who is stressed, so long as it is not physically or emotionally overtaxing.

- Eat foods containing the mineral magnesium which is often referred to as nature's tranquillizer.
- Always eat lightly when under stress. Foods which are simple and easy to cook are best as they are much less time- and energy-consuming.

ALMOND AND ROSE DATES

The nutritive value of the date is quite remarkable with high proportions of magnesium, phosphorus and calcium. The almond reinforces this, with the rose having a calming effect on the nervous system. The whole also has high contents of iron, vitamins B_1 and B_2, and vitamin A, which helps to fix the calcium.

The dates are also good for those who suffer from PMT and anaemia, and those who study and work late at night as they are a tonic and an excellent source of muscle and body energy.

1 lb (450 g) naturally dried dates, with no added sugar
1 lb (450 g) almonds
enough rosewater to cover the dates

To make your own rosewater, make an infusion of rose petals using 8 oz (225 g) petals to 600 ml (1 pint) water. Bring to the boil and simmer for 20 minutes. You may also use Greek distilled rosewater.

Leave the dates to steep overnight in the rosewater. In the morning, discard the rosewater and cut the dates in half. Remove the stones and replace with almonds.

(*See also* **depression, digestive system problems, fatigue, gout, headaches, insomnia, palpitations, menstrual cycle problems, skin problems** *and* **stiffness.**)

SUNBURN

This is an inflammation of the skin following exposure to the ultra-violet rays of the sun. Fair-skinned people have little protective pigmentation in their skins, and therefore burn more easily than darker-skinned people. Minor sunburn causes reddening of the skin and some discomfort, followed by increased pigmentation of the skin (i.e. a tan). More serious sunburn can cause the skin and tissue to swell painfully and to blister and peel.

It is now well known that sunbathing can cause skin cancer and this is a growing problem in northern countries because of the increased numbers taking brief holidays in the sun. Modern sun-screen products may only be superficially effective and the only answer would seem to be that fair-skinned people should avoid the direct rays of the sun whenever possible. Sun also causes skin to wrinkle and turn leathery.

When sunburnt, the skin needs to breathe, so wait until it has calmed down a little before applying any oils or lotions.

AROMATHERAPEUTIC TREATMENT

• A soothing and healing lotion can be made by adding 2 drops **lavender** oil to a tub of natural yoghurt. Mix well and apply to the skin while still tacky, cover the area with cotton (for example put on an old T-shirt if your shoulders or back are burnt). Go to bed like this, and repeat the application in the morning.

OTHER TREATMENTS

• If you must sunbathe, do so gradually. for the first few days, wear long sleeves and a shady hat to allow the skin to gently acclimatize. Lie in the sun for short periods only, using effective products, and try to avoid the midday sun, when it is at its hottest.
• If you suffer from sunburn, liquidize some potatoes or carrots, and apply the liquid on to affected areas for relief.

(*See also* **ageing skin** *and* **skin problems**.)

TEETHING PAINS

Teething can be painful for both baby and parents. The first signs may be a reddish gum, with a visible bumb, dribbling, red patches on the cheek and irritability.

AROMATHERAPEUTIC TREATMENTS

• To offer relief, give the baby something hard and cold to bite on. Chunks of **carrot**, cabbage or apple can be given, as these not only nourish, but contain soothing essential oils.
• Mix 1 drop of **chamomile** essential oil into a tablespoon of almond oil and rub directly on to the sore gums.

(*See also* **ear problems**.)

319

THROAT, SORE

A sore throat can be caused by many things – by colds, 'flu, bronchitis, laryngitis, tonsillitis, or by talking too much!

Laryngitis, one of the commonest causes of sore throats, is an inflammation of the larynx, part of the windpipe. It can be the result of viral or bacterial infection, and the acute version cause a painful, dry throat, but often with mucus, and a hoarse voice. Chronic laryngitis can occur in those who work in a dry dusty atmosphere, or in those who breathe through their mouths.

Tonsillitis is an inflammation of the tonsils which are glands of lymph tissue situated at each side of the back of the throat. Like laryngitis, it may be viral or bacterial in origin, and can occur when the body's resistance is lowered (after a cold, say), or by an improper diet which is high in carbohydrates and low in protein and other nutrients. Fever, redness and swelling in the back of the mouth, difficulty in swallowing, headaches, nausea and enlarged lymph glands throughout the body are only a few of the symptoms of tonsillitis. It is a disease which occurs mainly in childhood (particularly in the first years at school when children encounter viruses which they have not met before), and although once treated by removal of the tonsils, this is now deemed unnecessary because of its rareness after childhood.

AROMATHERAPEUTIC TREATMENTS

- To prevent infection in winter, gargle morning and night with a glass of boiled water and 1 drop of **cajuput, geranium, niaouli, pepper, rose, rosemary** or **tea tree**. Increase the drops of essential oil to 2 if a sore throat develops, and gargle five to six times a day. (**Celery, cinnamon, clove, cubeb, ginger, hyssop, myrrh, rose** and **clary sage** are also good.)
- Suck ice cubes made with boiled water mixed with fresh lemon and pineapple juices (the latter is good for clearing the mucus of many throat infections).
- Steam inhalations can help.

  (*See also* **lemon, marjoram** *and* **parsley**.)

OTHER TREATMENTS

- Keep in a warm but not dry atmosphere, drink plenty of fluids (avoiding tea and coffee), and do not talk too much.
- One of the best remedies is a glass of hot water with the juice of half a lemon and honey to taste.

- Avoid hard foods, which could hurt the throat.
- To help build up a resistance against all infections, eat a well-balanced diet which is adequate in protein, vitamins and minerals, with plenty of vitamin C-rich fruits.
- Do not smoke.

GARLIC SOUP *Serves 2*

This is an excellent soup for cold winter days, and it is particularly therapeutic for hangovers. It offers protection against colds, 'flu and bronchial problems. Serve it at the first sign of a sore throat.

4 garlic cloves, peeled
900 ml (1½ pints) water
1 tbsp tapioca
2 sprigs of thyme
1½ tbsp virgin olive oil
freshly ground black pepper
grated Gruyère or Parmesan cheese (optional)

Place the garlic and water in a stainless steel saucepan, and gently bring to the boil. Simmer for 20 minutes, then add the tapioca and thyme. Simmer for a further 10 minutes.

Remove the garlic cloves and crush them in a mortar or cup. Slowly add the olive oil and stir until you obtain a smooth paste. Stir this mixture gently into the hot soup. Serve with lots of black pepper and, if you like, grated cheese. This soup is best when served very hot.

(*See also* **bronchitis, colds, coughing** *and* **influenza.**)

THRUSH

The yeast-like fungus which causes thrush is known medically as *Candida albicans*, and the condition as candidiasis or moniliasis. The fungus is found normally in and on the body, but several changes in the body chemistry such as the taking of antibiotics, the contraceptive pill, pregnancy or menopause, and some diseases such as diabetes can encourage the fungus to grow. In women, the vagina is the most commonly affected area, causing itchiness, inflammation and a thick discharge. But it can occur elsewhere, in warm moist parts of the body like under the breasts or arms, or in the mouth. Nappy rash or napkin dermatitis in babies is probably associated with thrush. The condition can be sexually transmitted.

AROMATHERAPEUTIC TREATMENT

• Treat as for **leucorrhoea**.

(*See also* **marjoram, mint, orange, rose** *and* **sage**.)

TIREDNESS

(*See* **fatigue**.)

TONSILLITIS

(*See* **throat, sore**.)

TOOTHACHE

The process of tooth decay is really quite simple. Bacteria naturally present in the mouth rest on the teeth as plaque; this creates acids which eat into the enamel of the teeth. If good mouth hygiene and a sensible diet are followed, the saliva can remineralize the calcium of the enamel, and no further dental intervention need be necessary. Once the decay reaches through to the dentine under the enamel, however, the bacteria can wreak havoc, safely out of reach of brush and floss. The dentist would probably have to remove the decay at this stage and insert a filling. If this is ignored, though, the bacteria can eat through into the pulp, the nerve centre of the tooth, and pain results. Toothache is always severe and can persist. Like other body tissue, the pulp swells when inflamed, and as it is surrounded by a hard casing it presses on nerves resulting in acute pain.

If toothache developes, visit your dentist as soon as possible. Untended inflammation of the pulp could lead to an abscess, when the bacteria pour out of the cavity in the pulp into the bone holding the tooth. This can be extremely dangerous.

AROMATHERAPEUTIC TREATMENTS

• To alleviate the pain until you get to the dentist, use **mint** or suck a **clove** at the site of the pain. Both mint and clove (herb and spice as well as oil) have highly antiseptic as well as slightly anaesthetic properties.

(*See also* **coriander**.)

OTHER TREATMENTS
- Avoid toothache by keeping the mouth and teeth meticulously clean, and by omitting sugar and sugary foods from the diet.
- Avoid foods and drinks that are very hot or very cold.

(*See also* **ear problems, gum disease** *and* **neuralgia**.)

VARICOSE VEINS

Veins may become varicose in various parts of the body – in the rectum as haemorrhoids, for example – but the most familiar are those in the leg. If the flow of blood from the legs to the heart is interrupted, the blood can stagnate in the veins and these swell and twist, resulting in purple ropes of veins up the legs, and considerable discomfort. The condition occurs mainly in people who have to stand a lot – movement helps the leg muscles contract and pump blood upwards – but can also be caused by constipation, overweight and pregnancy. During pregnancy the expanding womb constricts the blood flow to the limbs and the extra weight carried makes it harder for the blood to return from the legs to the heart.

AROMATHERAPEUTIC TREATMENT

- Massage your legs every day with an oil consisting of 20 ml (4 tsp) almond oil, 2 drops wheatgerm and 4 drops each of **parsley** and **cypress**. Work up the legs from the feet towards the heart. Do this sitting on the floor rather than standing up.

(*See also* **lavender**.)

OTHER TREATMENTS

- Avoid standing as much as possible and try to lie with your feet higher than your heart (put blocks under the end of your bed to raise it a little).
- Do not sit with your legs crossed as the blood flow will be inhibited, and sit with your feet on something if on a long journey.
- Take as much exercise as possible.

- Eat a diet high in fibre, vitamins C and E and the bioflavinoids, which are all good for the circulatory system.
- Never take baths that are too hot, and finish with a cold shower on feet and legs.

(*See also* **broken veins and capillaries, cellulite, circulatory problems, constipation,** *and* **haemorrhoids**.)

GLOSSARIES

GLOSSARY OF MEDICAL TERMS

Amenorrhoea   Abnormal absence of menstruation
Anti-allergic   Preventing allergies
Anti-asthmatic   Preventing asthma attacks
Antirheumatic   Preventing inflammation and aching of the joints
Antiscorbutic   Preventing scurvy
Antiseptic   Ability to destroy undesirable microorganisms
Antispasmodic   Preventing spasms, convulsions and nervous
   disorders
Antiviral   Preventing the passage and acceptance of a virus into the
   body

Balsamic   Soothing, restorative properties
Bechic   Tending to cure or relieve a cough
Blennoragia   Inordinate discharge of mucus

Carminative   Having the quality of expelling wind
Cholagogue   That which benefits the liver
Citracizaton   The formation of mucus

Dermatitis   Inflammation of the skin
Depurative   Purifying the blood and other fluids
Diaphoretic   Having the property of promoting perspiration
Diuretic   Increasing the flow of urine
Dysmenorrhoea   Abnormally painful or difficult menstruation

Emmenagogic   Having the power to promote the menstrual discharge
Expectorant   That which clears the chest and lungs

Febrifuge   An anti-febrile agent, or one that has the power to dispel
   fever

Galactogogenic   Inducing the flow of breast milk

Haemostatic   Retarding or stopping bleeding
Hepatic   Relating to the liver
Hypoglycaemia   Less than normal blood sugar level

Leucorrhoea   A thick yellow-white vaginal discharge

Parasiticide   A preparation for destroying parasites

Pectoral   Good for diseases of the chest and/or lungs
Pediculosis   Parasitic infection of the feet

Scabies   Contagious skin disease
Sedative   A substance that reduces excitement or functional activity
Stimulant   A substance that increases the vital energy
Stomachic   Good for the stomach
Stupefacient   Producing stupor
Sudorific   Promoting or causing perspiration

Tonic   A substance that invigorates

Vaginitis   Inflammation of the womb, with a yellow or green
  discharge
Vaso-constrictor   That which causes dilation of a vessel
Vomitic   Causing vomiting
Vulnerary   Useful in healing wounds

GLOSSARY OF NAMES

Throughout the book I refer to doctors, scientists, herbalists, botanists and others, from ancient to modern times, who have all contributed through their research to today's greater awareness of the therapeutic properties of plants and essential oils. Many of these eminent people are referred to again and again in the pages of this book, so to avoid repetition their details are given below.

Avicenna (980 – 1037 AD)   Famous Arab philospher and physician often referred to as the Prince of Medicine. He was a remarkable author of many books. His medical work *Qanun* was the greatest single influence on medieval medicine.

J Chomel An eighteenth century French professor and pharmacist who became head of the Academy of Medicine in France in 1720. Wrote a *History of Common Plants* in three volumes in 1761 and in 1783 a book of medical formulations using plants that was then used by Parisienne hospitals.

Dioscorides Greek physician from the first century who wrote a medical treatise that remained a classic reference work until the Renaissance: *La Matière Medicale*.

Leonard Fuchs (1501 – 1566)   German scientist who became well known through his work on the Digitalis family of plants. The Fuchsia species of plants were named after him.

Galen (131-201 AD)   Greek physician, anatomist and physiologist. He wrote more than 100 medical treaties using plants and was referred to as The Oracle of Pergamo. He was the doctor of the gladiators, responsible for healing their wounds after fights.

Dr René Maurice Gattefossé (1881 – 1950)   One of the founders of modern aromatherapy, giving the therapy its name in 1900. Wrote many books on the subject which are still referred to today.

St Hildegarde (1098 – 1179)   Referred to as the Abbess of Bingen or Saint Healer. She belonged to the Benedictine monastery of Rupertsberg near Bingen in Germany. Wrote four treatises on medical plants, the most important is *Morborum Causae et Curae* which is still referred to today. She also translated texts from Theophrastes, Dioscorides, Galen and Pliny and gave the properties of over 250 plants.

Hippocrates (460 – 377 BC)   Greek physician commonly regarded as the father of medicine. One of his works, *Corpus Hippocratum* concerned the treatment of the body with plants and diet.

Dr Leclerc   Head of the Phytotherapy School in France earlier this century. Author of many books on aromatherapy and still considered an authority on the subject. His scientific research gained him many followers and helped in the recognition of the therapy as a serious one.

Dr Nicolas Lemery (1645 – 1715)   French doctor and chemist who wrote *Le Traité Universal des Drogues Simples* which became *the* authoritative work of reference for many doctors, particularily in France.

Linnaeus (1707 – 1778)   Swedish botanist who established the binomial system of biological nomenclature that forms the basis of modern classification.

P Matthiole (1500 – 1577)   Italian doctor and one of the most famous botanists of his time. Translated and brought back to life old texts, adding his own researches. He made valuable studies of lily of the valley and other medicinal plants. Founded the Florence Botanical Gardens for the Medicis.

Marguerite Maury (1895 – 1968)   Born in Austria. A pioneer of aromatherapy. In France she single handedly re-established the reputation of aromatherapy. She lectured and gave seminars on the subject and in 1961 wrote *Le Capital Jeunesse*. This book was republished in 1989 by C W Daniel and Co under the English title *The Secret of Life and Youth*. She opened aromatherapy clinics in Paris, Switzerland and England. She won two international prizes, in 1962 and 1967, for her research on essential oils and cosmetology.

Pliny (23 – 79 AD)   Known as Pliny the Elder. A Roman writer, author of the encyclopedic *Natural History* in 37 volumes. His descriptions of plants were valuable though not necessarily scientifically based.

School of Salerno   The first ever medical school, started in the Middle Ages in Naples and named after Roger de Salerne, an eminent surgeon. Naploeon the First closed the school in 1811. One of the first medical works written since ancient times was produced by the school – *Passionarium*. The book was rediscovered and its doctrines reintroduced in 1837 by a Dr Henschel.

BIBLIOGRAPHY

Many of my sources of reference are research papers and books published in France that have not been translated into English, hence the titles for these are given below in French. See also the Glossary of Names.

S Artault de Vevey *Le Myrtol en Injections Hypodermiques* (Revue de Therapie Medical 1986).

Dr Belaiche *Classification des Huiles Essentielles en Function de leur pouvoir Antiseptique Guide Familal, La Médecine par les Plantes* (Hachette 1982)

Bonnaure *Pouvoir Antiseptique des Lavandes* (1919)

C. Cadeac et A Meunier *Traveaux Divers, Comptes Rendus Sociobiology* (1889)

Jean Claude Bourret *Le Defi de la Médecine par les Plantes* (Editions France Empire 1978)

CCI (Centre du Commerce International, Genève) *Etude de Marché des Huiles Essentielles et Oleoresines* (1986)

F Caujolle et C Franck *Sur les Proprietés Epileplogenes de l'Essence d'Hysope* (1945)

P Coster *Phytotherapie des Affections Ortério-veinuses en Practique Phlebologique* (1963)

Couvreur *Plantes à Parfums et Plantes Aromatiques* (1930)

Dr F J Cazin *Traite Pratique et Raisonné des Plantes Médicinales* (1876)

Department of Agriculture, New South Wales, Australia, *Tea Tree Oil* (1989)

Dr Delioux de Savignac *Essence de Mente Analgesiante* (*Therapeutic Journal* 1875)

Dr Raymond Dextreit *La Cure Végétale* (Editions de la Revue, Vivre en Harmonie 1960)

Paul Faure *Parfums et Aromates de l'Antiquité* (Fayard 1987)

Dr René Maurice Gattefossé *Antiseptiques Essentials* (1931)
   Aromatherapie – Les huiles essentialles hormones végétales (1937)
   Distillation des Plantes Aromatiques et de Parfums (1926)
   Formulaire de Parfumerie et de Cosmetlogie (1938)
   Le Pouvoir Bactericide des Essences (1919)

E Gerard *Precis de Pharmacie Galenique* (1922)

H W Gerarde *De l'Ubiquité des Hydrocarbures* (1973)

Gilbert et Michel *Formulaire Practique de Thérapeutique et Pharmacologie* (1925)

Dr G Guibourt *Histoire Naturelle des Drogues Simples* (1876)

Wood Hutchinson MA MD *Health and Common Sense* (Cassel & Co Ltd 1909)

Hugh Johnson *The International Book of Trees* (Mitchell Beazley 1973)

F S Kahn *The Curse of Icarus* (Routledge 1990)

P Lechat *Abregé Pharmacologie Médicale* (Masson et cie 1969)

Dr Leclerc *Précis de Phytothérapie* (Masson et cie 1976)
> *Les Epices, Plantes Condimentaires* (1950)
> *Les Fruits de Grasse* (1952)
> *Les Legumes de France* (1955)

Brendan Lehane *Le Pouvoir des Plantes* (Hachette 1977)

Dr N Lemery *Le Traite Universal des Drogues Simples* (1699)

H F Macmillan *Tropical Planting and Gardening* (Macmillan & Co 1935)

Dr Maury *La Médecine par le Vin* (Edition Antulen 1988)

Maurice Messegué *C'est la Nature qui a Raison* (Robert Laffont 1972)

Y R Naves *Technologie et Chimie de Parfums Naturels* (Masson et cie 1974)

Mulgsch *Manual de Botonique Générale* (Masson et cie 1969)

Eugene Perrot *Matières Premieres Usuelles du Regne Végétal* (1940)
> *Les Plantes Médicinales* (1970)

E D Phillips *Aspects of Greek Medicine* (Charles Press 1973)

Dr Pomet *History of Drugs* (1694)

Rideal et Walker *Le Pouvoir Bactericide des Chaque Essence Aromatique* (1930)

Waverley Root *Food* (Simon & Schuster 1980)

Elenour Sinclair Rohde *A Garden of Herbs* (Herbert Jenkins 1706)

R Sarbach *Contribution à la Désinfection des Atmospheres*
> *Etude des Proprietes Antiseptiques de 58 Huiles Essentielles*

Shroeder and Messing *Discover a New Technique – The Aromatogramme* (1949)

Som Shuster *Dermatology in Internal Medicine* (OUP 1978)

Tom Stobart *Herbs, Spices and Flavourings* (Penguin 1979)
> *The Cook's Encyclopedia* (B T Batsford Ltd 1980)

Dr Jean Valnet *Docteur Nature* (Fayard 1980)

M Wong *La Médecine par les Plantes* (Edition Tchou 1976)

Eleventh International Congress of Essential Oils, Fragrances and Flavours, New Delhi, India 1989

9eme Dictionnaire des Parfums (Edition Sermadiras 1988)

INDEX

Page numbers in **bold** refer to main entries.

If you would like to receive more information about Danièle Ryman and her range of aromatherapy products, please write to

Danièle Ryman Ltd
Danièle Ryman Suite
Park Lane Hotel
Piccadilly
London
W1Y 8BX